Advances in Graves'
Disease and Other
Hyperthyroid
Disorders

McFarland Health Topics Series

Living with Multiple Chemical Sensitivity: Narratives of Coping.
Gail McCormick. 2001

Graves' Disease: A Practical Guide.
Elaine A. Moore with Lisa Moore. 2001

Autoimmune Diseases and Their Environmental Triggers.
Elaine A. Moore. 2002

Hepatitis: Causes, Treatments and Resources.
Elaine A. Moore. 2006

Arthritis: A Patient's Guide.
Sharon E. Hohler. 2008

*The Promise of Low Dose Naltrexone Therapy: Potential Benefits
in Cancer, Autoimmune, Neurological and Infectious Disorders.*
Elaine A. Moore and Samantha Wilkinson. 2009

Living with HIV: A Patient's Guide.
Mark Cichocki, RN. 2009

*Understanding Multiple Chemical Sensitivity:
Causes, Effects, Personal Experiences and Resources.*
Els Valkenburg. 2010

*Type 2 Diabetes: Social and Scientific Origins, Medical
Complications and Implications for Patients and Others.*
Andrew Kagan, M.D. 2010

*The Amphetamine Debate: The Use of Adderall,
Ritalin and Related Drugs for Behavior Modification,
Neuroenhancement and Anti-Aging Purposes.*
Elaine A. Moore. 2011

*CCSVI as the Cause of Multiple Sclerosis: The Science
Behind the Controversial Theory.* Marie A. Rhodes. 2011

*Coping with Post-Traumatic Stress Disorder: A Guide
for Families,* 2d ed. Cheryl A. Roberts. 2011

*Living with Insomnia: A Guide to Causes, Effects
and Management, with Personal Accounts.*
Phyllis L. Brodsky and Allen Brodsky. 2011

*Caregiver's Guide: Care for Yourself While You Care
for Your Loved Ones.* Sharon E. Hohler. 2012

*You and Your Doctor: A Guide to a Healing Relationship,
with Physicians' Insights.* Tania Heller, M.D. 2012

*Autogenic Training: A Mind-Body Approach to the
Treatment of Chronic Pain Syndrome and
Stress-Related Disorders,* 2d ed. Micah R. Sadigh. 2012

*Advances in Graves' Disease and
Other Hyperthyroid Disorders*
Elaine A. Moore with Lisa Marie Moore. 2013

Advances in Graves' Disease and Other Hyperthyroid Disorders

Elaine A. Moore and
Lisa Marie Moore

McFarland Health Topics Series

McFarland & Company, Inc., Publishers
Jefferson, North Carolina, and London

ALSO BY ELAINE A. MOORE
The Amphetamine Debate: The Use of Adderall, Ritalin and Related Drugs for Behavior Modification, Neuroenhancement and Anti-Aging Purposes (2011) • *Hepatitis: Causes, Treatments and Resources* (2006) • *Autoimmune Diseases and Their Environmental Triggers* (2002)

BY ELAINE A. MOORE AND LISA MOORE
Encyclopedia of Alzheimer's Disease; With Directories of Research, Treatment and Care Facilities, 2d ed. (2012) • *Encyclopedia of Sexually Transmitted Diseases* (2005; paperback 2009) • *Graves' Disease: A Practical Guide* (2001)

BY ELAINE A. MOORE AND SAMANTHA WILKINSON
The Promise of Low Dose Naltrexone Therapy: Potential Benefits in Cancer, Autoimmune, Neurological and Infectious Disorders (2009)

ALL FROM MCFARLAND

The information in this book is provided for educational purposes only. It is not intended as a substitute for medical treatment. The procedures and therapies described in this book should be discussed with a medical practitioner before being used.

LIBRARY OF CONGRESS CATALOGUING-IN-PUBLICATION DATA

Moore, Elaine A., 1948– author.
 Advances in Graves' disease and other hyperthyroid disorders / Elaine A. Moore and Lisa Marie Moore.
  pages cm. — (Mcfarland health topics series)
 Includes bibliographical references and index.

 ISBN 978-0-7864-7189-8
 softcover : acid free paper

 1. Graves' disease—Popular works. I. Moore, Lisa, 1973– author. II. Title.
 RC657.5.G7M664 2013
 616.4'43—dc23   2013035698

BRITISH LIBRARY CATALOGUING DATA ARE AVAILABLE

On the cover: scanning of a thyroid (iStockphoto/Thinkstock)

Manufactured in the United States of America

McFarland & Company, Inc., Publishers
 Box 611, Jefferson, North Carolina 28640
  www.mcfarlandpub.com

To Rick, Brooklyn, and Eli

Acknowledgments

I'm indebted to my daughter, Lisa Marie Moore, for agreeing to work with me on this project, and to Marv Miller for his insightful illustrations.

Thanks also to Valerie Sosnow for teaching me about the new sensory therapies used to treat hyperthyroidism indirectly, and to Marian Dyer for her careful proofreading and suggestions. Thanks also to Doctors Burch and Stewart for providing me with copies of their publications. At this time I'd also like to thank Lisa Reynolds for her generosity in sharing photos and to my thyroid friends from around the world who keep me in the game, especially Jody, Lolly, Doris, and Judy. Thanks also to the many visitors to my website who keep me connected to and intrigued by the subject of hyperthyroidism. — E.A.M.

Table of Contents

Acknowledgments vi
Preface 1
Introduction 3

  1. Hyperthyroidism and Its Signs and Symptoms 5
  2. Causes of Hyperthyroidism 27
  3. Graves' Disease: When the Autoimmune Response
     Goes Awry 47
  4. Genetic and Environmental Factors and Influences 69
  5. Coexisting Conditions in Graves' Disease and
     Hyperthyroidism 87
  6. Diagnosing Hyperthyroidism and Graves' Disease 106
  7. Conventional Treatment Options for Hyperthyroidism 131
  8. Complementary and Alternative Treatments for
     Hyperthyroidism 160
  9. Hyperthyroidism in Pregnancy and the Postpartum Period 187
10. Hyperthyroidism in Children and Adolescents 196
11. Graves' Ophthalmopathy and Other Extrathyroidal
     Manifestations 211

Glossary 233
References 255
Resources 265
Index 271

Preface

In *Advances in Graves' Disease and Other Hyperthyroid Disorders* I describe the various disorders of hyperthyroidism along with their causes, diagnoses, and treatments based on current guidelines and recommendations of the American Thyroid Association, American Association of Clinical Endocrinologists, and the Endocrine Society.

In addition, I describe the special concerns of hyperthyroidism in pregnancy and in children and adolescents. I also explain the relationship of hyperthyroidism with other disorders, including nodular disease and vitamin B12 deficiency, and I describe the extrathyroidal manifestations of Graves' disease such as Graves' ophthalmopathy, euthyroid Graves' disease, pretibial myxedema, and thyroid acropachy.

In other chapters I describe the environmental and genetic causes of hyperthyroidism, the role of diet in both contributing to and treating hyperthyroidism, and the role that alternative and complementary medicine play in the healing process. While my focus is on new treatment trends, genetic mutations that cause hyperthyroidism, the autoimmune process in Graves' disease, and other pertinent discoveries, I also describe new research pathways and future treatments as well as basic information. For instance, I explain how iodine can cause both hypothyroidism and hyperthyroidism and I describe the discovery of goitrogens in the 1940s and the application of goitrogenic properties in today's anti-thyroid drug therapies.

As an educator and laboratory consultant, I am frequently asked for information on hyperthyroidism and laboratory tests. Thus, another of my goals was to address the facets of hyperthyroidism and its causes and treatments that most often confuse patients. My expertise is in the clinical laboratory, and I also emphasized (and attempted to clarify) the sometimes confusing role thyroid function and thyroid antibody tests play in predicting one's clinical course. — E.A.M.

1

Introduction

In the 12 years since *Graves' Disease: A Practical Guide* (2001), much new information has emerged. For instance, the mainstay anti-thyroid drug (ATD) propylthiouracil (PTU) has been given a black box warning, making methimazole the ATD of choice. Worldwide, anti-thyroid drugs continue to be the most widely used treatment for hyperthyroidism, and now they are the most commonly used treatment used for hyperthyroidism in North America.

In addition, herbs proven effective for the treatment of hyperthyroidism have become available in the form of patent tonics. Researchers have also made gains in discovering the defects in the immune response and the metabolism that contribute to autoimmune disease, making the underlying origins of Graves' disease much clearer. In addition, several new drugs used to reduce pro-inflammatory cytokines and reduce thyroid antibody production are now available for treating Graves' ophthalmopathy and pretibial myxedema. Low dose naltrexone is now used off label in both Graves' disease and Graves' ophthalmopathy to promote immune system healing. These are just a few of the advances that indicate a newfound interest in hyperthyroid disorders.

Hyperthyroid disorders have always been unique and rather mysterious because they typically cause symptoms that vary in severity over time; the disease course is also characterized by periods of remission that alternate with periods of symptoms. In autoimmune hyperthyroid disorders, remission is possible and so is relapse. This new book describes the reasons why hyperthyroid disorders are unique in each individual and explains how environmental factors, including diet, influence thyroid hormone production.

Also addressed are the special concerns of hyperthyroidism brought about by hereditary mutations, nodules, thyroiditis and other causes, as well as the special concerns that occur during pregnancy and in children. As always, the underlying goal is to educate and empower patients so that they can take charge of their own health.

1

Hyperthyroidism and Its Signs and Symptoms

Chapter 1 focuses on thyroid function and what one can expect in hyperthyroidism. Conditions of hyperthyroidism occur when normal thyroid function goes awry, causing the thyroid gland to produce and release excess thyroid hormone. Hyperthyroidism can cause thyrotoxicosis. Thyrotoxicosis is a clinical, physiologic, and biochemical condition that occurs when the body's tissues are exposed to and respond to excess thyroid hormone. Thyrotoxicosis can also occur in other conditions of thyroid dysfunction that do not cause hyperthyroidism. In thyroiditis, for example, rather than producing excess thyroid hormone, damaged thyroid cells release excess thyroid hormone directly into the blood circulation.

Specifically, this chapter describes normal thyroid function and hyperthyroidism. It includes the physical and neurological changes that can occur in Graves' disease, toxic multinodular goiter (TMG), and other disorders of hyperthyroidism or other conditions that cause thyrotoxicosis, such as the ingestion of excess thyroid replacement hormone or the hyperthyroid phase of Hashimoto's thyroiditis.

An overview of the thyroid gland's anatomy and physiology is also provided in this chapter to explain what the thyroid gland is and how it normally functions to produce adequate thyroid hormone to cover the body's needs. Readers will also learn how conditions of excess thyroid hormone affect other organs and bodily systems to produce a wide variety of signs and symptoms.

Above all, readers will discover what it means to be diagnosed with conditions of hyperthyroidism, including subclinical hyperthyroidism as well as controlled euthyroid (normal thyroid function) thyrotoxic states. In addition they'll learn what signs and symptoms are associated with the severe condition of thyrotoxicosis known as thyroid storm.

Endocrine Glands

Endocrine glands include the thyroid, adrenals, parathyroid, pituitary, ovaries, testes, thymus, pineal, and the islet of Langerhans in the pancreas. Endocrine glands secrete chemical messengers known as hormones. Hormones exert their intended effects by reacting with protein receptors located on the cells throughout the body. During this reaction, the reactor is activated, causing changes in DNA with specific effects. For instance, when thyroid hormone activates receptors on cardiac cells, the cells of the heart are prompted to beat faster. This is just one of the functions of thyroid hormone. Each hormone has a variety of effects, which are influenced by several factors, including the body's general health, activity level, temperature and other factors, including the number of available thyroid hormone receptors.

Endocrine Hormones

Endocrine glands produce, store, and release specific hormones that they release directly into the blood circulation as needed. For instance, the thyroid gland produces various thyroid hormones, and the adrenal glands produce cortisol and other adrenal hormones. Hormones also affect the function of other glands and organs under their control. For instance, the thyroid gland influences the activity of the ovaries and the production of various sex hormones. Hyperthyroidism can alter levels of sex hormones and cause conditions of amenorrhea (absent or scant menstrual periods) in women and breast enlargement in men. Production of endocrine hormones can be disrupted when there is damage to glands or when normal regulatory mechanisms fail. This is the case in autoimmune endocrine disorders.

Endocrine hormones are released directly into the bloodstream to provide adequate hormones as required. In the bloodstream, hormone molecules link to carrier or transport proteins. These protein-linked, inactive hormones travel through the blood and lymphatic system until they reach their target destinations. Consequently, the effects of hormones are slower and subtler than reactions involving the nervous system.

However, if normal hormone levels change and become chronically diminished or increased (as in hypothyroidism or hyperthyroidism), the subsequent effects are sustained until the blood levels are corrected with appropriate treatment or the condition itself resolves. In hyperthyroidism, for instance, although associated symptoms persist during the course of the illness, their severity can vary, typically increasing (becoming exacerbated) in times of stress and dissipating when blood levels return to the normal or reference range.

The Thyroid Gland

The largest of the endocrine glands, the thyroid gland is situated in the neck and suspended directly below the larynx or Adam's apple. The thyroid has the same consistency as muscle tissue, and it follows the movement of the larynx. When the thyroid gland is enlarged, it is readily visible as it follows the movement of the larynx when swallowing. A home test to detect thyroid enlargement involves observing one's neck while drinking a glass of water and watching for the rising movement of an enlarged thyroid.

Thyroid Anatomy

Normally weighing about 20 grams (two-thirds of an ounce), the thyroid gland is usually larger in women than men. It is protected from injury by a shield-shaped cartilage covering. The word *thyroid*, meaning shield, is derived from the characteristic appearance of the cartilage rather than the gland. The gland itself has a butterfly shape and is covered by a reddish-brown fibrous capsule with projections (pseudolobules) that extend like fingers wrapping around nearby organs.

The thyroid gland consists of a right and a left lobe attached on either side to the trachea. Each lobe is about 4 cm in length with a 2 cm thickness, and the lobes are connected together near the top by a thin band of connective

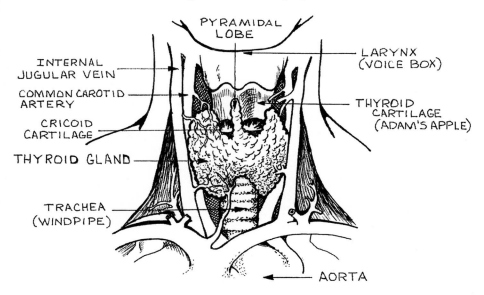

The thyroid gland (courtesy Marvin G. Miller).

tissue called the isthmus. Some people also have a small pyramidal lobe situated between the right and left lobes. The pyramidal lobe is generally present in Graves' disease.

Because thyroid hormone can affect and influence the function of every cell in the body, the thyroid gland's blood circulation per unit weight exceeds that of the kidney. Occasionally, when the gland is enlarged (forming a goiter), the excessive pounding blood flow in the gland may be heard with a stethoscope. The sound is known as a bruit, and the feel of excess blood flow upon palpation of the gland is known as a thrill.

THE THYROID GLAND VIEWED MICROSCOPICALLY

Thyroid lobes can be further divided into lobules. Lobules contain 20–40 microscopic follicles or sacs of varying sizes. The adult male contains about 3 million thyroid follicles. Spaces between the follicles allow for the elasticity needed to accompany the constantly changing follicle size.

The various thyroid cells, nerve fibers, lymphatic tissue, blood vessels, and immune system cells are enclosed in a stroma or sheath of connective tissue. After periods of hyperactivity, especially in the early stages of Graves' disease, the connective tissue may expand to enclose isolated follicles, forming thyroid nodules or pseudoadenomas (Hoffman 1961, 505–06).

Blood to the thyroid is supplied from four thyroid arteries. Lymphatic vessels are also present. They line the borders of each follicle and form a net-

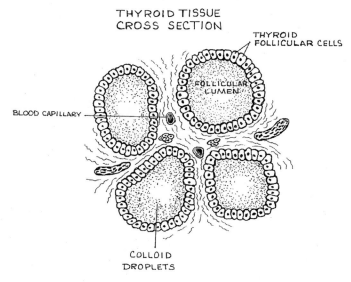

Microscopic view of thyroid cells (courtesy Marvin G. Miller).

work between the follicles. Thyroid lymph vessels ultimately drain into the deep cervical and pretracheal lymph glands. These lymph glands are occasionally enlarged in individuals with Graves' disease.

Thyroid Hormone Production

The thyroid gland produces and releases thyroid hormone. Thyroid hormone results from a combination of iodine and the amino acid tyrosine. In a process of organification, iodide ions are concentrated in the thyroid gland into organic iodine by hydrogen peroxide or oxygen. Thus, thyroid hormone production is limited by available iodine stores. The iodine taken up by the active thyroid cells binds (iodinates) with tyrosine resulting in the formation of monoiodotyrosine (MIT) and diiodotyrosine (DIT). The enzyme thyroid peroxidase (TPO, thyroperoxidase) is required for this reaction. MIT and DIT molecules combine to form the hormone triiodothyronine (T3), whereas two DIT molecules combine to form T4.

Thyroid Physiology: The Site of Thyroid Activity

The functional unit of the thyroid gland is the follicle, which is a hollow sac. Each follicle is composed of a roughly spherical group of cells arranged around a protein-rich storage material called colloid. Thyroid epithelial cells that secrete the gelatinous colloid material line the border of each individual follicle, and the follicle itself is enclosed by a basement membrane. Thyroglobulin is the most important protein found in colloid. Thyroglobulin serves as the matrix for thyroid hormone production and as a warehouse for stored thyroid hormone.

Thyroid Cells

Thyroid tissue is composed of thyroid tissue (epithelial) cells, follicular cells, parafollicular cells, and oxyphil cells. In hyperthyroidism there is an increase in the size (hypertrophy) of follicular cells and an increase in the number of cells (hyperplasia) caused by increased thyroid hormone production.

THYROID FOLLICULAR CELLS

The basement membrane of the follicle consists of follicular cells that trap iodine from the blood circulation and transport it to the follicular lumen, where it is used for the production of thyroid hormone. Thyroid follicular cells are considered the most important because of their dual role in thyroid metabolism and in the production of both colloid and thyroid hormone.

PARAFOLLICULAR (C) CELLS AND OXYPHIL CELLS

Parafollicular or C cells are found in the upper poles of thyroid lobes located within the follicular wall, which is situated beneath the basement membrane or in the spaces between follicular cells. C cells produce and secrete the hormone calcitonin, which helps to regulate blood calcium levels. Increased levels of calcitonin serve as a marker for parafollicular and other thyroid neoplasms.

Oxyphil cells, which include oncocytes, Askanazy, and Hürthle cells, are abnormally enlarged follicular cells with granular cytoplasm, swollen mitochondria and large nuclei. Oxyphil cells are commonly seen in irradiated thyroid tissue, autoimmune thyroiditis, Hashitoxicosis, long-standing Graves' disease, thyroid neoplasms and some adenomatous thyroid nodules. Askanazy cells are seen in inflammatory thyroid conditions such as Hashimoto's thyroiditis.

To describe how thyroid antibodies exert their effects, the following sections describe the role of cell receptors.

Cell Receptors

Receptors are proteins found on the cell surface, cell mitochondria, or nucleus in which hormones and drugs react to modulate gene expression. These changes in gene expression result in physiological changes such as an increase in body temperature or a reduction in pain. Specific receptors, for instance for thyroid hormone or for opiates, can be found on various cells throughout the body. Receptors can be compared to locks where hormones or drugs can react as if they were keys. Receptor sites can be opened or closed depending on the cells' needs. The number of receptor sites affects how much of an effect hormones and drugs can produce.

Receptors can also malfunction or have genetic mutations that alter the ways in which hormones or drugs can react. Various drugs can also interfere with the function of receptors. The anticonvulsant drug phenytoin (Dilantin) has been shown to interfere with the binding of T3 thyroid hormone to thyroid receptors in the pituitary gland. Nonsteroidal anti-inflammatory drugs (NSAIDs) and excess free fatty acids also prevent T3 from binding to nuclear receptors.

In addition to specific receptors, the body contains several orphan receptors, cell receptors whose target hormones haven't yet been discovered. It's unknown if any of the orphan receptors can be activated by thyroid hormone.

Hormonal Disruptors

Receptor sites can also be blocked or activated by chemicals known as hormonal disruptors. Because of their ability to bind to foreign (not their usual target receptor) receptors, hormonal disruptors can be used therapeutically. When blockage of estrogen is desired, for example, a plant substance with mildly estrogenic effects such as red clover can be administered, minimizing estrogen stimulation. However, hormonal disruptors rarely act beneficially.

Numerous environmental hormonal disruptors, primarily industrial chemicals, have been identified. Although many hormonal disruptors, such as PCB and DDT, are no longer produced, they're still prevalent since they don't degrade well. The list of known and suspected hormonal disruptors includes organic pesticides, phthalates, heavy metals, plastics, phenolic compounds and styrene dimers and trimers. The organ most affected by hormonal disruptors is the adrenal gland, which produces stress hormones, followed by the thyroid gland (Colborn 1996, 85).

The Thyroid Hormone Receptor

When receptor sites on thyroid cells are blocked, the intended hormonal message can't be relayed. When the wrong message or no message is sent, thyroid function is affected. In *Screaming to Be Heard, Hormonal Connections Women Suspect ... and Doctors Ignore*, Elizabeth Vliet explains how environmental endocrine disruptors prevent thyroid hormone from exerting its intended effects. Consequently, laboratory values may stay normal for months or years while the patient suffers from the effects of thyroid hormone deficiency (Vliet 1995, 57–61).

Mammalian thyroid hormone receptors are encoded by two genes designated alpha and beta. Each of these genes can be spliced, resulting in four different thyroid hormone receptors: alpha-1, alpha-2, beta-1, and beta-2. Like other members of the nuclear receptor family, thyroid hormone receptors encapsulate three functional domains: a transactivation domain; a DNA-binding domain; and a ligand-binding and dimerization domain. The different forms of thyroid receptors found in different tissues vary depending on the type of tissue and the developmental stage.

Thyroid hormone receptors bind to short, repeated sequences of DNA called thyroid or T3 response elements (TREs) as monomers, homodimers, or as heterodimers, with heterodimers having the highest binding affinity. A greater response is seen when the thyroid hormone receptor has already bound to T3, forming a complex. These are the reasons for the variable response of thyroid hormone seen among different individuals. Genetic mutations in thyroid hormone receptors cause the condition of resistance to thyroid hormone.

THE SUPERFAMILY OF RECEPTORS

Cell receptors for steroid hormones, thyroid hormones, vitamin D and the retinoids (vitamin A and its derivatives) regulate the transcription of specific genes on the cells where they're located. These receptors are all part of a larger family of transcription factors regulated by similar chemical processes. The TSH receptor is a member of the family of G protein–coupled receptors and is structurally similar to the receptors for the pituitary hormones, luteinizing hormone (LH) and follicle-stimulating hormone (FSH), which are reproductive hormones capable of binding to each others' receptors.

Hyperthyroidism

Hyperthyroidism is a condition of increased thyroid hormone production and secretion by the thyroid gland. Similar to other conditions of thyroid dysfunction, hyperthyroidism can be a temporary condition that runs its course and resolves. Alternately, hyperthyroidism can spontaneously move on as it does in thyroiditis and eventually lead to hypothyroidism. In another variation, hyperthyroidism can be episodic with periods in which variable symptoms alternate with periods of remission. This is especially common in the early phase of Graves' disease.

The severity and the associated symptoms associated with hyperthyroidism can vary over time. Hyperthyroidism is often associated with other conditions such as celiac disease that are described in Chapter 5. Although Graves' disease is the most common cause of hyperthyroidism, hyperthyroidism has a number of different causes, which are described in Chapter 2.

Conditions of hyperthyroidism, especially Graves' disease, are often characterized by phases, including an initial period of hypothyroidism that occurs before hyperthyroidism develops. Similarly, in Hashimoto's thyroiditis, an autoimmune hypothyroid disorder, rapid thyroid cell destruction can release high levels of thyroid hormone, resulting in a hyperthyroid phase that occurs during the early course of the disease. In autoimmune thyroid disorders, it's also not uncommon to have more than one disorder in one's lifetime. Individuals with Hashimoto's hyperthyroidism often develop Graves' disease after many months or years. About 20 percent of individuals with Graves' disease move into conditions of hypothyroidism that are often transient.

Duration of Hyperthyroid Symptoms and Age-Related Symptoms

In hyperthyroid disorders caused by thyroiditis, symptoms usually emerge suddenly, appearing over the course of a few weeks. In Graves' disease, symptoms are more likely to develop over many months. Compared with younger patients, older patients have fewer symptoms and signs associated with stimulation of the sympathetic nervous system, such as anxiety, tremor and hyperactivity, and they're less likely to have a palpable thyroid gland. Among younger patients, the presence of goiter and exophthalmos is more common, although before midadolescence, severe ophthalmopathy is rarely seen. Children with thyrotoxicosis are typically tall for their age and tend to be taller at full growth than predicted. In addition, their bone ages are advanced. Children are also more likely to have movement disorders such as jerking and hyperkinetic movements that may be confused with symptoms of attention deficit hyperactivity disorder (ADHD).

Older patients are more likely to have signs and symptoms of cardiovascular dysfunction, such as atrial fibrillation and shortness of breath, and they're more likely to complain of anorexia and constipation (Braverman and Utiger 2000, 515). Elderly patients with severe hyperthyroidism may have cognitive dysfunction, delirium or coma (Bunevicius and Prange 2006, 901). Apathetic hyperthyroidism, which is seen in patients with Graves' hyperthyroidism, presents with symptoms of depression, apathy, somnolence or pseudodementia. Although these symptoms have been described in young adults and adolescents, apathetic symptoms are more common in elderly patients.

While the severity of symptoms and signs observed in thyrotoxicosis do not usually correlate with blood thyroid hormone levels or radioiodine uptake results, symptom severity is considered a better indicator of disease severity.

Thyrotoxicosis

The term *thyrotoxicosis* is sometimes used synonymously with hyperthyroidism. However, according to the medical literature, thyrotoxicosis refers to a distinct syndrome that differs from conditions of hyperthyroidism. "Toxicosis" in the word *thyrotoxicosis* refers to the effects of elevated thyroid hormone and not to the common meaning of toxicity, caused by drugs or poisons. Thyrotoxicosis refers to the changes caused when the body's tissues are stimulated by and respond to excess thyroid hormone.

Although thyrotoxicosis is technically not the same as hyperthyroidism, for practical purposes and following the example of the prominent thyroidologist Leslie DeGroot, in this book the terms *hyperthyroidism* and *thyrotoxicosis* are used synonymously (DeGroot 2010, 1).

Many Graves' disease patients are incorrectly told that they're thyrotoxic on the basis of a low TSH level in the presence of low or normal thyroid hormone levels. However, the problem with interpretation is more than that of semantics. Elevated thyroid hormone levels, not a low TSH level, are responsible for the symptoms associated with thyrotoxicosis.

Thyrotoxicosis has traditionally been regarded as a clinical syndrome with a wide variety of signs and symptoms resulting from the hypermetabolic state, which is caused by increased levels of either free thyroxine (measured with the FT4 blood level) or free triiodothyronine (measured with the FT3 blood level).

Thyrotoxicosis Versus Hyperthyroidism

Whereas hyperthyroidism refers to conditions in which the gland produces and releases excess thyroid hormone, thyrotoxicosis can occur whenever thyroid hormone levels rise into the abnormal range. Thyrotoxicosis can be caused by a release or "dumping" of thyroid hormone into the blood circulation when thyroid cells are destroyed in conditions of thyroiditis (for instance the hyperthyroid phase of Hashimoto's thyroiditis), or it can be caused by an excessive intake of exogenous thyroid hormone.

Writing in the online thyroid textbook *Thyroid Manager*, Dr. Peter Koop emphasizes that the elevation of free thyroid hormone levels does not always result in thyrotoxicosis in all tissues (Koop 2010, 1). In the syndrome of resistance to thyroid hormone (RTH), for instance, dominant negative mutations in the thyroid hormone receptor subunit b (TRb) result in decreased thyroid hormone action in tissues where TRb is the predominant receptor, for example in the liver and the pituitary, whereas other tissues such as the heart, which express mainly TRa (the subunit a of the thyroid hormone receptor), show signs of increased thyroid hormone action.

Signs and Symptoms of Thyrotoxicosis

Signs refers to the objective findings noted by practitioners or patients or that are discovered with the aid of diagnostic tests. Signs can usually be measured or evaluated and include elevated systolic blood pressure or fluid retention (edema). Some signs may occur for reasons other than thyrotoxicosis, particularly when patients have other conditions associated with hyperthyroidism. For instance atrial fibrillation and also long QT syndrome (which causes increased risk for ventricular fibrillation and sudden death) may occur because of genes associated with thyroid dysfunction. In one recent study, two gene products, the proteins KCNE2 and KCNQ1, which are involved in human cardiac arrhythmias, were linked to thyroid dysfunction and the formation of a thyroid stimulating hormone (TSH)–stimulated potassium channel within the thyroid gland (Purtell 2010).

In addition, some signs are associated with gender or age. For instance, goiter is more likely to be seen in elderly patients, and weight gain is more likely to occur in young women. Although hyperthyroidism is ten times more common in women, men typically have more severe symptoms at the time of diagnosis and their cardiovascular and nervous systems are more likely to be affected. Men are also more likely to develop amiodarone-associated thyrotoxicosis.

Symptoms refers to subjective findings that are usually noticed by patients. Common symptoms in thyrotoxicosis include headache, anxiety and dizziness. There is considerable overlap with some symptoms such as weight loss that may also be considered measurable signs. There is also considerable overlap with a number of symptoms known to occur in both hypothyroidism and hyperthyroidism. These include palpitations, sleep disturbances, anxiety and weight changes. Symptoms in thyrotoxicosis may also be caused by associated conditions and are described in Chapter 5. There is no one symptom that defines hyperthyroidism.

Individuals with hyperthyroidism typically develop several predominant signs and symptoms rather than the entire spectrum of symptoms. Both signs and symptoms can change over time, as can their severity. Most symptoms seen in thyrotoxicosis are common and can occur alone or in other conditions. Before being diagnosed with hyperthyroidism, many patients are misdiagnosed, and frequently are erroneously treated for anxiety or depression.

Signs and symptoms in hyperthyroidism and thyrotoxicosis such as an elevated heart rate or nervousness are directly caused by excess thyroid hormone. In autoimmune hyperthyroid conditions, symptoms can also occur as a result of autoimmunity; these are further discussed with Graves' disease in Chapter 3. Many of the signs and symptoms related to autoimmunity are extrathyroidal (occurring away from the thyroid) manifestations and include thyroid acropachy, pretibial myxedema, which primarily causes swelling and scaling of the lower legs, and the eye condition Graves' ophthalmopathy (thyroid eye disease). These manifestations are described in Chapter 11.

SIGNS SEEN IN THYROTOXICOSIS

- Abnormal liver function tests, e.g., low albumin, increased globulins, increased bilirubin and liver enzymes (alanine transaminase [ALT], aspartate transaminase [AST], and alkaline phosphatase due to nutrient deficiencies and increased metabolism
- Arrhythmia, primarily atrial fibrillation and sinus tachycardia (increased heart rate)
- Bruit (audible sign of turbulence associated with increased thyroid blood flow)
- Elevated blood levels of free thyroxine (FT4) and/or free triiodothyronine (FT3) and low levels of the pituitary hormone thyrotropin (also known as thyroid stimulating hormone or TSH)

- Enlarged lymph nodes
- Enlarged thymus gland
- Enlarged thyroid gland (goiter)
- Increased drug metabolism — the metabolism and excretion of many drugs are accelerated in the thyrotoxic state; consequently, a number of medications require an increase in dosage to work effectively
- Increased systolic blood pressure; decreased diastolic blood pressure
- Enlarged lymph nodes
- Enlarged thymus
- Histological thyroid changes, i.e., lymphocytic hyperplasia
- Hyperkinesis (increased and sometimes involuntary erratic muscle movement) exemplified in table drumming, tapping feet and jerky, exaggerated, aimless movements or frenetic (frenzied) behavior, thought and speech patterns
- Increased alcohol and drug metabolism
- Increased red blood cell volume (due to increased oxygen consumption)
- Increased systolic blood pressure; decreased diastolic blood pressure
- Increased tendon reflex (hyperreflexia)
- Low blood cholesterol level
- Malabsorption
- Muscle weakness (myopathy)
- Nutrient deficiencies, particularly low levels of omega 3 essential fatty acids, the oil-soluble vitamins A, D, E, CoQ10, and B vitamins
- Rhabdomyolysis (in severe conditions, e.g., thyroid storm)
- Seizures occur more often in individuals with convulsive disorders
- Steatorrhea (increased stool lipids)
- Thrill (palpable sign of turbulence associated with increased thyroid blood flow)
- Tremor

SIGNS SPECIFIC TO HYPERTHYROIDISM CAUSED BY GRAVES' DISEASE

- Serological changes including the presence of stimulating TSH receptor antibodies (also known as thyroid stimulating immunoglobulins or TSI) and, in most cases, thyroglobulin and thyroid peroxidase (TPO) antibodies; rarely, antinuclear (ANA) and DNA antibodies are seen.
- Eye changes (common changes include upper eyelid lag on down-gaze, upper eyelid retraction, diplopia, incomplete and frequent blinking, palsy or paralysis of extraocular muscle, and unilateral eye edema; less common signs are described in Chapter 11).
- Antibodies to megalin (the thyroglobulin receptor on thyroid cells) and to the thyroidal iodide symporter (DeGroot 2010, 1)

- Circulating immune (antigen-antibody) complexes
- Elevated levels of ICAM-1, and IL-6 and IL-8 cytokines
- Diffusely enlarged gland with increased iodine uptake
- Increased prevalence of mitral valve prolapse (Klein and Levery 2000, 602)

SYMPTOMS IN THYROTOXICOSIS

The following list includes the more common symptoms that can occur in thyrotoxicosis. Because thyroid hormone affects so many of the body's organs, symptoms related to specific organs and bodily systems that are commonly affected follow the symptom list.

- Anxiety
- Depression
- Edema, peripheral
- Elbow redness
- Emotional lability
- Euphoria, exhilaration
- Fast, jerky movements
- Fast speech
- Fatigue
- Flushing of the face and neck
- Goiter, diffuse or nodular
- Gynecomastia (breast enlargement) in men
- Hair changes (hair loss, increased growth, fine texture, diffuse nonscarring alopecia)
- Headaches
- Heat intolerance
- Hyperpigmentation (especially facial with patchy areas)
- Inattention
- Increased appetite and thirst
- Increased bowel movements
- Increased sweating
- Increased urination
- Irritability
- Mental alertness
- Menstrual abnormalities (absent or scant periods)
- Mood disturbances
- Muscle weakness (often related to CoQ10 deficiency)
- Nail changes (onchylosis, increased growth, ragged margins, Plummer's nails)

- Nausea, vomiting
- Restlessness
- Shortness of breath (dyspnea)
- Skin of the hands may be reddened, hot or moist
- Sleep disturbances
- Tremor, fine
- Weakness
- Weight loss and occasionally weight gain

Metabolic Symptoms

Metabolism is increased in hyperthyroidism. Excess thyroid hormone affects glucose homeostasis via its effects on several different organs, including increased output of the liver's stored glycogen and increased clearance by the kidneys. Although carbohydrate absorption is increased, glucose moves quickly through the intestines causing blood glucose levels to fall faster. This can cause symptoms of hypoglycemia, insulin resistance and increased insulin levels in some patients. Patients with Graves' disease may also develop insulin autoimmune syndrome (Hirata's disease), which is described in Chapter 3.

DIABETES AND THYROTOXICOSIS

Diabetes may be temporarily activated or intensified, although these transient conditions of diabetes resolve when the thyrotoxicosis is treated (DeGroot 2010, 1). In patients with type 2 diabetes, diabetic ketoacidosis can develop if thyrotoxicosis remains untreated. It's recommended that all diabetic patients be screened for thyroid dysfunction because correcting hyperthyroidism can profoundly affect glucose homeostasis. Similarly, patients with diabetic ketoacidosis should have thyroid function tests (Potenza 2009).

KIDNEY FUNCTION IN THYROTOXICOSIS

Thyrotoxicosis increases both renal (kidney) blood flow and glomerular filtration rate. By lowering the plasma creatinine level, the increased extracellular fluid volume induces substantial muscle wasting. Blood urea nitrogen (BUN) levels are typically elevated, causing an increased BUN:creatinine ratio.

Urination may be increased in thyrotoxicosis and some patients may have an impaired urinary concentrating ability (Scheinman and Moses, 2000, 617) resulting in fluid retention. Pitting edema is a common symptom and usually involves the ankles, legs, and sacrum. In hyperthyroidism caused by Graves' disease, the uric acid level may be elevated.

THYROTOXIC PERIODIC PARALYSIS

Thyrotoxic periodic paralysis, which is sometimes called hypokalemic thyrotoxic periodic paralysis, is a condition characterized by generalized attacks of muscle weakness, including flaccid paralysis, which may occur for a few hours to several weeks. This condition is more common in men and can occur even when thyrotoxicosis is mild. Low potassium levels are usually present, although levels may not be abnormally low. Thyrotoxic periodic paralysis is more common in Asian patients, although cases have been reported in patients of all ethnicities. Sugar and alcohol consumption, performing strenuous exercise in hot weather, and the administration of insulin or acetazolamide are reported to precipitate attacks. Changes in the movement of potassium ions in thyrotoxicosis are thought to be responsible (Moore 2000, 22).

LIVER FUNCTION

Although the exact cause is unknown, the liver is often affected in thyrotoxicosis, with a minority of patients having abnormal thyroid function tests. Tissue examinations show that liver cells of these patients develop changes characteristic of nonspecific liver injury, which presumably is caused by excess thyroid hormone (Sellin and Vasilopoulou-Sellin 2000, 623). Liver function tests return to normal when thyrotoxicosis is corrected.

WEIGHT LOSS AND WEIGHT GAIN

Thyrotoxicosis often causes a loss of lean body mass. This is primarily due to loss of muscle protein rather than loss of body fat (Franklyn 2000, 669). While protein synthesis and degradation are increased in thyrotoxicosis, the greater effect on degradation results in a net breakdown of protein. This leads to a loss of muscle fiber volume and impaired exercise capacity. A minority of thyrotoxic patients, usually teenagers and young adults, gain weight. This is especially likely when FT3 is higher relative to FT4 levels. The increased appetite that occurs in hyperthyroidism can lead to cravings for sugar and fat, which lead to weight gain.

Cardiac Symptoms

Common cardiac symptoms in thyrotoxicosis include tachycardia (prevalence 95 percent); palpitations (prevalence 85 percent); widened pulse pressure (prevalence 75 percent); exercise intolerance (prevalence 65 percent); cardiac flow murmurs (prevalence 50 percent); shortness of breath on exertion (prevalence 45 percent); atrial fibrillation (prevalence 5–10 percent); and angina pectoris (prevalence 3–5 percent) While atrial fibrillation is associated with increased mortality, less than 5 percent of all cases of atrial fibrillation are caused by thyrotoxicosis (Klein and Levey 2000, 599–600).

Thyrotoxicosis causes decreases in systemic vascular resistance (one of the earliest signs) and increases in cardiac output, systolic blood pressure, heart rate, left ventricular ejection fraction, cardiac contractility and mass and red blood cell volume. Decreased vascular resistance, which may be as high as 70 percent, causes increased blood flow to the skin, muscles, kidney and heart (Klein and Levey 596).

Both thyroxine (T4) and triiodothyronine (T3) affect the cardiac cell (myocyte) nucleus and other cellular components by binding to specific receptors that direct specific DNA sequences. Although sensitivity to catecholamines (epinephrine, norepinephrine) is usually normal in thyrotoxicosis, sensitivity to these compounds may be somewhat increased, particularly during infectious states. Elderly patients may only experience tachycardia presumably due to lowered adrenergic activity, although an increase in systolic blood pressure is also more common in the elderly due to reduced blood vessel elasticity (Klein and Levey 2000, 600). Congestive heart failure is rare and more likely to occur in elderly patients with atrial fibrillation, higher levels of systemic vascular resistance and a disproportionate increase in vascular resistance with exercise or chronic thyrotoxicosis.

Respiratory Symptoms

Shortness of breath is the most common respiratory symptom in thyrotoxicosis and is thought to be caused by respiratory muscle weakness, heart failure causing an engorged pulmonary capillary blood vessel bed, increased ventilator drive to breathe, increased airway resistance, and tracheal compression resulting from an enlarged thyroid gland (Ingbar 2000, 606).

Other changes that may be seen in thyrotoxicosis include increased oxygen consumption, increased carbon dioxide production, respiratory muscle weakness, decreased lung compliance, and pulmonary artery dilation and hypertension.

Psychiatric and Neural Symptoms

Mental changes are common in patients with thyrotoxicosis and include insomnia, poor concentration, episodic anxiety, irritability, hyperactivity, and behavioral changes ranging from whimsical behavioral changes to severe disturbances in cognitive function and behavior (Boyages 2000, 633). Less common changes include agitated delirium, confusion, apathy, depression and mania. Overall, higher rates of panic disorder, simple phobia, obsessive-compulsive disorder, major depressive disorder, bipolar disorder, depression and cyclothymia (condition of alternating periods of depression and expansiveness/irritability/hallucinations) are seen in patients with thyroid dysfunction, including hypothyroidism, even when they are receiving appropriate treatment for their condition. Patients with thyroid storm, which is described later in this chapter, can show symptoms of confusion, agitation and delirium. Rarely, these patients have seizures, psychosis, stupor or coma.

Increased motor activity in thyrotoxicosis can cause patients to appear agitated. Although this can mimic mania, the fully developed syndrome of mania is surprisingly rare in thyrotoxicosis (Whybrow and Bauer 2000, 673). When true mania and hypomania occur in patients with thyrotoxicosis, the patients typically have a previous diagnosis of bipolar disorder or a family history of that disorder.

The effects of stimulants and alcohol are pronounced in thyrotoxicosis and this can also contribute to behavioral changes. Nutrient deficiencies, particularly deficiencies of B vitamins and magnesium, can also contribute to irritability and depression. Patients with hyperthyroidism may also feel fatigued and distracted, compounding the problem. Emotional lability is often a predominant symptom in thyrotoxicosis, with patients complaining of mood swings. Moods can quickly change from euphoria to despair. Patients may appear irritable, jittery and easily moved to tears, and some patients report having feelings of paranoia and experiencing disjointed, rambling speech disturbances. Mania in thyrotoxicosis is manifested by rapid speech, quick movements, and disorganization of thought content.

In a study of patients diagnosed with hyperthyroidism, Bunevicius and Prange note that antithyroid drugs combined with beta-adrenoreceptor antagonists are the treatment of choice for hyperthyroidism, as well as for the psychiatric disorders and mental symptoms caused by hyperthyroidism. They also note that psychiatric symptoms may persist after euthyroidism is restored and they describe an association between heightened stress and high levels of TSH receptor antibodies in patients with Graves' disease (Bunevicius and Prange 2006, 898).

GRAVES' RAGE

Graves' rage is a temporary condition in which the behavioral changes associated with thyrotoxicosis become extreme. Paranoia and psychosis can manifest, and patients show exaggerated reactions to stress. Graves' rage appears to occur when thyroid hormone levels change abruptly, with psychosis more likely to occur in patients given aggressive treatment that causes a sudden swing from hyperthyroidism to hypothyroidism.

Stress is considered an important precipitating factor in Graves' rage.

Several studies have been conducted in an attempt to show that patients with Graves' disease demonstrate a heightened reaction to stress. Although these studies have been inconclusive, a genetic tendency toward the neuroendocrine response has been recently proposed (Whybrow and Bauer 2000, 676).

Diagnostic Problems

Because patients with thyroid disorders have a considerable overlap between mental and physical complaints including loss of energy and tremulousness, the true incidence of psychiatric symptoms in patients with thyroid disorders is hard to estimate. Overall, about 10 percent of patients with hyperthyroidism are suspected of having neuropsychiatric symptoms. In addition, about 31 percent of patients have depression and 62 percent have anxiety disorders (Whybrow and Bauer 2000, 673). Patients with subclinical hyperthyroidism are also reported to show increased anxiety and irritability and decreased vitality and activity when compared to normal subjects. Panic disorders are rarely seen in hyperthyroidism although they are likely to occur in hypothyroid patients.

Reproductive and Adrenal Symptoms

Although sexual maturation and the onset of menses may be delayed, children with thyrotoxicosis do not suffer reproductive system effects (Loncope 2000, 653). In women, the menstrual period may become scant or absent. An increase in the transport protein sex hormone-binding-globulin (SHBG) can lead to increased estrogen levels in women and men. Testosterone levels in women are typically low, but despite fertility being slightly depressed, pregnancy can develop. Although the miscarriage rate is increased in thyrotoxicosis, symptoms of thyrotoxicosis typically are ameliorated or resolved as pregnancy progresses. By the second half of pregnancy, the immune system slows down its activity and changes in other sex steroid hormones cause a fall in thyroid hormone levels.

Men with thyrotoxicosis can also have high serum estradiol levels due to increased conversion of androstendione to estradiol. This may lead to breast enlargement (gynecomastia). Because of an increase in transport proteins, levels of testosterone may also increase in men. In one study of hyperthyroid men, low sex drive was seen in 17.6 percent of subjects, delayed ejaculation was seen in 2.9 percent, premature ejaculation in 50 percent, and erectile dysfunction in 14.7 percent (Carani et al. 2005, 673–4).

While cortisol levels are typically lower because of decreased clearance in thyrotoxicosis, there may be an exaggerated response to catecholamines (adrenaline, noradrenaline).

Subclinical Hyperthyroidism

Subclinical hyperthyroidism is a condition defined by a low TSH level in the presence of normal thyroid hormone (T4/FT4) levels (Woeber 2005, 687) The most common causes of subclinical hyperthyroidism are Graves' disease and toxic multinodular goiter. Although symptoms can occur when thyroid hormone levels rise higher than usual, conditions of subclinical hyperthyroidism are not typically treated with anti-thyroid drugs as this can cause thyroid hormone levels to fall too low. In one small study, it was shown that in cases of subclinical hyperthyroidism caused by Graves' disease, most cases resolve spontaneously within 19 months (with TSH levels rising and levels of TSH receptor antibodies falling) whereas in subclinical hyperthyroidism caused by toxic multinodular goiter, low TSH levels are more likely to persist (Woeber 2005, 687–88). Another recent study showed that less than 1 percent of individuals with subclinical hyperthyroidism developed hyperthyroidism during an observation period of seven years (Vadivello et al. 2011). Although anti-thyroid drug treatment isn't needed for subclinical hyperthyroidism and could cause levels to fall too low, patients should be regularly monitored because subclinical hyperthyroidism causes an increased risk for cardiovascular disease.

Euthyroid Hyperthyroxinemia

Euthyroid hyperthyroxinemia is defined as a condition in which the serum total or, rarely, the free thyroxine (T4) concentrations are abnormally elevated without evidence of clinical thyroid disease. These changes may be transient or persistent and may be associated with normal, low, or high triiodothyronine (T3) levels. The usual cause is a genetic mutation that can cause increased levels of binding or transport proteins. These proteins have an affinity for thyroid hormone and form complexes of bound hormone. In this form, thyroxine (measured by the total T4 level) is inactive. This can lead to a form of resistance to thyroid hormone and conditions of hypothyroidism causing learning disabilities in children as well as symptoms of attention deficit hyperactivity disorder (ADHD).

Drugs associated with the development of euthyroid hyperthyroxinemia include: oral contraceptives or estrogen replacement, amiodarone, propranolol, heparin, perphenazine, clofibrate, 5-fluorouracil, heroin and methadone (Singh 2011, 5).

In addition to presenting with elevated serum thyroxine levels, many of these syndromes of euthyroid hyperthyroxinemia are also accompanied by abnormalities in triiodothyronine and free thyroid hormone levels, as well as unresponsiveness of thyroid-stimulating hormone to thyrotropin-releasing hormone (causing a low TSH), all of which further erroneously indicate a diagnosis of thyrotoxicosis, which can lead to inappropriate treatment. Cases include acquired and inherited abnormalities of serum thyroid-hormone-binding proteins, peripheral resistance to thyroid hormones, acute nonthyroidal illness, acute psychiatric illness, and some drug-induced conditions associated with nonthyrotoxic elevations of serum thyroxine.

Controlled Euthyroid Thyrotoxic States

Patients with hyperthyroidism are considered euthyroid when medical treatment brings their FT4 level into the normal range. If their FT3 level, however, remains above the normal range, thyrotoxicosis can develop. In newly diagnosed patients with elevated levels of both FT4 and FT3, anti-thyroid drugs typically return FT4 levels to the reference range within 6–8 weeks. FT3 can take up to an additional 6–8 weeks to fall within the reference range.

Thyroid Storm

Thyroid or thyrotoxic storm or crisis is a rare life-threatening syndrome characterized by exaggerated clinical manifestations of thyrotoxicosis. Because there are no established diagnostic criteria, its incidence is unknown, but it's thought to occur in 1–2 percent of all cases of hyperthyroidism (Schraga 2012, 2). In thyroid storm, the usual physiological mechanisms that deal with excess thyroid hormone fail and thyrotoxicosis is considered uncompensated.

Thyroid hormone levels in thyroid storm are not exceptionally high and, in fact, are similar to those of many people with mild to moderate hyperthyroidism. Thyroid storm is generally presumed to be caused by bodily changes such as infection that cause heightened sensitivity to excess thyroid hormone or to a sudden increase in thyroid hormone secretion. Adult mortality rate from thyroid storm is approximately 10–20 percent, but it has been reported to be as high as 75 percent in hospitalized populations (Schraga 2012, 2). Underlying precipitating illness may contribute to high mortality.

MANIFESTATIONS OF THYROID STORM
- Fever, usually above 102°F
- Tachycardia out of proportion to fever

- Atrial fibrillation (the most common cardiac arrhythmia associated with thyroid storm). Other arrhythmias such as atrial flutter and, less commonly, ventricular tachycardia may also occur.
- Gastrointestinal symptoms (diarrhea, nausea, vomiting)
- Jaundice and liver enlargement
- Central nervous system dysfunction (anxiety, agitation, emotional lability, mania, psychosis, tremor, weakness, confusion, obtundation or coma)
- Recent excessive weight loss (usually 40 lbs or more)
- Profuse sweating
- Hyperglycemia
- Muscle weakness and rigidity
- Rhabdomyolysis
- Pulmonary edema

EVENTS ASSOCIATED WITH THE ONSET OF THYROID STORM

- Infection
- Acute medical illness; in diabetics, ketoacidosis, hyperosmolar coma, and insulin-induced hypoglycemia may produce thyroid storm, although it is very rare for diabetic ketoacidosis and thyroid storm to develop simultaneously (Osada et al. 2011).
- Acute emotional stress
- Acute psychosis
- Surgery
- Childbirth
- Trauma
- Radioiodine ablation (due to high concentrations of thyroid hormone and thyroid antibodies released from dying thyroid cells; risk for up to 12 weeks following ablation)
- Thyroidectomy without appropriate pre-treatment to appropriately lower thyroid hormone levels (The advent of appropriate preoperative preparation of patients undergoing thyroidectomy for hyperthyroidism has led to a dramatic reduction in the prevalence of surgically induced thyroid storm)
- High dose iodine administration
- Iodinated radiographic contrast agents
- Abrupt cessation of anti-thyroid drug therapy
- Vigorous palpation of the thyroid gland

TREATMENT OF THYROID STORM

Untreated, thyroid storm may progress to congestive heart failure, refractory pulmonary edema, circulatory collapse, coma and death within 72 hours.

Thyroid storm is a medical emergency and typically treated in an emergency room setting. Supportive therapy such as antipyretics to reduce fever and intravenous fluids to replace fluid volume are used. Specific treatment consists of anti-thyroid drugs to reduce the production and secretion of thyroid hormone; ionorganic iodide (strong solution of potassium iodide or SSKI, Lugol's solution) to inhibit the secretion of thyroid hormone; propylthiouracil and iodine contrast agents to inhibit the conversion of T4 into T3; and propranolol or other beta adrenergic blocking agents to reduce the systemic effects of excess thyroid hormone. In extreme cases, plasmapheresis or peritoneal dialysis are used to quickly lower blood concentrations of thyroid hormone (Wartofsky 2000, 682).

Diagnostic Scoring for Thyroid Storm and Impending Storm

As mentioned, there are no universally accepted criteria or validated clinical tools for diagnosing thyroid storm. However, in 1993, Burch and Wartofsky introduced a scoring system using precise clinical criteria for the identification of thyroid storm based on body temperature and other symptoms that may be associated with thyroid storm.

According to Burch and Wartofsky's guidelines, a body temperature between 99 and 99.9°F has a score of 5 points, whereas a temperature equal or higher than 104°F counts as 30 points. A heart rate between 90 and 109 beats per minute (bpm) yields 5 points and a heart rate equal or higher than 140 bpm counts as 25 points. Symptoms such as unexplained jaundice count as 20 points, although jaundice is rare in thyroid storm and is likely to have other causes. According to these criteria, a score of 45 or more is highly suggestive of thyroid storm, whereas a score below 25 makes thyroid storm unlikely. A score of 25 to 44 is suggestive of impending storm. While this scoring system is deemed by some experts to likely be sensitive, it is not very specific and it is rarely used or relied on today.

2

Causes of Hyperthyroidism

Hyperthyroidism has a number of different causes. Graves' disease, an autoimmune disorder, is the most common. Although both women and men of all ages can develop Graves' disease, its incidence is especially high in women ages 30 to 50 years. Among people older than 50 years, toxic multinodular goiter (TMG) is the most common cause of hyperthyroidism. Hyperthyroidism can also result from a number of other causes including thyroiditis, genetic mutations, excess iodine intake, tyrosine supplements, malignancies, medications, resistance to thyroid hormone, excess thyroid replacement hormone, thyroid booster supplements, food that has been contaminated with thyroid hormone, and pituitary disorders.

Thyroid hormone is the product of a complex interaction or axis between the pituitary gland, the hypothalamus in the brain, and the thyroid gland. This chapter describes the feedback axis and the role played by the pituitary hormone thyrotropin (also known as thyroid stimulating hormone or TSH) in regulating thyroid hormone levels.

Various thyroid abnormalities lead to excess thyroid hormone. Excess thyroid hormone is the cause of hyperthyroidism and thyrotoxicosis. An understanding of how thyroid hormone is normally produced helps determine how these abnormalities can be corrected, while an understanding of how the thyroid gland normally functions provides insight into the aberrations that can lead to hyperthyroidism. The various disorders that cause hyperthyroidism together with a description of the conditions that can lead to thyrotoxicosis are the main focus of this chapter. Because the disease course, associated conditions, symptoms and complications, as well as treatment considerations, depend on the specific cause of hyperthyroidism, a careful investigation into the exact cause of hyperthyroidism is necessary to produce a successful outcome.

Ensuring a Correct Diagnosis

Years ago, before the autoimmune nature of Graves' disease was discovered, many people with hyperthyroidism from other causes were erroneously diagnosed with Graves' disease on the basis of a high radioiodine uptake scan or an absence of palpated nodules. How many of them had other hyperthyroid conditions, such as toxic multinodular goiter, thyroiditis, or TSH receptor mutations, is unknown.

Some individuals were not given the essential diagnostic tests and were treated with radioiodine ablation, which can cause and increase the production of thyroid stimulating immunoglobulins (TSI, the antibodies that cause hyperthyroidism in Graves' disease). These individuals have no way of later knowing if they originally had Graves' disease or if they developed these antibodies as a result of their radioiodine ablation. Patients should keep copies of laboratory reports, make sure the needed diagnostic tests are done, and ensure that their diagnosis is accurate.

The Thyroid-Pituitary-Hypothalamic Axis

Thyroid hormone production is normally regulated by the pituitary hormone thyrotropin (TSH). TSH reacts with the TSH receptor, a protein on thyroid cells, ordering these cells to grow and produce thyroid hormone. Normally, the pituitary gland secretes small pulses of TSH throughout the day, and it secretes the highest amounts at night. This ensures that adequate thyroid hormone can be produced the following day to keep blood levels stable despite various demands, for instance sudden drops in temperature that increase our need for thyroid hormone.

The hypothalamus monitors our thyroid hormone levels, and it takes action when levels begin to change. The hypothalamus orders the pituitary to produce and secrete more or less TSH depending on changes in our blood levels of the thyroid hormones T4 and T3.

T4 and T3 are best measured through blood levels of free hormone using free T4 (FT4) and free T3 (FT3) blood tests. Similar to the natural catecholamines epinephrine and norepinephrine, thyroid hormone is synthesized from the amino acid tyrosine. When iodine reacts with tyrosine, thyroid hormone is produced.

Normally, when blood levels of FT4 and FT3 begin to fall, the hypothalamus acts to raise these levels and maintain stable thyroid hormone levels by producing increased amounts of the regulatory hormone called thyrotropin-releasing hormone (TRH). In response to increased TRH, the pituitary gland is directed to secrete more TSH.

Likewise, when thyroid hormone levels begin to rise, the hypothalamus directs pituitary cells to dampen their response to TRH. This signals the pituitary gland to secrete less TSH in an attempt to keep thyroid hormone levels from rising too high. In summary, excess thyroid hormone (both T4 and T3) inhibits the production and release of TSH, with low TSH levels seen in hyperthyroidism.

The TSH Molecule

The TSH molecule consists of alpha and beta subunits that are tightly bound together. These subunits are also found in other hormones including the hormone beta human choriogonadotropin (beta HCG) that rises in pregnancy. This explains why other hormones, particularly beta HCG, can affect the production of thyroid hormone. In the disorders described later in this chapter such as hyperemesis gravidarum, familial HCG hypersensitivity, and malignancies that secrete HCG, hyperthyroidism can occur.

The alpha subunit is found in TSH, follicle stimulating hormone (FSH), luteinizing hormone (LH), and human chorionic gonadotropin (HCG). The beta subunit adds specificity to TSH because this subunit reacts with the TSH receptor on thyroid cells. On its own the beta subunit is inactive and requires the alpha subunit to exert its intended effects (thyroid cell growth, production and release of thyroid hormone). The alpha subunit is regulated by a gene located on chromosome 6, while the beta subunit is regulated by a gene on chromosome 1.

The TSH Blood Level

Among the general population, blood levels of TSH normally reflect the thyroid gland's status. That is, in most cases, a TSH level that falls into the normal or reference range indicates that the thyroid gland is functioning normally. This makes TSH a good basic test for thyroid function and provides a simple, inexpensive tool for screening the general population for thyroid disease. In this sense, the TSH test is considered the gold standard for screening thyroid disorders. In most people, a low TSH indicates hyperthyroidism and a high TSH indicates hypothyroidism. However, as we'll learn in Chapters 3 and 6, the TSH test result can be misleading in people who have certain thyroid disorders, and the result can be affected by other factors including medications and other non-thyroidal conditions.

The Feedback Mechanism

Similar to the way TSH normally reflects thyroid status, the feedback mechanism between TSH, TRH, and thyroid hormone normally prevents hyperthyroidism from developing. In the conditions of hyperthyroidism described in the following sections, this feedback mechanism is overcome by other factors that cause the thyroid gland to produce excess thyroid hormone regardless of a drastic drop in the TSH level.

Graves' Disease

Graves' disease stands out as the most common cause of hyperthyroidism, accounting for approximately 80 percent of all cases (Nussey and Whitehead 2001, 6). The autoimmune mechanism is described briefly here and the disease process in Graves' disease is addressed in Chapter 3. Factors influencing the

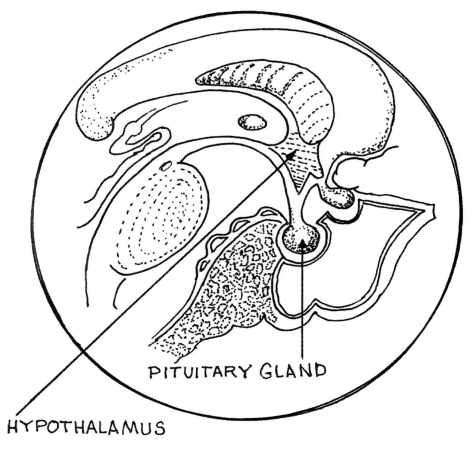

Regulation of thyroid hormone (courtesy Marvin G. Miller).

development of Graves' disease are found in Chapter 4. Because Graves' disease is an autoimmune disorder, its development is more complex and its manifestations more extensive than those seen in other forms of hyperthyroidism. Graves' disease is caused by a defect in the immune system that leads to the production of stimulating TSH receptor antibodies.

These thyroid antibodies, also known as thyroid stimulating immunoglobulins or TSI, act in place of TSH. In doing so, they react with TSH receptors on thyroid cells, ordering the cells to continue producing and releasing thyroid hormone levels. Even when TSH levels become undetectable, TSI antibodies cause thyroid hormone levels to escalate, bypassing the normal feedback axis. Thyroid antibodies are described in greater detail in Chapter 6; hyperthyroidism in Graves' disease as well as its environmental triggers, its genetic associations, and its coexistence with other disorders are described in Chapters 3, 4, and 5.

Marine-Lenhart Syndrome

Graves' disease accompanied by functioning thyroid nodules is known as Marine-Lenhart syndrome. Marine and Lenhart initially described this rare disorder in 1911, and it is now considered a distinct subentity of Graves' disease, occurring in about 2.7 percent of patients with Graves' disease. Technetium scans in this syndrome show an increased homogeneous uptake throughout the gland with an area of intense focal uptake where nodules are present.

Thyroid Nodules

Nodules are clusters of thyroid cells (thyrocytes) with increased growth and proliferation. Thyroid nodules are generally classified as functioning (hot), nonfunctioning (cold), or photo-deficient depending on their unique imaging tracer activity. However, classifying nodules as hot or cold can be misleading. Unless oblique views of the gland are imaged, the presence of activity concentration cannot be definitively determined (Khan 2012). In addition there can be influences from adjacent tissue.

Although thyroid nodules are reported to be present in half of the population, they're only palpable on examination in about 4–7 percent of cases (Khan 2012). Most hot nodules are benign adenomas. Nodules are more common in women and more prevalent in parts of the world that are deficient in iodine. Nodules are considered toxic when they begin to produce excess thyroid hormone. See Chapter 6 for more information on nodules and their differential diagnosis.

Autonomously Functioning Thyroid Nodule (AFTN)

Autonomously functioning nodules may remain stable in size, grow, degenerate or, less commonly, become gradually toxic, usually over a period of years. Nodules lose their usual regulatory control and can produce thyroid hormone at a dramatically increased rate. In studies of hyper-functioning thyroid nodules, TSH receptor mutations have been found in approximately 45–80 percent (Arturi, et al. 2003, 342; Kopp 2010).

Adenoma

Thyroid adenomas are usually benign neoplasms composed primarily of follicular or papillary cells and represent hot nodules. According to Dr. Daniel Kelley, only 5–20 percent of thyroid nodules are true neoplasms compared to the majority, which are hyperplastic nodules (Kelley and Meyers, 2011). Most toxic adenomas are equal to or greater than 3 cm and are easily palpated. Follicular adenomas are the most common type and arise from the follicular epithelium within the thyroid gland. Follicular adenomas are typically homogeneous, solitary, and encapsulated tumors that are histologically distinct from adjacent thyroid tissue.

In one study of 159 patients with nodules, ultrasound testing evaluated changes in nodular size during a period of 1 to 15 years. An increase in size was seen in only 10 percent of nodules, whereas in 4 percent, the size of nodules decreased. In addition, a loss of function (move into hypothyroidism) due to degenerative changes was observed in 4 nodules. Eight percent of

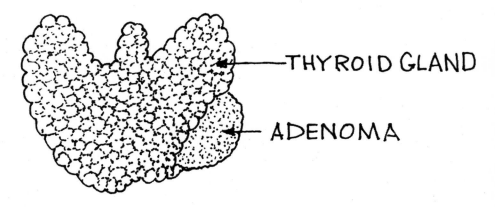

THYROID GLAND

ADENOMA

A thyroid adenoma is a type of tumor that may affect the function of the thyroid gland. In some cases it causes the production of excessive thyroid hormone, and results in hyperthyroidism (courtesy Marvin G. Miller).

patients developed overt thyrotoxicosis during a follow-up of 3 to 5 years, while 3 percent of patients developed subclinical hyperthyroidism (Hamburger 1980, 1090–1091).

Adenomas that cause low TSH levels are considered toxic adenomas. Symptoms of overt or subclinical hyperthyroidism often emerge quickly and are similar to those seen in other forms of hyperthyroidism. However, the eye signs and symptoms of Graves' disease are absent. Similar to the laboratory profile in Graves' disease, about 30 percent of patients can have levels of FT3 that are relatively higher than levels of FT4.

Follicular adenomas can be further classified according to their cellular architecture and relative colloid content into fetal (microfollicular), colloid (macrofollicular), embryonal (atypical), and Hürthle (oxyphil) cell types. Colloid adenomas have no potential for microinvasion, while the fetal, embryonal, and Hürthle cell adenomas all have the potential for microinvasion. The incidence of thyroid cancer remains low, representing about 1 percent of all newly diagnosed cases of cancer (Kelley and Meyers, 2011).

A hyperfunctioning solitary adenoma is suggested by its presence on imaging tests or palpation and by atrophy of the remainder of the thyroid. On scintiscan, preferential accumulation of radioiodine is demonstrated in the nodule, indicating hyperfunction. In some adenomas, constitutive activation of the TSH second-messenger cascade is demonstrated, indicating increased cAMP production. Mutations in the gene encoding the stimulatory alpha subunit of the G protein, Gs-alpha, have also been implicated.

Toxic Multinodular Goiter (TMG)

Up to 5 percent of the population is reported to have toxic multinodular goiter (TMG) although autopsy studies reveal that multinodular goiter is much more common, occurring in 50 percent of autopsies (Nussey and Whitehead 2001, 13). Nussey and Whitehead also report that women are affected 10 times more than men, and that multiple nodules are 4 times more common than solitary nodules.

In TMG, multiple nodules have cumulative effects that result in hyperthyroidism. The usual symptoms of hyperthyroidism occur; the most common features include: dysphagia (difficulty in swallowing), shortness of breath, and hoarseness. The word *toxic* in TMG refers to the development of thyrotoxicosis. Early studies show that 30 percent of patients with differentiated thyroid cancer have coincidental multinodular goiters (Gemsenjager and Girard 1981, 1563).

Sarcoidosis of the Thyroid Gland

Sarcoidosis of the thyroid gland is a rare cause of thyrotoxicosis, which may occur in individuals with Graves' disease and toxic multinodular goiter. Although this condition is most likely to affect affect young and middle-aged females, males and females of all ages may be affected. Because of the development of fibrosis, hypothyroidism is the most common result, although sarcoidos may also cause thyroiditis as well as hyperthyroidism. When sarcoidosis occurs in thyrotoxic patients who show resistance to treatment with I131 ablation or anti-thyroid drugs, an evaluation for sarcoidosis is indicated. In cases where thyroidectomy surgery was used to treat hyperthyroidism that didn't respond well to other treatments, sarcoidosis of the thyroid gland has been reported as an incidental finding in postoperative tissue studies.

On imaging scans (RAI-uptake and scan) the granulomas of sarcoidosis may easily be misidentified as cold thyroid nodules. Sometimes these lesions are also mistaken for thyroid cancer. Patients with conditions of systemic sarcoidosis without any evidence of thyroid disease may also develop sarcoid lesions in various organs, including the thyroid gland.

Often, symptoms related to sarcoidosis such as pulmonary changes or skin lesions are the first indications of thyroid sarcoidosis. The granulomas of sarcoidosis, which can, on palpation, be confused with thyroid nodules, can cause elevated levels of both circulating 25 OH vitamin D and also 1, 25 OH vitamin D. Other laboratory changes that may occur in sarcoidosis include a low white blood cell count, elevated urine and plasma calcium levels, and a low uric acid level.

In addition, sarcoidosis can affect the eye, causing a condition distinct from Graves' ophthalmopathy characterized by symptoms of proptosis and orbital swelling that may be confused with euthyroid Graves' disease or Graves' ophthalmopathy (Giovinale et al. 2009, 37–40).

Genetic Causes of Hyperthyroidism

In the last two decades researchers have discovered a number of different genetic mutations that can cause hyperthyroidism as well as thyrotoxicosis resulting from thyroid hyperfunctioning adenomas. Besides genetic mutations, several familial disorders described in the next section can cause hyperthyroidism.

TSH Receptor Mutations

Somatic mutations in the TSH receptor gene have been found in hot nodules, hyperfunctioning areas within multinodular goiters and in thyroid carcinomas, particularly those associated with hyperthyroidism (Arturi et al. 2003, 341). Both autoimmune and non-autoimmune familial conditions of hyperthyroidism occur as a result of mutations to the TSH receptor.

FAMILIAL AUTOIMMUNE HYPERTHYROIDISM

Genetic mutations of the TSH receptor have been detected that lead to constitutive activation of the cyclic adenosine monophosphate (cAMP) signaling pathway found in many cases of familial autoimmune hyperthyroidism. In addition, de novo germline TSH receptor mutations have been documented in rare cases of recurrent diffuse thyroid hyperplasia, a condition of increased thyroid cell growth associated with severe hyperthyroidism (Arturi et al. 2003, 341). Considered "gain of function" mutations, these TSH receptor mutations are heterozygous and transmitted in an autosomal dominant fashion in familial cases.

FAMILIAL NON-AUTOIMMUNE HYPERTHYROIDISM

Autosomal dominant familial hyperthyroidism without evidence of an autoimmune etiology was first described in 1982. The hyperthyroidism that occurs in this condition is caused by monoallelic gain-of-function germline mutations in the TSH receptor. Ultimately, the diagnosis requires sequence analysis of the TSH receptor gene in order to evaluate it for the presence of a monallelic mutation. If the mutation is unknown, functional in vitro analyses are needed to demonstrate that the mutated allele confers constitutive activity to the receptor.

FAMILIAL HYPERSENSITIVITY TO HCG IN PREGNANCY

A germ-line activating mutation in the TSH receptor gene can cause an unusual form of familial gestational hyperthyroidism with increased sensitivity to activation by the pregnancy hormone beta-human chorionic gonadotropin (beta–HCG). This can result in transient conditions of HCG-induced gestational hyperthyroidism during pregnancy.

In one of the first reported cases, a patient had a history of two miscarriages that were accompanied by hyperemesis. Subsequently, she had two pregnancies that were complicated by hyperthyroidism, severe nausea and vomiting and no evidence of thyroid antibodies. The patient's first-semester HCG levels, determined during the second pregnancy, were in the normal range. The patient and also the patient's mother had a history of one miscarriage and two pregnancies that were complicated by hyperemesis gravidarum. Sequence analysis of the *TSH receptor* gene in both the patient and her mother revealed the presence of a genetic mutation resulting in the substitution of K183R. Functional studies in cells transfected with the mutated receptor documented no differences in membrane expression, and similar levels of basal and TSH stimulated cAMP accumulation. In contrast to the wild-type TSH receptor, which reacts only minimally to high doses of HCG, the K183R TSH receptor mutant is hypersensitive to HCG, although it still is 1000 times less responsive to HCG than the luteinizing hormone/chorionicgonadotropin receptor. The K183R TSH receptor mutation is unique because sensitivity is increased for HCG but remains unaltered for TSH. This observation also supports the possibility of an HCG-independent connection between hyperthyroidism and hyperemesis gravidarum (Kopp 2010).

HYPEREMESIS GRAVIDARUM

Hyperemesis gravidarum is a transient condition of thyrotoxicosis that can occur during pregnancy. Hyperemesis gravidarum is characterized by severe nausea, vomiting, dehydration, the presence of urinary ketones, and weight loss of more than 5 percent by 6 to 9 weeks' gestation. This condition is usually associated with an elevated FT4, low TSH, and occasionally an elevated FT3 result and accompanied by exaggerated morning sickness. Familial conditions with fetal loss have been reported.

Anti-thyroid drugs are poorly tolerated in this condition and, even when thyroid hormone levels fall, vomiting persists. Management includes intravenous fluids for severe cases. Most cases resolve and thyroid hormone levels return to normal by 16–20 weeks gestation, although TSH levels may be suppressed longer.

Sporadic Non-Autoimmune Neonatal Hyperthyroidism

Autoimmune neonatal hyperthyroidism is a rare condition caused by the transplacental passage of thyroid stimulating immunoglobulins (TSI, stimulating TSH receptor antibodies). This condition occurs in less than 2 percent of newborns born to mothers with a history of Graves' disease, especially mothers who have been treated with radioiodine ablation. Once they are produced, TSI antibodies remain intact for 2–3 months before they're broken down into amino acids and excreted. This can cause sporadic TSI levels and subsequently sporadic thyroid hormone elevations and sporadic symptoms of hyperthyroidism before the condition spontaneously resolves in 2–3 months.

Autoimmune Neonatal Hyperthyroidism

Autoimmune neonatal hyperthyroidism is a more common and transient autoimmune form of neonatal hyperthyroidism. Affected infants have pronounced hyperthyroidism, which requires a more aggressive therapeutic approach that may necessitate surgery and ablative radiotherapy early in life. In one study, several children with severe neonatal hyperthyroidism were reported to have mild mental retardation, suggesting that high levels of thyroid hormone may have a negative impact on brain development (Kopp 2010). Alternatively, mental development may have been impaired because of premature closure of the cranial sutures. A subset of these children had proptosis. Computer tomography of the retro-orbital tissue in one of these children did not, however, demonstrate infiltration of the eye muscles (Kopp 2010).

Hyperthyroidism in Tumors and Malignancies

Thyroid malignancies and also other trophoblastic (hormone-secreting) tumors can rarely cause conditions of hyperthyroidism.

Choriogonadotropin-Mediated Thyrotoxicosis

As described earlier in this chapter, high levels of or sensitivity to the hormone known as beta-human chorionic gonadotropin (beta–HCG) can cause hyperthyroidism. Beta-HCG is secreted in women during pregnancy and in individuals with various gonadotropin-secreting malignancies, including hydatidiform moles, choriocarcinomas, and rarely seminomas (type of testicular germ cell tumor).

Hydatidiform mole refers to a rare mass or growth that forms inside the uterus at the beginning of a pregnancy. Most women with hydatidiform moles present with uterine bleeding in the first half of pregnancy, and their uterine size is large for the duration of gestation. Many women with molar pregnancies have nausea and vomiting and occasionally pregnancy-induced hypertension or preeclampsia. Hydatidiform mole is a type of gestational trophoblastic disease (GTD) that results from overproduction of the tissue that is supposed to develop into the placenta. Partial molar pregnancies show some fetal development, whereas in complete molar pregnancies a fetus is absent. HCG-induced hyperthyroidism is a common feature.

Choriocarcinoma is a quick-growing form of cancer that occurs in a woman's uterus (womb). Abnormal cell growth starts in the tissue that would normally become the placenta. Although it is most often associated with a complete hydatidiform mole, the cancer may develop after a normal pregnancy. In addition, the abnormal tissue supporting the mole can continue to grow even after the mole is removed and it can turn into cancer. About half of all women with a choriocarcinoma had a hydatidiform mole, or molar pregnancy.

Choriocarcinomas may also occur after an abortion, miscarriage, ectopic pregnancy or genital tumor. High levels of HCG can cause an HCG-induced form of hyperthyroidism.

Similar in structure to the alpha-subunit of TSH, beta–HCG can cause thyroid cells to secrete excess thyroid hormone. Women with trophoblastic disease typically show signs of hyperthyroidism when beta–HCG levels exceed 100,000 IU and thyrotoxicosis when levels exceed 300,000 IU (Cain et al. 1991, 1129).

HCG-Induced Thyrotoxicosis in Men

Various tumors and trophoblastic diseases can cause increased secretion of beta–HCG. An article published in *Clinical Chemistry* describes a 38-year-old man with a metastatic tumor of unknown primary origin that resulted in high levels of beta–HCG and thyroid hormone. The patient was reported to have cardiac symptoms associated with thyrotoxicosis (supraventricular tachycardia and hypertension) but no lid lag, exophthalmos, or bilateral proximal myopathy (muscle weakness) during his hospitalization when the thyrotoxicosis was detected.

After an initial course of chemotherapy, levels of both beta–HCG and free thyroxine decreased and the patient became euthyroid. After a second course of chemotherapy, the patient declined further treatment and died one month after returning home. An autopsy was not performed, and the patient was presumed to have gonadotropin-secreting-metastatic tetracarcinoma (Cain et al. 1991, 1128). The authors describe several other cases of HCG-secreting tumors in men who had either extensive choriocarcinoma or embryonal carcinoma.

Struma Ovarii

Struma ovarii is an extremely rare cause of thyrotoxicosis. This condition, which results in a low radioiodine uptake test, is seen when more than 50 percent of the mass of an ovarian teratoma is composed of functioning thyroid tissue. First described in 1899, struma ovarii comprise 1 percent of all ovarian tumors.

Several variants of struma ovarii are found. The symptoms of struma ovarii are similar to other ovarian tumors and are nonspecific in nature. The majority of tumors are benign and the presence of carcinoid tumors is extremely rare.

Although struma ovarii is predominately composed of thyroid tissue, thyrotoxicosis is seen in only 5 percent of all cases. Rarely, hyperthyroidism is the presenting symptom, and it's seen in 5–8 percent of patients with struma ovarii. Most cases occur during the reproductive years with peak incidence occurring in the fifth and sixth decades of life although rare cases have been seen before puberty (Kelly 2012).

Follicular and Papillary Thyroid Carcinoma

Rarely, follicular cancer can cause thyrotoxicosis, and up to 200 cases have been reviewed in the medical literature with a smaller number of cases seen in papillary cancer. In hyperthyroidism associated with thyroid cancer, T3 thyrotoxicosis is a common feature (higher elevation of FT3 relative to FT4) and thyroglobulin levels are elevated. Age and sex distribution in affected patients does not differ from that of patients with follicular carcinoma without thyrotoxicosis (Kopp 2010).

Malignant Thyroid Lymphoma

Subclinical hyperthyroidism is reported to occur in up to 40 percent of patients with malignant thyroid lymphoma (Gemsenjager 1981, 1563).

Metastatic Thyroid Cancer

Secondary thyroid cancer that has metastasized from primary cancer in a different organ, especially the lung, liver, or bone, can rarely cause thyrotoxicosis. The radioiodine uptake test is low in this condition.

Conditions of Excess TSH production

Through the thyroid-hypothalamic-pituitary feedback mechanism described earlier in this chapter, it's clear that TSH causes thyroid cells to produce and release thyroid hormone. In certain disorders, the pituitary gland may deviate from this axis and produce excess amounts of thyroid hormone.

Pituitary Tumors (TSHomas)

About 2 percent of all pituitary tumors lead to excess TSH production and cause thyrotoxicosis. When enlarged, these tumors, which are known as TSHomas) can cause deficiencies in other hormones, pressure symptoms, or expansion of the sella turcica. In diagnostic tests, after TRH stimulation, the TSH level may remain unchanged or show modest elevations, and MRI studies show the presence of a pituitary tumor. The characteristic findings include an elevated TSH level, elevated thyroid hormone levels, and an elevated alpha subunit of TSH, measured by specialized laboratory procedures. Although TSHomas have been found in children, they are more common in elderly patients.

Excess TRH Production

Another disorder that causes excess TSH production and thyrotoxicosis is the rare condition of excess thyrotropin releasing hormone (TRH), which is also known as pituitary T3 resistance. TRH hypersecretion is characterized by an absence of pituitary tumor, elevated TSH levels and failure to respond to TRH administration. Additional features include mild thyrotoxicosis, elevated TSH levels, no excess TSH alpha subunit secretion and TSH suppression if large doses of T3 replacement hormone are administered. This condition is caused by a genetic mutation on the thyroid hormone gene.

Excess Iodine

Administration of large amounts of iodine (exceeding 150 mcg daily) used in contrast dyes for imaging tests, foods, medications such as amiodarone, dietary supplements including thyroid and metabolic boosters, and contaminated meat can result in thyrotoxicosis especially in patients with multinodular goiter, latent Graves' disease, and adenomas. In addition, excessive iodine can trigger Graves' disease and other autoimmune thyroid disorders in genetically predisposed individuals.

Approximately 150 mcg of iodine is needed for the body's daily needs. Higher amounts generally do not cause problems except for individuals at risk, including people with latent Graves' disease who have achieved remission using antithyroid drug therapy or alternative medicine.

In individuals who have had aggressive treatment for Graves' disease (thyroidectomy surgery or radioiodine ablation) the situation is reversed. In these patients, iodine excess causes overt clinical hypothyroidism. Patients with a history of Graves' disease treated with radioiodine or partial thyroidectomy, partial thyroidectomy for thyroid nodules, or autoimmune thyroiditis are particularly predisposed to iodine-induced hypothyroidism. Even relatively small excessive doses of 750 mcg daily may be sufficient to induce hypothyroidism due to reduced thyroid volume (Kopp 2010).

Amiodarone-Induced Hyperthyroidism and Thyrotoxicosis

The heart medication amiodarone can cause both hyperthyroidism and thyrotoxicosis. Amiodarone-induced thyrotoxicosis has two subtypes:

Type I is characterized by the synthesis and release of excess thyroid hormone, making it a hyperthyroid disorder. This subtype is more often seen in patients with preexisting subclinical thyroid disorders and causes increased thyroid blood flow. Type I is treated with anti-thyroid drugs, sometimes with the addition of potassium perchlorate to lower iodine uptake by the thyroid gland.

Type II is a destructive thyroiditis that causes the release of preformed thyroid hormone from the damaged thyroid gland and is associated with reduced thyroid blood flow. Type II amiodarone-induced thyrotoxicosis is treated with corticosteroids (Pearce et al. 2003).

Causes of Thyrotoxicosis

Thyrotoxicosis refers to the symptoms caused by excess thyroid hormone. Thyrotoxicosis can be caused by other conditions besides hyperthyroidism, including conditions of thyroiditis and thyrotoxicosis factitia.

Thyroiditis

Thyroiditis is a condition of thyroid gland inflammation. Damage to thyroid cells can result in the release of excess thyroid hormone into the blood circulation. Ensuing temporary conditions of thyrotoxicosis are often followed by hypothyroidism, which can be permanent. Thyroiditis can also result from autoimmunity in postpartum thyroiditis (PPT) or occur as a consequence of infection. Acute thyroiditis (acute suppurative thyroiditis, bacterial thyroiditis, pyogenic thyroiditis) is an uncommon disorder, usually bacterial in origin, although it may be caused by fungi, parasitic organisms or *Pneumocystis carinii* (usually in patients with HIV infection).

In painless sporadic thyroiditis, postpartum thyroiditis, and painful subacute thyroiditis, inflammatory destruction of the thyroid gland may lead to transient thyrotoxicosis, which is usually mild, as preformed thyroid hormones are released from the damaged gland. In thyroiditis, serum T4/FT4 concentrations are proportionately higher than T3/FT3 levels, reflecting the ratio of stored hormone in the thyroid gland (Pearce et al. 2003).

POSTPARTUM THYROIDITIS (PPT)

Postpartum thyroiditis is a transient condition causing a small painless goiter and a very low radioiodine uptake test result. PPT occurs within one year after childbirth, miscarriage or other termination of pregnancy. Thyroglobulin and thyroid peroxidase antibodies, if present, are low and there may be a family history of autoimmune thyroid disease. Considered a variant of Hashimoto's thyroiditis, it primarily occurs in young adults and may occur 3–12 weeks after delivery as an immunologic rebound from the normal immunosuppression that occurs in pregnancy.

A period of hypothyroidism may follow the hyperthyroid phase and several cycles of alternating hyperthyroidism and hypothyroidism can develop. However, only a minority of women fit the classic pattern. Most women with PPT have only a thyrotoxic or a hypothyroid phase, which may become permanent in about 25 percent of patients. In PPT, thyrotoxicosis is caused by an inflammation-induced release of preformed thyroid hormone. Patients with PPT may occasionally go on to develop Graves' disease. Also see the sections headed Hyperemesis gravidarum and Familial Hypersensitivity to HCG in Pregnancy described earlier in this chapter with causes of hyperthyroidism.

PAINLESS SPORADIC THYROIDITIS

Painless sporadic thyroiditis is indistinguishable from postpartum thyroiditis except that there is no association with the former to pregnancy. Both PPT and sporadic thyroiditis may represent subacute forms of Hashimoto's thyroiditis. Painless sporadic thyroiditis accounts for about 1 percent of all cases of thyrotoxicosis (Pearce et al. 2003). In this condition, thyroid dysfunction spontaneously resolves in most cases, although about 20 percent of patients will have residual conditions of chronic hypothyroidism. High titers of TPO antibodies are typically present, although the levels are not as high as those typically seen in Hashimoto's thyroiditis.

RIEDEL'S THYROIDITIS (INVASIVE FIBROUS THYROIDITIS, RIEDEL STRUMA)

Riedel's thyroiditis, a very rare form of thyroiditis also known as Riedel struma or invasive fibrous thyroiditis, was first described by Riedel in 1896. Only 37 cases were noted among 56,700 thyroidectomies performed at Mayo Clinic between 1920 and 1984 (Singer 1991, 61–62). Women are affected three times more often than men, and the peak incidence occurs between 30 and 60 years of age.

Riedel's thyroiditis is characterized by the replacement of normal thyroid tissue with dense fibrous tissue. Patients typically complain of a painless neck enlargement ranging in duration from several weeks to several years. Symptoms include difficulty swallowing, pressure and occasionally respirator obstruction. Early in the disease course, patients may have symptoms of thyrotoxicosis resulting from increased thyroid hormone released from damaged thyroid cells. Most patients, however, are euthyroid unless their entire gland is affected. This results in hypothyroidism.

SUBACUTE THYROIDITIS (SAT)

Subacute painful thyroiditis (SAT), which is also known as DeQuervain thyroiditis and granulomatous painful thyroiditis, was first described by DeQuervain in 1940. SAT causes granulomatous-type changes and giant cells in thyroid glands of those affected. SAT is fairly common and may account for as many as 5 percent of all visits to physicians for thyroid abnormalities (Singer 1991, 63). Thought to have a viral origin, SAT frequently follows a respiratory infection and is most often seen in the summer and fall. SAT is associated with outbreaks of mumps as well as adenovirus, Coxsackie, influenza and infectious mononucleosis.

Individuals with SAT may have TSH receptor antibodies making it sometimes confused with Graves' disease (Singer 1991, 64). Similar to Graves' disease, most cases of SAT develop in women and the peak incidence is between 40 and 50 years of age. There's also evidence to suggest a genetic predisposition to the development of SAT. An association between SAT and the genetic marker HLA-Bw35 has been reported in two-thirds of both Chinese and Caucasians (Singer 1991, 64). For this reason, SAT is also seen in siblings, and new familial cases typically develop within a two-year period.

SAT causes an initial hyperthyroid phase that lasts for about 4–10 weeks. This is frequently followed by a hypothyroid phase of similar duration, although the illness can persist for a year or longer, with most patients eventually becoming euthyroid. SAT often develops after a viral upper respiratory infection and neck pain is characteristic. SAT is the most common cause of hyperthyroidism accompanied by a low radiation uptake test result, with the 24-hour uptake commonly less than 2 percent (Daniels 1999, 6). Usual laboratory findings include a mild normochromic, normocytic anemia (normal size of red blood cells), an elevated erythrocyte sedimentation rate (ESR, sed rate), a high T4 level relative to T3, and mild to moderate hypothyroidism. Ultrasonography shows the gland to be edematous, which is reflected as hypoechogenicity. Because the gland may not be affected uniformly, this finding can be regional.

Individuals with SAT complain of substantial pain and tenderness in their thyroid gland along with the usual symptoms of thyrotoxicosis. Treatment is aimed at reducing symptoms. Beta-blockers such as propranolol are typically used in the hyperthyroid phase of the illness along with nonsteroidal anti-inflammatory agents, which are used to reduce pain and inflammation.

SUPPURATIVE THYROIDITIS (ACUTE THYROIDITIS, BACTERIAL THYROIDITIS, PYOGENIC THYROIDITIS)

Suppurative thyroiditis is a potentially fatal condition if diagnosis and treatment are delayed. Usually caused by bacterial infection, its origins may also lie in fungal, mycobacterial, or parasitic infections, and it can occur after sinus surgery or respiratory infections. Because a firm capsule encloses the thyroid gland, infectious agents are rarely able to penetrate thyroid tissue.

Consequently, this condition is rare and most often seen in elderly, immunosuppressed or debilitated individuals, particularly those with AIDS and coexisting *Pneumocystis carinii* infection; in patients with preexisting thyroid disease, especially thyroid cancer, Hashimoto's thyroiditis, or toxic multinodular goiter; and children with congenital anomalies such as pyriform sinus fistula. The most common etiologic agents are *Streptococcus pyogenes*, *Staphylococcus aureus*, and *Pneumococcus pneumoniae*, although other bacterial causes include *Escherichia coli*, *Hemophilus influenza*, and meningococcal organisms (Singer 1991, 61).

Suppurative bacterial thyroiditis causes an acute illness with fever, dysphagia, dysphonia, anterior neck and erythema (redness), and a tender thyroid mass. Thyroid function is usually normal but episodes of both hypothyroidism and thyrotoxicosis can occur. The white blood cell count and erythrocyte sedimentation rate tests are elevated in this condition, and suppurative areas appear "cold" with radioactive iodine assisted thyroid scans. Treatment consists of appropriate antibiotics and drainage of any abscesses if present.

SILENT THYROIDITIS (LYMPHOCYTIC THYROIDITIS, SUBACUTE LYMPHOCYTIC THYROIDITIS)

Silent thyroiditis is one of the least common types of thyroiditis. Although silent thyroiditis wasn't recognized until the 1970s, according to James Norman, M.D, it probably existed and was treated as Graves' disease before then (Norman 2012).

Silent thyroiditis has elements of Hashimoto's thyroiditis because of the lymphocytic infiltration noted in the thyroid gland. It also resembles postpartum thyroiditis in that the majority of patients have been young women following pregnancy and it is a painless type of thyroiditis. Symptoms are typically milder than those seen in Graves' disease and treatment is rarely needed. Approximately 80 percent of patients show complete recovery and become euthyroid after 3 months (Norman 2012). Later symptoms may be of an underactive thyroid until the thyroid recovers. Recurrent episodes of hyperthyroidism and hypothyroidism may also occur before the condition resolves, typically within one year.

Treatment usually consists of bed rest or reduced activity with beta blockers occasionally prescribed to control palpitations. Radioactive iodine, surgery, or antithyroid drugs are never needed. Rarely, patients develop permanent hypothyroidism.

HYPERTHYROID PHASE OF HASHIMOTO'S THYROIDITIS

Hashimoto's thyroiditis is an autoimmune thyroid disorder of hypothyroidism that can have a thyrotoxic phase as thyroid hormone is released from damaged thyroid cells. This phase typically lasts 3–4 months. Treatment consists of propranolol or other beta blockers to reduce symptoms.

Females with Turner's and Down's syndromes often have Hashimoto's thyroiditis and may experience transient episodes of thyrotoxicosis during the hyperthyroid or discharge thyroiditis phase of Hashimoto's thyroiditis (Idris and O'Malley 2000, 272).

HASHITOXICOSIS

Patients with Hashimoto's thyroiditis who develop the stimulating TSH receptor antibodies seen in Graves' disease can have transient bursts of excess thyroid hormone, causing temporary episodes of thyrotoxicosis. Known as Hashitoxicosis, this condition can occur during the transition in which patients move from one autoimmune thyroid disorder to another.

THYROTOXICOSIS FACTITIA

Thyrotoxicosis factitita is a condition caused by intentional or accidental self-administration of excess thyroid replacement hormone from overuse of pharmaceutical preparations or contaminated dietary supplements and foods. Patients with thyrotoxicosis factitia typically present with thyrotoxicosis, a small thyroid gland, a low thyroid uptake and a low serum thyroglobulin level. In addition, they show a lack of response to anti-thyroid drugs.

A number of dietary supplements sold as dietary or metabolic boosters have been found to contain thyroid hormone derivatives. Accidental cases of thyrotoxicosis factitia have occurred in patients using various dietary supplements. In a recent study, researchers found T4 and T3 contaminants in 9 out of 10 products they sampled. Detectable amounts of triiodothyronine ranged from 1.3 to 25.4 mcg per tablet, while some products contained double the amount of T4 found in prescription products (Kang 2011).

RESISTANCE TO THYROID HORMONE (RTH)

The syndrome of resistance to thyroid hormone (RTH) is defined by a normal or elevated TSH level with elevated circulating levels of free thyroid hormone resulting from an underlying condition of reduced target tissue responsiveness. Most patients with RTH have a goiter, and their thyroid status is variable, with patients appearing euthyroid, hypothyroid or hyperthyroid. RTH is most commonly caused by monoallelic mutations of the *TR* gene.

The mutation can be inherited in an autosomal dominant manner or it can occur as a new mutation. The mutant receptors act in a dominant negative fashion to block the activity of the normal allele, thereby explaining the dominant inheritance. The gene defect remains unknown in about 15 percent of subjects with a RTH phenotype. It is likely that mutations in cofactors required for normal thyroid hormone function are involved in the pathogenesis of RTH in these patients (Donovan 1997).

In RTH, symptoms are of variable severity, with common features including goiter, tachycardia, and hyperactivity. Thyroid hormone levels are elevated in the presence of a normal TSH level, which causes this disorder to be occasionally missed when TSH alone is used to screen for thyroid disease. There are reports of children diagnosed with attention deficit hyperactivity disorder (ADHD) who were later found to have RTH.

Decreased TBG Production

Mild, temporary elevations of FT4 may occur after transient reductions in thyroxine-binding-globulin (TBG) production, for instance when medications containing estrogens are stopped. This is especially common in the hospital setting when hormone replacement therapy may be stopped during hospitalization. Estrogen withdrawal can cause decreased levels of TBG and a transiently elevated FT4 lasting for 2–3 weeks. Because of the many changes to thyroid function that occur during nonthyroidal illness, thyroid function tests are not recommended for hospitalized patients.

3

Graves' Disease:
When the Autoimmune
Response Goes Awry

Graves' disease is a self-limiting autoimmune disorder and the most common cause of hyperthyroidism. Besides its potential to cause hyperthyroidism, Graves' disease can also cause extrathyroidal manifestations (affecting other organs besides the thyroid gland).

These manifestations can occur either alone or in conjunction with the thyroid disorder. Among these manifestations, which are described in Chapter 11, Graves' disease can affect the eyes, causing Graves' ophthalmopathy (thyroid eye disease or TED); the skin, causing pretibial myxedema; and the soft muscles of the extremities, causing thyroid acropachy. In addition, Graves' disease can cause a variety of symptoms associated with its autoimmune origins, and patients with Graves' disease are susceptible to developing several coexisting conditions that are described in Chapter 5. Chapter 3 describes the history, autoimmune nature, disease course, and the unique features and characteristics that make Graves' disease more than just a hyperthyroid disorder.

The History of Graves' Disease

In the late 1700s, the British physician Caleb Hiller Parry discovered a link between an enlarged thyroid gland, a racing pulse, and cardiovascular symptoms. He reported his findings in an article, "Eight Patients with Diffuse Goiter and Hyperthyroidism," but the article wasn't published until 1825, three years after his death. Around the same time, the Italian doctors Giuseppe Flajani and Antonio Giuseppe Testa also published articles describing this connection.

In 1835 the Irish physician Robert Graves went on to describe another important feature of Graves' disease, bulging eyes or proptosis. This caused him to gain renown for discovering the disorder now known as Graves' disease. He described the condition now known as Graves' ophthalmopathy in his article "Three Females with Goiter, Palpations, and Exophthalmos."

In 1840, in Wurzburg, Germany, the physician Karl Adolph von Basedow was also treating several patients with Graves' disease and went on to describe their symptoms of nervousness and weight loss. Basedow described the "Wurzburg triad" in Graves' disease, which consisted of exophthalmos, stroma or goiter, and palpitations of the heart. Based on his observations, Basedow theorized that excess iodine contributed to Graves' disease. In Europe, Graves' disease is referred to as Basedow's disease.

Despite these descriptive early reports from several different sources, it took more than 100 years for researchers to discover the immunological dysfunction that lies at the root of Graves' disease. In 1956 Adams and Purves discovered a large protein molecule in the serum of Graves' disease patients. They called this molecule long-acting thyroid stimulator (LATS), and blood tests for LATS were developed. In the 1970s researchers discovered that LATS was an IgG immunoglobulin, which they called thyroid stimulating immunoglobulin (TSI), and proposed that Graves' disease was an autoimmune disorder.

Who Gets Graves' Disease?

Women are 8 times more likely than men to be affected by Graves' disease. The peak incidence occurs between the ages of 20–40 years although people of all ages can be affected. Graves' disease occurs more often in individuals with a family history of autoimmune disease, and it occurs less frequently in regions where iodine deficiency is endemic. Worldwide, the distribution of Graves' disease appears to be relatively equal, affecting all countries and races. The prevalence of Graves' disease is reported to be 1.0 percent (Huber et al. 2008).

Subclinical Graves' Disease

In subclinical Graves' disease, thyroid hormone levels (FT4 and FT3) are within the reference range, the TSH level is low, and elevated levels of TSH receptor antibodies are present, although they're generally below the laboratory cut-off. Treatment with anti-thyroid drugs is not used as it can cause thyroid hormone levels to fall too low. However, patients are regularly monitored with blood levels and they're treated with beta adrenergic blocking agents if symptoms of hyperthyroidism occur.

A recent large study showed that less than 1 percent of patients with subclinical hyperthyroidism develop overt hyperthyroidism within a 7-year observation period (Vadiveloo et al. 2011). This study involved more than 2000 patients and showed that patients with subclinical hyperthyroidism have an increased risk of cardiovascular disease and dysrhythmia. There is an association with fracture and dementia that is not related to TSH concentration and therefore is less likely to be causally related. No association was found between TSH and cancer. This study included patients with both subclinical Graves' disease and subclinical hyperthyroidism caused by nodular goiter. The disease course in subclinical nodular goiter is typically more severe than that seen in subclinical Graves' disease.

Pathology in Graves' Disease

Graves' disease shares a number of immunologic features with autoimmune hypothyroidism, including elevated levels of thyroglobulin and thyroid peroxidase (TPO) antibodies. Thyroglobulin antibodies are seen in about 50 percent and TPO antibodies in about 80 percent of Graves' disease patients. These antibodies may modify the effects of stimulating TSH receptor antibodies (Weetman 2000, 1236).

Hyperthyroidism in Graves' disease is characterized by the presence of specific white blood cells, both B and T lymphocytes, that are sensitized to several thyroid protein antigens. These antigens primarily include the TSH receptor and, to a lesser degree, thyroglobulin, thyroid peroxidase, and the sodium/iodide co-transporter (Davies 2000, 18). In thyroid tissue studies in patients with Graves' disease, lymphocytic infiltration primarily comprised of T lymphocytes is apparent, and thyroid follicular cells are larger and more abundant.

The immune system defect that leads to thyroid antibody production lies in the immune system's surveillance rather than the protein antigens. In the immune response to these antigens, lymphocytes produce several different thyroid antibodies that target these cellular proteins. The most significant is the stimulating TSH receptor antibody (stimulating TRAb, TSI), which directs thyroid cells to grow and produce excess thyroid hormone. Consequently the thyroid gland in Graves' disease patients has a columnar and folded epithelium with little colloid, along with hypertrophy and hyperplasia in the thyroid follicles. This causes the characteristic diffuse goiter sometimes seen in Graves' disease patients.

The lymphocytic infiltration in Graves' disease is primarily composed of T lymphocytes, the soldiers in the immune system army intended to fight foreign antigens such as infectious agents. T lymphocytes consist of two subtypes: helper (CD4) and suppressor (CD8) cells. Both subtypes secrete proteins known as cytokines, which regulate the immune response. The CD4 lymphocytes can further be divided into Th1 and Th2 subtypes, which differ in the types of cytokines they express and secrete. Th1 cells usually secrete interferon-gamma and other cytokines, whereas Th2 cells secrete interleukin-4. Disruptions in the usual proportions of Th1 and Th2 cells promote autoimmune disease development.

The Th1 response promotes cell-mediated immunity, which is required to clear infectious organisms and generally involves interferon-gamma (IFN-γ). In contrast, a Th2 response enhances humoral (or antibody) immunity and is seen in allergy and generally involves the interleukins IL-4, IL-5, and IL-13. The Th2 response is implicated in Graves' hyperthyroidism, which is associated with elevations of IL-4 and IL-5.

Hygiene or Counterregulation Hypothesis

However, an association in Graves' disease with the gene CTLA-4 responsible for downregulating T-cell responses could prevent normal counter-regulatory mechanisms, also promoting enhanced autoimmune and allergic responses. Normal counter-regulatory mechanisms may also be reduced in individuals without adequate exposure to normal infectious agents, commonly referred to as the hygiene or counterregulation hypothesis (McLachlan and Rapoport 2003). A number of studies have shown that excessive use of antibiotics, antibiotic cleaners, vaccines, and limited exposure to foreign antigens can weaken the immune system, causing an erratic immune response that leads to autoimmunity.

Variability in Graves' Disease

The considerable variation in the pathology of Graves' disease is dependent on a number of different factors. These include the number of TSH receptors available to react with thyroid antibodies; the immunoreactivity of an individual's specific TSI antibodies; and the effects of blocking TSH receptor antibodies, which prevent TSI from reacting with thyroid cells. Consequently, a TSI level can't gauge disease severity or predict the disease course (Weetman 2000, 1236). Symptoms are more important than the TSI or thyroid hormone levels and are generally relied on to evaluate disease severity.

The Disease Course in Graves' Disease

The onset of hyperthyroid symptoms in Graves' disease is usually gradual, with patients most often complaining of increased nervousness, irritability, fatigue, weight loss and menstrual irregularity over a period of several months or longer. Early on, symptoms typically wax and wane, as do blood levels of thyroid hormone, making a correct diagnosis elusive.

In older patients, cardiovascular and myopathic (muscle involvement) features may predominate while the more typical characteristics may be mild or absent, leading to the term *apathetic hyperthyroidism.* This term can also refer to the symptoms of withdrawal, listlessness, weakness, or depression sometimes seen in this age group. In Graves' disease, these symptoms may be accompanied by small goiters, modest tachycardia, occasionally cool and even dry skin, and few eye signs. Long-standing thyrotoxicosis in these patients causes extreme fatigue. Congestive heart failure may also be the initial manifestation in older patients, especially if there is underlying cardiac disease.

Graves' disease is a chronic disorder. Once Graves' disease develops, it persists for life, although remission (absence of active disease) is a natural step in the disease course. With the introduction of antithyroid drug therapy, the natural disease progression is difficult to estimate. However, it's known that, untreated, hyperthyroidism in Graves' disease can spontaneously improve and result in a fairly quick return to normal, with spontaneous remission estimated to be 10 to 25 percent each year (Felz and Stein 1999). Remission occurs when the immune system heals and stops producing TSI antibodies at a rate capable of causing hyperthyroidism.

Anthony Weetman, M.D., reports that about 20 percent of patients with mild hyperthyroidism who are treated with beta adrenergic antagonists (beta blockers such as propranolol) for one year will become clinically and biochemically euthyroid, but the frequency of permanent euthyroidism is unknown (Weetman 2000, 1243).

Most, if not all, individuals with Graves' disease have an initial hypothyroid phase. Hypothyroidism in this phase is usually mild and not diagnosed, although prior clinical records may show an elevated TSH level. Alternately, newly diagnosed Graves' disease patients remark that they had early symptoms of hypothyroidism. In addition, some patients are diagnosed with Hashimoto's thyroiditis and are on replacement hormone for months or years before developing Graves' disease.

The active phase of Graves' disease is variable and tends to depend on environmental influences. It's not unusual for symptoms to become exacerbated during times of stress, particularly the stress accompanying bereavement. It's also not unusual in the early stage of Graves' disease for symptoms to wax and wane, with periods of remission alternating with periods of symptoms. Predominant symptoms and also symptom severity can also change over time. Lifestyle changes, particularly avoiding known triggers such as excess dietary iodine, frequently lead to a reduction in symptoms and earlier remission.

The active phase of Graves' hyperthyroidism can range from several months to several years with most patients on anti-thyroid drugs achieving remission within 2 years. However, it's important to evaluate remission with laboratory tests rather than using an arbitrary timeframe.

While most patients experience alternating periods of relapse/flares and remission/mild symptoms, some patients have a single episode of hyperthyroidism, sometimes followed by the development of hypothyroidism 10–20 years later. Thyroid failure in hypothyroidism is thought to result from the presence of blocking TSH receptor antibodies, which causes atrophic thyroiditis or primary myxedema, and from tissue destruction by cell-mediated immunity and cytotoxic antibodies (Kasagi et al. 1993).

Legal Issues and Mortality

In the United States, thyroid disease is included under the Americans with Disabilities Act of 1990. For general information, visit the web site at www.ada.gov/pubs/ada.htm.

The estimated mortality rate from untreated Graves' disease has been reported to be as high as 11 percent. However, death attributable to untreated thyrotoxicosis is rarely seen today and is primarily associated with the elderly. Heart problems, such as myocardial infarction, arrhythmia and heart failure, have been responsible for most deaths associated with Graves' disease.

The Autoimmune Nature of Graves' Disease

Autoimmunity in Graves' disease is caused by a combination of genetic and environmental factors that are described in Chapter 4. Working in tandem, these factors cause the immune system to produce thyroid autoantibodies that lead to the development of Graves' disease. Further evidence of ongoing autoimmunity in Graves' disease is the elevation of ICAM-1, and IL-6 and IL-8 cytokines seen in hyperthyroid patients who have achieved remission (DeGroot 2010, 1).

The TSH Receptor

Receptors for TSH located on thyroid cells are the primary target of TSI antibodies. TSI antibodies cause hyperthyroidism by reacting with the TSH receptor on thyroid cells, acting in place of TSH and causing thyroid cells to grow and produce excess thyroid hormone. When TSI antibodies rise high enough, typically to 125 percent activity in most people, hyperthyroidism develops.

However, the TSI level associated with hyperthyroidism can vary. People vary in the number of TSH receptors found on their thyroid cells and the reactivity of these receptors. It's thought that subtypes of TSI exist with some subtypes having a stronger influence on thyroid hormone production. In addition, blocking TSH receptor antibodies, which are described in the next section, can block TSI from reacting with the TSH receptor. Tests for TSI are important for confirming Graves' disease and follow-up tests after 6–12 months are used to show treatment response. Once TSI antibodies are produced, they remain in the blood circulation for 2–3 months before being broken down into amino acids and excreted. For this reason, TSI levels change slowly.

Autoimmune Factors

The immune system in patients with Graves' disease leans towards a Th2 rather than a Th1 response. The Th2 response promotes autoimmunity and is characteristically seen in many autoimmune diseases, including Graves' disease and type 1 diabetes.

Graves' disease is considered an antibody-mediated autoimmune disorder. Here, stimulating TSH receptor antibodies (also known as thyroid stimulating immunoglobulins or TSI) react with the TSH receptor protein on thyroid cells, ordering these cells to produce excess thyroid hormone.

While the immediate goals in treating Graves' disease are to reduce thyroid hormone levels and lessen the effects of hyperthyroidism, the long-term goals are to heal the immune system and reduce the production of TSI. There is some variation in TSI antibodies and their reactivity to the TSH receptor. This explains why Graves' patients with very high TSI levels can have mild symptoms and Graves' patients with moderate TSI levels can have severe symptoms. It's suspected that there are several subtypes of TSI. Presumably, these subtypes determine the type of epitopes or binding sites on the TSH receptor that TSI can bind to. TSI may bind to epitopes that result in stimulation of thyroid cells or they may bind to epitopes that are less potent. In addition, many patients with Graves' disease also have blocking TSH receptor antibodies that block both TSH and TSI from reacting with the TSH receptor, thereby preventing thyroid cells from producing excess thyroid hormone.

The intrathyroidal inflammatory lymphocytes that produce TSI also produce immune system chemicals known as cytokines, such as interleukin-1, tumor necrosis factor alpha, and interferon-gamma, that induce the expression of adhesion molecules such as CD 54, regulatory molecules, and HLA class II molecules. HLA class II antigens are human leukocyte antigens that regulate what foreign antigens we'll react with as well as the severity of the reaction. These cytokines also induce thyroid cells to synthesize cytokines that help perpetuate the autoimmune process. Anti-thyroid drugs reduce the production of thyroidal cytokines, which helps to explain the immunomodulatory effects, contributing to remission in some patients with Graves' disease (Weetman 2000, 1238).

Thyroid Antibodies in Graves' Disease

TSI antibodies are also implicated in the development of Graves' ophthalmopathy, pretibial myxedema and thyroid acropachy. Individuals with autoimmune thyroid disease develop specific thyroid conditions depending on what type of thyroid antibody predominates at the time. It's not unusual for individuals with one autoimmune thyroid disorder to develop different thyroid disorders at different times in their lifetime.

Up to 80 percent of patients with Graves' disease also have moderately increased levels of thyroid peroxidase (TPO) antibodies, which are markers of thyroid inflammation, and 50–60 percent of patients have moderately increased levels of thyroglobulin antibodies. Most individuals with Graves' disease also have blocking TSH receptor antibodies. Blocking TRAb reduces the effects of TSI, and when they predominate, they contribute to the development of hypothyroidism. At any given time, the type of TSH receptor antibodies that predominate determines the specific thyroid status of the individual. About 20 percent of individuals with Graves' disease spontaneously move into hypothyroidism, which can be a temporary condition, when blocking TRAb antibodies predominate. This form of hypothyroidism is usually mild and capable of resolving, although it requires treatment with replacement hormone when thyroid hormone levels are too low for the body's needs.

Immune System Health

The immune system is a complex network of organs and cells working together to promote good health. Immune system cells react to the presence of foreign protein antigens, including infectious agents and allergic substances. In the immune response, the immune system attacks foreign antigens and produces antibodies that ward off subsequent attacks. These antibodies can also serve as markers of past infection or allergic reactions.

When the immune system is crippled by constant infections and exposure to allergens or its function is compromised by overuse of antibiotics and vaccines, it becomes weakened. A weakened immune system is ineffective. Without the ability to respond appropriately to foreign antigens, it reacts erratically and begins targeting the body's own tissues and cells. Consequently, the immune system produces autoantibodies, that is, antibodies that attack the body's own tissues, causing autoimmune disease. First termed "horror autotoxicus" by the German physician Ehrlich in 1900, autoimmune diseases are now known to be caused by immune system defects and include some of the most common chronic disorders affecting mankind.

The Endocrine, Immune, and Nervous Systems

The endocrine glands, the immune system, and the nervous system all work together in a process known as homeostasis, which promotes optimal health. Anything that affects one of these three systems affects the other two systems. The effects of psychological stress, for instance alterations in levels of neurotransmitters such as dopamine and serotonin, alter the levels of the immune system's white blood cells and of the immune system's modulatory chemicals known as cytokines. Changes in these cells and chemicals can affect the levels of hormones that are produced by endocrine glands. The field of study of this interaction between the three systems is known as psychoneuroimmunology.

Studies in psychoneuroimmunology show why low levels of thyroid hormone can increase resistance to infection, cause anxiety and depression and increase the risk of developing peripheral neuropathy. From the opposite end of the spectrum, increased levels of thyroid hormone can cause muscle weakness, mood disturbances, euphoria, and tremor. The many varied signs and symptoms caused by thyrotoxicosis described in this chapter are directly related to the effects of excess thyroid hormone on the body's various organs and systems.

Autoimmune Thyroid Disorders

Most thyroid diseases, whether they cause hypothyroidism, hyperthyroidism or thyroid eye disease (TED), are autoimmune disorders. Here, a defect in the immune system's response leads to diminished or excessive thyroid function or characteristic eye changes. The specific disorder that someone develops depends on the particular thyroid antibodies produced during this faulty immune response. The particular disorder can change over time and it can also improve, stabilize, or resolve when the immune system heals.

Many people with autoimmune hypothyroidism, either Hashimoto's thyroiditis or atrophic thyroiditis, later develop Graves' disease. Autoimmune thyroid disorders occur in people with specific immune system and thyroid regulatory genes that predispose them to developing thyroid disease in the presence of certain environmental triggers. Many people have these predisposing genes, but only a fraction of them develop autoimmune thyroid diseases. Certain environmental triggers are known to trigger or induce thyroid disease in these people. The genetic and environmental influences of Graves' disease are described in Chapter 4.

Overlapping Autoimmune Thyroid Diseases

Patients with autoimmune thyroid disease (AITD) may have features of both Hashimoto's thyroiditis and Graves' disease in a condition known as Hashitoxicosis. In Hashitoxicosis, patients are primarily hypothyroid and have the stimulating TSH receptor antibodies characteristic of Graves' disease, which causes transient symptoms of hyperthyroidism. Conditions of Hashimoto's encephalopathy, a form of dementia, may also overlap with other autoimmune thyroid disorders, particularly Hashimoto's thyroiditis, although individuals with Graves' disease may be affected. Individuals with Graves' disease and high concentrations of thyroglobulin antibodies may also develop some features characteristic of Hashimoto's thyroiditis.

Hashitoxicosis

Hashitoxicosis is an autoimmune disorder in which patients with Hashimoto's thyroiditis or autoimmune atrophic thyroid disease have transient hyperthyroid episodes.

Hashitoxicosis is an autoimmune thyroid condition that can occur for long periods, causing transient symptoms periodically. Alternately, it can occur as a transitional phase as patients move from autoimmune hyperthyroidism to autoimmune hypothyroidism or from autoimmune hypothyroidism to autoimmune hyperthyroidism.

Individuals with Hashitoxicosis can have thyroglobulin, TPO, or blocking TSH receptor antibodies, but they always have TSI antibodies, although their levels typically do not reach the high levels (1.3 or 130 percent activity) that cause hyperthyroidism in patients with Graves' disease.

In Hashitoxicosis, patients exhibit variable signs and symptoms of hyperthyroidism that may change over time. Common symptoms include headache, hot flashes, irritability, increased appetite, weight loss, muscle weakness, increased heart rate, increased systolic blood pressure, atrial fibrillation, increased hair and nail growth, nervousness, tremor, nausea, mood disturbances, hives, and palpitations. However, hives and palpitations may also occur as a symptom of hypothyroidism.

The Graves' Disease Family

Graves' disease shares many features with other autoimmune disorders that share a common embryological origin. Graves' disease is associated statistically with a group of autoimmune diseases including pernicious anemia, atrophic gastritis, vitiligo, alopecia, angioedema, myasthenia gravis, and idiopathic thrombocytopenic purpura (DeGroot 2010, 3). A weak association is also suspected with rheumatoid arthritis and systemic lupus erythematosus (SLE). Graves' disease is an example of an organ specific autoimmune disease, and it appears not to be statistically more common among individuals who have the systemic autoimmune disorders dermatomyositis or scleroderma.

Autoimmune Endocrine Disorders

Autoimmune endocrine disorders include: Hashimoto's thyroiditis, Graves' disease, Addison's disease (adrenal gland insufficiency), autoimmune hypophysitis (pituitary gland insufficiency), autoimmune oophritis (ovarian insufficiency), insulin dependent (type 1) diabetes mellitus (IDDM), autoimmune hypoparathyroidism, testicular insufficiency, and premature ovarian failure.

Multiple Endocrine Disorders

Patients with organ-specific autoimmune endocrine disorders such as type 1 diabetes or Graves' disease are more likely to develop a second autoimmune endocrine disorder than other people. Some of these people may have two coexisting glandular disorders and others may go on to develop one of the autoimmune polyglandular syndromes, which are described in Chapter 5.

Autoimmune thyroid disorders are the most common autoimmune endocrine disorder, and they are also the disorder most likely to occur in people with other autoimmune endocrine disorders. For instance, it's not unusual for people with Addison's disease or type 1 diabetes to develop Hashimoto's thyroiditis years later. Even in the absence of autoimmune thyroid disease, a large number of patients with other endocrine disorders have high titers of thyroid antibodies.

Symptoms in Autoimmune Endocrine Disease

The body's endocrine glands produce hormones that help regulate various functions including growth, metabolism, and reproduction. Autoimmune endocrine disorders usually damage endocrine glands thereby causing hormone deficiencies. The exception is Graves' disease, a disorder of excess thyroid hormone production. Symptoms of endocrine disease vary considerably depending on the particular gland affected. In type 1 diabetes, for instance, destruction of the insulin-producing cells of the pancreas results in diminished insulin production. Without adequate levels of insulin, blood glucose levels rise. Graves' disease can occur as one of multiple autoimmune disorders in Schmidt's syndrome and in multiple autoimmune syndrome (MAS).

Overall, endocrine deficiencies and excesses of hormones affect all of the body's systems and consequently cause a wide range of symptoms. Most people with Graves' disease, for instance, will have several predominant symptoms that can change over time, rather than all symptoms associated with the disorder. Similar to most other autoimmune conditions, symptoms in endocrine conditions wax and wane, periods of remission frequently alternating with periods of variable symptoms.

More Than a Hyperthyroid Disorder — Signs and Symptoms

Besides having the typical signs and symptoms of hyperthyroidism, pretibial myxedema, acropachy and Graves' ophthalmopathy, patients with Graves' disease can also develop a number of different symptoms related to autoimmunity or as manifestations of Graves' disease.

For instance, Graves' disease can also cause several metabolic changes and atypical symptoms such as hives, muscle wasting, and weight gain. Psychiatric symptoms are also not uncommon. It's important to recognize that these symptoms can be part of the Graves' disease spectrum rather than indications of a newly emerging illness.

Dermal Symptoms

Graves' disease can cause a number of dermal symptoms, particularly rashes and hives related to hypersensitivity reactions, and vitiligo.

HYPERSENSITIVITY REACTIONS

Hypersensitivity reactions occur when the immune system responds in an exaggerated fashion to foreign antigens such as pollen or food proteins. In both hypersensitivity reactions and Graves' disease, the immune system is ineffective and erratically launches an exaggerated immune response against innocent proteins.

Hypersensitivity reactions are common in people with autoimmune diseases. Some hypersensitivity reactions are also known to trigger autoimmune disease development and exacerbate symptoms in individuals with autoimmune disorders. Furthermore, individuals with autoimmune disease are more likely to experience one or more different types of hypersensitivity reactions. The specific environmental substances someone will react to and the severity of these reactions are under the control of immune system and organ-specific genes. Hypersensitivity reactions include:

- Type I or immediate hypersensitivity
- Type II or cytotoxic (capable of destroying cells) hypersensitivity
- Type III or immune complex hypersensitivity
- Type IV or delayed hypersensitivity

Each subtype plays a role in autoimmune disease, with the type of reaction triggering the type of disorder that occurs. For instance, in immune complex reactions, complexes of antigens and antibodies lodge into kidney tissue, which leads to kidney damage.

Type I Hypersensitivity. In type I hypersensitivity reactions, the reaction is immediate and related to the production of immunoglobulin E. Immunoglobulin E, upon entering the blood circulations, latches on to mast cells, which produce histamine. Histamine then induces allergy-associated symptoms. Examples include reactions to penicillin, insect bites and molds. Common symptoms include hives, itching (urticaria) and swelling of the larynx. Individuals with hypersensitivity to specific allergens may develop anaphylactic reactions when they're exposed to significant amounts of these allergens. Reactions may be more intense during times of stress or during exercise. While type I hypersensitivity reactions don't cause autoimmune diseases directly, they stimulate the immune system. Chronic immune stimulation, over time, impairs its effectiveness.

For instance, about 42 percent of patients with autoimmune thyroid disease are likely to have type I hypersensitivity reactions compared to 32 percent of normal subjects. When Type I hypersensitivity reactions occur, symptoms in autoimmune disease flare or worsen. For instance, studies show that when

IgE levels rise due to pollen allergies, symptoms in Graves' disease worsen, with higher IgE levels correlating with more severe disease states.

Type II Hypersensitivity. Type II hypersensitivity or cytotoxic hypersensitivity is caused by antibody-mediated reactions. When the immune system reacts to antigens, it produces various immunoglobulins or antibodies, usually long-lasting immunoglobulin G (IgG) antibodies. In type II hypersensitivity reactions, K-cells rather than mast cells are involved, and production of the immune system chemical known as complement increases. These changes injure tissue cells. Autoimmune diseases most often mediated by type II hypersensitivity reactions include pemphigus, autoimmune hemolytic anemia (AIHA) and Goodpasture's syndrome.

Type III Hypersensitivity. Type III or immune complex hypersensitivity is characterized by circulating autoantibodies that are linked to targeted antigens. These immune complexes can lodge between tissue cells and interfere with the function of the affected organ. Immune complexes are responsible for lupus nephritis in several autoimmune conditions, including systemic lupus erythematosus and can rarely cause kidney disease in Graves' disease patients.

Type IV Hypersensitivity. Type IV hypersensitivity reactions are delayed reactions in which the immune system's response to specific antigens is slow, typically occurring 1–2 days after the antigenic exposure. An example is the delayed rash that can occur 2 days after receiving an inoculation of tuberculin in the tuberculosis skin test.

CHRONIC URTICARIA AND ANGIOEDEMA

Persons with autoimmune disorders, especially thyroid disorders, systemic lupus eythematosus, and Sjogren's, are at risk for urticaria (rashes), angioedema (hives) and urticarial vasculitis. Urticaria is defined by the presence of rashes characterized by a raised swelling of the skin with itching that typically lasts no longer than 24–48 hours. Angioedema presents as a deeper, nondependent swelling without itching. In certain types of urticaria and angioedema, the underlying cause is autoimmunity related to the presence of thyroid antibodies or an acquired C1 inhibitor deficiency.

The cumulative lifetime incidence of urticaria is estimated to be as high as 20 percent in the general population. The most common cause is IgE mediated (allergic) reactions to food or drugs. The cause is mast cell degeneration with release of histamine caused by the formation of IgE antibodies. When the offending trigger is identified and removed, the urticaria resolves.

When the solution isn't as simple and urticaria persists for longer than 6 weeks, the condition is known as chronic urticaria. Approximately 50 percent of patients with chronic urticaria also have conditions of angioedema.

When both conditions are present the condition is seldom related to allergy and it is known as chronic idiopathic urticaria/angioedema.

The Role of Thyroid Antibodies. Several groups of researchers have described a relationship between chronic urticaria and thyroid disease, primarily Hashimoto's thyroiditis and to a lesser extent Graves' disease. These patients typically had high levels of thyroid peroxidase antibodies and severe chronic urticaria/angioedema with no other signs of thyroid disease although some patients were reported to have a slight goiter. Treatment with levothyroxine caused improvement in the urticaria and angioedema. When treatment was stopped the symptoms returned and then subsided with the continuation of treatment. In the patients without evidence of thyroid antibodies, levothyroxine had no effect. The pathogenic relationship between thyroid antibodies and the chronic urticaria hasn't yet been determined (Zuraw 1997, 59–61). Low levels of vitamin A caused by malnutrition in hyperthyroidism have also been reported to contribute to the development of hives.

VITILIGO

About 7 percent of patients with Graves' disease develop white or blanched patches of skin in a condition known as vitiligo. Vitiligo is characterized by a loss of brown pigment from areas of skin, resulting in irregular smooth white patches that usually affect both sides of the body equally. Lesions in vitiligo primarily affect the face, elbows and knees, hands and feet, and genitals.

Vitiligo occurs when immune cells destroy the cells that produce brown pigment (melanocytes). This destruction is related to autoimmunity and is associated with Addison's disease, pernicious anemia and Graves' disease. Vitiligo may appear at any age. There is an increased rate of the condition in some families. The condition affects about 1 out of every 100 people in the United States.

DERMATITIS HERPETIFORMIS

Dermatitis herpetiformis, an autoimmune disorder characterized by chronic, intensely pruritic (itchy) symmetric groups of vesicles, blisters, waxy lesions, papules, and wheals (hives), can affect the elbows, knees, arms, legs, shoulders, scalp, buttocks, neck, and face. Clinical signs are often highly variable, ranging from groups of papulovesicles with excoriations or eczema-like lesions to minimal variants of discrete redness with small water blisters or areas of small purpura (purple bruise-like lesions).

Also known as Duhring's disease, Brocq-Duhring disease, or dermatitis multiformis, herpetiformis multiformis usually occurs in people with celiac disease as well as milder forms of gluten sensitivity and, less often, in people with autoimmune thyroid disorders including Graves' disease. Dermatitis herpetiformis has a typical onset in the late teens and early twenties, or in the third or fourth decades of life, although it can affect people of all ages. Males are affected twice as often as females, and it occurs more often in whites than in people of Asian or African descent.

Although lesions in the oral mucosa are rare, there are reports of oral lesions occurring early in the stages of dermatitis herpetiformis. These lesions may also be mistaken for the apthous ulcers (oral blisters) that frequently occur in people with celiac disease.

Environmental triggers include gluten, which is found in wheat, rye, and barley and other grains that are contaminated with wheat during harvest. Gluten is also found in hydrolyzed vegetable protein, artificial colorings, malts, malt ales, beer, hydrolyzed plant protein, monosodium glutamate, preservatives, modified food starches, vegetable gum, and vinegar. Iodide in iodized salt and foods high in iodine and halide are suspected of causing disease flares. Untreated, dermatitis herpetiformis tends to wax and wane, although with a constant diet of gluten, symptoms persist. It can take a few weeks to several years for symptoms to clear with a gluten-free diet with longer periods required for patients who have had symptoms for a long time before restricting gluten.

ERYTHEMA ANNULARE CENTRIFIGUM

Erythema annulare centrifugum (EAC) is classified as one of the figurate or gyrate erythemas (causing redness). The rash in EAC is characterized by a scaling or nonscaling, reddened eruption that spreads from the edges outward while the center area of the lesion clears. An exact trigger hasn't been determined for the hypersensitivity reaction in EAC. In scaling lesions, a trail of scales may follow the rash's periphery as it spreads. There are several varieties of EAC, some associated with itching. EAC tends to recur in times of stress, and the condition may persist for several months to many years. Besides its association with Graves' disease, EAC may occur in patients with liver disease, hypereosinophilic syndrome, appendicitis, systemic lupus erythematosus (SLE) and Sjogren's syndrome.

BLISTERS AND EROSIONS

Skin and mucous membrane blisters and erosions can occur in Graves' disease as well as coexisting conditions, especially herpes gestationis, which can occur in pregnancy and during the postpartum period. In Graves' disease the development of blisters and erosions may be confused with an anti-thyroid drug reaction.

Metabolic Signs and Symptoms

Graves' disease is associated with several different metabolic and hematological signs and symptoms that stem from autoimmunity.

Blood Sugar Disturbances

Hypoglycemia, a condition of low blood sugar, can occur as a transient condition in patients with Graves' disease. The hypoglycemia that occurs in patients with Graves' disease is caused by the presence of insulin antibodies that cause a condition of insulin autoimmune syndrome, which is described in Chapter 5.

In addition, thyrotoxicosis promotes an insulin-resistant state similar to type 2 diabetes. To meet its increased glucose demands, the body uses whatever sources are available. Glucose utilization by thyroid cells is also enhanced in thyrotoxicosis and contributes to the diminished reserves. With its own demands, the thyrotoxic body becomes insensitive to the normal regulatory effects of insulin, resulting in a state of insulin resistance. Compensatory increases in insulin secretion (in response to the rise in blood glucose) are a result of the body's efforts to maintain a normal blood glucose level.

Hyperglycemia, a condition of elevated blood sugar, can occur in patients with Graves' disease as part of a hyperglycemic hyper-osmolar state, similar to dehydration.

Weight Gain

Weight gain occurs in 10–15 percent of patients with Graves' disease, usually younger patients. The reasons are unclear but appear to be due to inflammation and to deficiencies of free fatty acids. Sedentary changes related to fatigue may also be responsible.

Myopathy

Patients with muscle frequently exhibit muscle weakness (myopathy) and fatigue. Thyrotoxic myopathy, the muscle involvement that resembles wasting, is generally limited to proximal muscle (proximal thigh as compared to distal calf), and its severity appears out of proportion to overall loss of weight. Weakness is most pronounced in the pelvic and shoulder girdles and the proximal limb muscles. The shoulder and hand muscles undergo the most obvious atrophy, although the facial muscles may also be affected. Patients with Graves' disease often have trouble climbing stairs because of weak leg muscles.

Some reduction in the power of muscle contraction is thought to occur in nearly all patients with Graves' disease. One of the earliest physiologic measurements of muscle function, the deep tendon reflex test, is increased in Graves' disease. In recent years, skeletal muscle has been found to be a site of thyroid hormone metabolism and contains TSH receptors. CoQ10 deficiency in hyperthyroidism is a known cause of muscle weakness in Graves' disease.

Digestive Disturbances

Digestion in Graves' disease is usually accelerated. Bowel movements tend to be increased (hyperdefecation), although rarely to the extent that causes diarrhea. Rapid digestion causes malabsorption (nutrients aren't absorbed from food) and steatorrhea (excess undigested fat in stools). Weight loss is caused by both increased caloric requirements and malabsorption. Malabsorption with its subsequent nutrient deficiencies also triggers food cravings.

Elevated liver enzymes are common in hyperthyroidism, and coexisting autoimmune liver diseases can occur. Celiac disease and its milder variation, gluten sensitivity, are seen in patients with autoimmune thyroid disorders more frequently than in the normal population.

Inflammation

Graves' disease can cause a persistent low-grade inflammation. Manifestations include periodontal disease, enlargement of the spleen, and enlarged lymph nodes. Levels of inflammatory blood markers, such as the erythrocyte sedimentation rate (ESR, sed rate), and C-reactive protein (CRP), generally fall within the reference range.

Rhabdomyolysis

Rhabdomyolysis, a potentially fatal condition of muscle destruction typically seen in cocaine and amphetamine overdoses, has been reported to rarely occur in patients with severe Graves' disease. In Graves' disease, rhabdomyolysis is caused by increasing energy consumption associated with depletion of muscle energy and muscle substrate stores.

Hypokalemia

Hypokalemia, a condition of low potassium, is occasionally seen in patients with Graves' disease, especially Asian males, and it can lead to thyrotoxic periodic paralysis. This condition leads to muscle weakness and temporary paralysis and tends to be exacerbated by the ingestion of alcohol and foods with a high glucose content.

Immune Complex Nephritis

Patients with Graves' disease, including those whose who have radioiodine ablation, may have slight proteinuria (elevated urine protein) even in the absence of thyrotoxicosis. Rarely, patients may also develop circulating immune complexes, usually of thyroglobulin with thyroglobulin antibodies that can lead to glomerulonephritis (Scheinman and Moses 2000, 619).

Mitral Valve Prolapse

Mitral valve prolapse, as diagnosed by echocardiography, is also more common in individuals with Graves' disease and is thought to be related to autoimmunity as well as genetic influences. Mitral valve dysfunction may decrease left ventricular performance in patients with thyrotoxicosis.

Hematological Changes

A small number of patients with hyperthyroidism caused by Graves' disease are reported to have increased Factor VIII activity, which can cause increased clotting and cerebral venous thrombosis.

Patients with Graves' disease, especially those with ophthalmopathy, are more likely than other people to have antiphospholipid or anticardiolipin antibodies, which cause increased blood clotting. Antiphospholipid syndrome is the primary cause of miscarriages and strokes in young women. Fortunately, blood clots, antiphospholipid syndrome, and recurrent miscarriages are rare occurrences in patients with Graves' thyrotoxicosis, and the presence of these antibodies may be a nonspecific marker of immune system activation (Porter and Mandel 2000, 629).

Platelet Deficiencies

Occasionally, patients with Graves' disease develop thrombocytopenia, a condition of platelet deficiency. Usually, thrombocytopenia is mild, although, rarely, severe conditions of thrombocytopenia occur. The cause is typically platelet antibodies and coexisting conditions of autoimmune thrombocytopenic purpura, a condition that may precede the development of thyrotoxicosis.

Neurological Changes

In their article titled "Psychiatric Manifestations of Graves' Hyperthyroidism," Bunevicius and Prange write,

> The vast majority of patients with hyperthyroidism, certainly including those with Graves' hyperthyroidism, meet criteria for some psychiatric disorders. A few patients may not meet these criteria but they are probably not free of mental symptoms such as tension, anxiety or depression [Bunevicius and Prange 2006, 95].

Bunevicius and Prange also report that a substantial proportion of patients with hyperthyroidism have psychiatric disorders or mental symptoms and decreased quality of life even after successful treatment of their hyperthyroidism. Treatment based on TSH results can be misleading, however since TSH levels remain typically suppressed in Graves' disease patients even when thyroid hormone levels fall too low for the body's needs. Depression, anxiety and panic disorder are also commonly seen in hypothyroidism.

The mental symptoms of hyperthyroidism may precede the physical symptoms, and they may be more pronounced, confusing diagnosis. Hyperthyroidism is often associated with elation, which can reach manic proportions and cause hallucinations. The transition from slightly manic (hypomanic) to manic behavior may be gradual or abrupt. Its onset may concur close to the initial diagnosis of Graves' disease or be delayed until long afterward.

In rare cases of hyperthyroidism, severe psychic disturbances may occur. Rarely, bipolar and mood swing disorders, and schizoid or paranoid reactions, may emerge. Other psychiatric symptoms reported in Graves' disease include schizophreniform psychosis, cognitive defects, psychological distress, poor stress tolerance, mood disturbances, obsessive-compulsive disorder and social phobia. Mania tends to occur only in patients with a family history of bipolar disorder.

However, not all studies have shown consistent results. In a nonclinical setting, patients with subclinical hyperthyroidism were reported to have better moods compared to euthyroid subjects. In addition, psychiatric symptoms were reported to cease in patients treated with either anti-thyroid drugs or beta adrenergic blocking agents when thyroid hormone levels returned to the reference range (Bunevicius and Prange 2006, 97).

Persistent psychiatric symptoms have also been found to occur more often in patients with Graves' ophthalmopathy. These patients also score lower on quality-of-life rating scores.

Elderly patients are also more likely to have psychiatric symptoms than younger patients. A condition known as rapid consciousness disturbance, which is similar to dementia, can occur in Graves' disease, especially in elderly patients. Apathy is a similar presentation in the elderly Graves' patient. Apathetic hyperthyroidism presents with symptoms of depression, apathy, somnolence or pseudodementia in the absence of the usual signs of hyperthyroidism.

Headache is a rare occurrence in Graves' disease and can be an early warning sign of cerebral venous thrombosis. Six reports of cerebral venous thrombosis have been reported in Graves' disease patients and appear to be related to recurrent inflammation. Of these six patients, one was a male and the other five were females. All the females were using oral contraceptives.

Hashimoto's encephalopathy has been reported to occur in a small number of patients with Graves' disease, primarily middle-aged and elderly patients. Seizures and a condition of multifocal motor status epilepticus have also been reported in a small number of patients with Graves' disease.

Hashimoto's Encephalopathy

Hashimoto's encephalopathy (HE), which has recently been designated "steroid-responsive encephalopathy associated with autoimmune thyroiditis" (SREAT), is an autoimmune disorder that can cause memory impairment, cognitive changes, dementia and associated neurological symptoms. HE can occur in patients with Hashimoto's thyroiditis or Graves' disease, and in patients with normal thyroid function in the presence of thyroid antibodies.

TPO antibodies are the cause of HE. However, in SREAT, rather than affecting thyroid tissue, these antibodies cause brain inflammation. Most experts believe that SREAT is underdiagnosed and that many patients thought to have Alzheimer's disease actually have SREAT, which is a treatable disorder. Hashimoto's encephalopathy has been reported worldwide, and cases have been documented in patients ranging from 12 to 82 years with women more likely to be affected than men.

Encephalopathy is a general term referring to an inflammatory brain disease that alters the brain's structure or function. Encephalopathy is suspected in patients showing signs of an altered mental state. Common symptoms of encephalopathy include stroke-like symptoms of memory loss, difficulty concentrating, hallucinations, irritability, restlessness, amnesia, diminished cognitive ability, myoclonus (involuntary muscle twitching), tremors, nystagmus (rapid, involuntary eye movement), muscle weakness, dementia, seizures, convulsions, difficulty swallowing, impaired speech, confusion, disorientation, psychosis, headache, right-sided hemiparesis or partial paralysis, and fine motor problems, including incoordination of arms, hands and fingers.

HE is diagnosed in patients with high titers of thyroid peroxidase (TPO) antibodies who show signs of cognitive impairment responsive to corticosteroids. Lymphocytic vasculitis of the veins and venules of the brain stem in

HE supports the notion that HE may be an autoimmune vascular disorder. Vasculitis as a contributing factor to HE is also supported by the presence of anti-alpha-enolase antibodies in HE. These antibodies are also seen in other conditions of vasculitis, including systemic lupus erythematosus (SLE) and ANCA-associated vasculitis.

HE may, like multiple sclerosis, also cause a relapsing form of encephalopathy with imaging test results varying depending on whether the disease is in active or relapsing mode. Relapsing white-matter edema is the usual presentation. Most patients have elevated titers of TPO antibodies and some patients have thyroglobulin antibodies. However, because 20 percent of the older population, especially women, may have these antibodies, antibody test results must be interpreted with caution.

Patients with HE are also reported to occasionally have antinuclear antibodies (ANA) and anti-parietal cell antibodies. Fine needle aspiration (FNA) studies in patients with HE show lymphocytic thyroiditis. Patients with SREAT show a good response to corticosteroids such as prednisone and related immunosuppressants because of the ability of these medications to reduce thyroid antibody production and reduce inflammation. Researchers in India report a case of SREAT that did not respond to corticosteroids but showed a very favorable response to plasma exchange, a technique used to remove circulating antibodies.

4

Genetic and Environmental Factors and Influences

Autoimmune thyroid disorders arise from a combination of environmental and genetic factors. About 20 percent of the population has genes that make them susceptible to developing one or more autoimmune disorders. However, only about 5 percent of the population goes on to develop autoimmune disorders, presumably depending on their exposure to environmental triggers. Graves' disease is associated with a number of different immune system and organ-specific genes and a variety of known and suspected environmental triggers.

Comparing Genetic and Environmental Factors

Among monozygotic twins the rate of concordance for Graves' disease is about 20 percent while the rate among dizygotic twins is much lower at 3 percent. This indicates that genes make only a moderate contribution to susceptibility (Brix et al. 1998). More recent studies, however, suggest that genes may play a larger role in the development of Graves' disease. Although this is still a matter of debate, DeGroot estimates that genes account for 79 percent of Graves' disease risk (DeGroot 2010).

Evaluating data from the National Health and Nutrition Examination Survey (NHANES) III study, researchers showed that siblings of individuals with hyperthyroidism were 9.7 times more likely (sibling risk ratio) to develop hyperthyroidism than people without affected siblings. However, the causes of hyperthyroidism in the NHANES study participants weren't studied. In addition, 75 percent of the subjects in the study were Caucasian, which isn't a true representation of the general population. Hispanics and African Americans have a lower prevalence of autoimmune thyroid disease than Caucasians and Asians (Villanueva et al. 2003).

Autoimmune Thyroid Disorders

Most thyroid disorders are autoimmune in nature. Even if initial thyroid hormone imbalances are triggered by lithium or excess iodine, the immune system can go on to launch a response that leads to the development of thyroid antibodies. Thyroid antibodies, depending on their nature, can destroy thyroid tissue, promote inflammation, interfere with thyroid hormone production or stimulate thyroid cells to produce excess thyroid hormone.

The Genetic Component

There are three generally accepted ways to prove the genetic basis of autoimmune disease. The first is family clustering. About 15 percent of patients with Graves' disease have a relative with this disorder, and about 50 percent of relatives of Graves' disease patients have low levels of circulating thyroid autoantibodies, indicating thyroid autoimmunity but not autoimmune thyroid disease (Greenspan 1991, 221). The second is a proven genetic component, and a number of genes have been found to be associated with Graves' disease. The third is that similar autoimmune diseases can be found in the progeny of animals experimentally induced to develop autoimmune thyroid disease.

Genetic Factors in Graves' Disease

In 2002, Dr. Shamael Waheed and colleagues at Bart's and the Royal London Hospital used molecular genetic technology to examine the genes of people with Graves' disease. These researchers found that the genes that control programmed cell death or apoptosis in thyroid cells are switched on in people with Graves' disease. This causes these cells to survive longer and consequently become more vulnerable to attack by the immune system (BBC News 2002).

Another gene, one that controls vitamin D absorption and transport by binding proteins, has also been found to be defective in patients with Graves' disease. This leads to the characteristically low vitamin D levels seen in Graves' disease. Low vitamin D levels in Graves' disease lead to poor absorption of calcium and symptoms of muscle wasting, bone loss, cardiovascular disease, and nervous system disorders.

A polymorphism to the CYP27B1 transporter gene has been demonstrated in a Polish population of Graves' disease patients. Polymorphisms in the CTLA-4 gene and in several genes for other specific cytokines have also been demonstrated in Graves' disease. The high incidence of genetic changes seen in Graves' disease may account for the considerable variability seen in symptoms, signs, disease severity, and the disease course of patients with Graves' disease.

Susceptibility Genes in Graves' Disease

Several autoimmune thyroid disease susceptibility genes have previously been identified: CD40, CTLA-4, thyroglobulin, TSH receptor, and PTPN22. Some of these susceptibility genes are specific to either Graves' disease or Hashimoto thyroiditis, while others confer susceptibility to both conditions. The genetic predisposition to thyroid autoimmunity is thought to interact with environmental factors or events, which are described later in this chapter, to precipitate the onset of Graves' disease (DeGroot, 2010).

Two new susceptibility loci have also been found: the RNASET2-FGFR1OP-CCR6 region at 6q27 and an intergenic region at 4p14. Moreover, strong associations of thyroid-stimulating hormone receptor and major histocompatibility complex class II variants with persistently thyroid stimulating hormone receptor autoantibodies (TRAb)-positive Graves disease have been identified. The major histocompatibility complex is involved in presenting foreign particles to T-cells during the immune response. This is the first step in the development of autoreactive T-cells in autoimmune disease.

In a recent study published in the *Journal of Immunology*, Shanghai researchers have found that a process of polarization, along with the secretion of the cytokine interferon-alpha, impairs T regulatory cell-mediated regulation in lymphoid organs. In other words, polarization and cytokine imbalances interfere with the normal immune response. This, similar to the apoptosis-induced decrease in T regulatory cells, ultimately triggers the activation of autoreactive Th and B cells, which leads to the generation of large amounts of TSH receptor antibodies and the development of Graves' disease (Mao et al. 2011).

In addition, Graves' disease patients have a higher rate of peripheral blood mononuclear cell conversion into CD34+ fibrocytes compared with healthy controls. These fibrocytes may contribute to the pathophysiology of Graves' ophthalmopathy by accumulating in orbital tissues and producing inflammatory cytokines, including TNF-alpha and IL-6 (Yeung 2011).

Genes of the Major Histocompatibility Complex

Molecules that mark a cell as being "self" or part of the body are encoded by a group of genes located on the short arm of chromosome 6 called the major histocompatibility complex (MHC). The immune system normally recognizes "self" antigens (the body's naturally occurring cellular proteins) and tolerates their presence. The prefix "histo" refers to the body's tissues. This system was first discovered when attempts were made to find compatible tissue donors for organ transplants. Researchers discovered that the MHC genes and the molecules they encode vary from one person to another and control the immune response. These genes must be compatible for successful organ transplants or the donor tissue will be rejected.

Human Leukocyte Antigens

In humans, the MHC is called the human leukocyte antigen or HLA system. The genes expressed on the body's cells are HLA antigens. The MHC complex consists of a series of genes that code for proteins expressed on the cell surface of all nucleated cells, particularly lymphocytes. Their principal function is to protect the body from disease by controlling the immune system's response to specific antigens. These genes are located within the HLA region on the short arm of chromosome 6 in man.

Within the MHC complex, there are three subsets known as Class I, Class II, and Class III antigens or genes, which are described in the following two sections. In the immune reaction, certain events are limited to antigens expressed in only one particular subset. Although Class II antigens are generally associated with Graves' disease, other MHC genes, such as those encoding the tumor necrosis factor, also have an association.

Gene Locus and Haplotypes

The MHC loci (positions of genes on chromosome, singular = locus) are closely linked. The complex of linked genes that are inherited as a group on the same chromosome are known as haplotypes. (For instance, the allele B8 and the allele D3 are often inherited as a couple.) Each individual inherits two MHC haplotypes, one from each parent, and has two alleles for each of the loci. Thus there are four possible MHC genes in the offspring of parents ab and cd, known as ac, ad, bc and bd.

LINKAGE DISEQUILIBRIUM

Linkage disequilibrium refers to the tendency for certain alleles at two linked loci to occur together as haplotypes significantly more often than would be expected based on chance (for example, if all the children of ab/cd parents were ac). Haplotypes seen in certain diseases frequently occur more often than expected, especially in certain ethnic groups.

Regulation in the MHC

MHC markers regulate the immune response by determining which specific antigens an individual can respond to as well as the strength of the response. MHC markers also allow immune cells (macrophages, B cells and T cells) to communicate with one another. For instance, in an infection, the invading microorganism infects cells unless it is engulfed by immune cells such as monocytes. Inside the cell that becomes infected, MHC Class I antigens alert T lymphocyte cells to the presence of "self" cells and also cells that have been detrimentally altered by infection or mutation. These molecules alert killer T cells to the presence of damaged or infected cells.

Class II molecules, which are found on B lymphocytes, macrophages and other immune system cells, act as receptors for antigen fragments. Once these fragments have bound to the MHC molecules and have been translocated to the cell surface, the MHC Class II complex alerts the helper T cells. Receptors on T cells interact with the antigen MHC complex, triggering both humoral (antibody producing) and cellular (cell, particularly T cell initiated) immune responses.

Specifically, the Ia (immune response associated) molecules are encoded by the HLA-D region and are called HLA-DR (d related) antigens. The activated B lymphocyte (responsible for antibody production) presents antigens through these HLA-DR molecules to T or B cells.

Class I molecules are coded by three loci of chromosome 6, the HLAA, B and C regions that are expressed on most nucleated cells of the body and also platelets. The central function of Class I molecules is to recognize and oust virally infected or tumor cells. Class II antigens include the Ia molecules (HLA-DR, HLA-DQ, and HLA-DP, DC/MB, SB subregions) and are expressed on macrophages, B lymphocytes and activated T lymphocytes. Class III includes the MHC linked complement components, (C2, C4 and BF), 21-hydroxylase (21-OH), and tumor necrosis factor (TNF).

Antigenic Recognition

Peptide antigens presented by MHC molecules are derived from two distinct sources:

1. Exogenously (originating outside the body) derived antigens, such as bacteria, that are taken into cells and ultimately presented by Class II

MHC molecules to CD4 T helper cells. Here, they capture, process and present antigens for future use in delayed hypersensitivity reactions or the production of antibodies.

2. Endogenous antigens that originate in the internal environment of the cell. Endogenous peptides may include peptides from self-antigens or peptide fragments derived from early viral proteins produced in a virus-infected cells. These peptides are presented primarily by Class I MHC molecules and are recognized by CD8 positive T suppressor cells.

T-Cell Activation

The immune response has two stages. First, the nonspecific effectors, including cytokines, macrophages, natural killer cells, polymorphonuclear leukocytes and complement, attack potential pathogens, such as infectious molecules. The second stage involves T cell activation and antibody production.

The first step in T cell activation occurs when B lymphocytes are stimulated by an antigen causing multiplication of the cell line. Macrophage cells are then activated to produce a soluble product called lymphocyte activating factor (LAF) or interleukin-1 (IL-1), a type of cytokine needed for T cell growth. The elevated levels of IL-6 and IL-8 cytokines seen in hyperthyroid patients are evidence of the ongoing autoimmune process in Graves' disease.

IL-1, produced in the first step, is required for the second step in T cell activation. IL-1 induces a subpopulation of T cells with specific receptors for another soluble factor called T cell growth factor (TCGF) or interleukin-2 (IL-2). Helper T cells are then activated by a complex of antigen plus IL-1 to produce receptors (binding sites) for IL-2.

The binding of IL-2 molecules to the specific receptor sites on T cells induces cell proliferation. Once T cells acquire the receptors for IL-2, they no longer require the presence of antigen for continued proliferation. Thus, once the process has begun and T cell activation is complete (autoreactive T cells are formed), an antigenic response is no longer required for autoantibody production.

Loss of Tolerance in Autoimmunity

Normally, the immune system has self-tolerance, meaning it tolerates its own cells and doesn't react with them. Autoimmunity is related to a loss of self-tolerance. Three basic mechanisms normally prevent autoreactive lymphocytes from developing.

These are (1) clonal deletion or physical elimination, (2) clonal anergy that reduces cell responsiveness, and (3) suppression or destruction of autoreactive lymphocytes by other cytotoxic lymphocytes such as natural killer lymphocytes (NK cells). Cytotoxic cells normally are able to prevent autoimmunity by secreting certain cytokines with negative regulatory effects. This results from cross linking of surface receptors, or by the creation of anti-autoantibodies (anti-idiotypes).

THYROID CELL ANTIGENS

Normally, thyroid epithelial cells do not express Class II antigens. However, Class II antigens are expressed in the thyroid glands of patients with Graves' disease because of the increased number of lymphocytes present in the thyroid gland. According to current theories, a local viral infection or a persistent allergic response could lead to the lymphocytic infiltration of the thyroid gland seen in Graves' disease patients. Consequently, this lymphocytic infiltration can lead to the increased production of interferon or other cytokines within the thyroid gland. The increase in cytokines and lymphocytes, in turn, would induce Class II expression, inducing step 2 of T cell activation. This reaction ultimately leads to the production of TSH receptor antibodies.

HLA Genes Associated with Graves' Disease

HLA-DR3 and HLA-B8 genes have long been linked to the development of Graves' disease. The relative risks (likeliness of developing a disease) are highest for HLA-D and DR alleles because the Class II HLA-DR3 molecule appears to be a stronger link. The association between Graves' disease and HLA-B8 and HLA-DR3 genes is seen in Caucasians as well as South African blacks. Other genes conferring susceptibility include CTLA4, HLA-DRB1, and HLA-DQB1. In addition, some genes offer protection against disease development. HLA-B7 confers protection against developing Graves' disease. HLA genes, while not the direct cause of Graves' disease, are reported to increase risk 5–7 fold (DeGroot 2010). HLA genes show disease susceptibility but they are not used to diagnose specific autoimmune disorders, with the exception of HLA-B27, which is used to help diagnose ankylosing spondylitis.

In addition, Graves' disease is associated with different Class I and II HLA antigens in other ethnic groups, and within different ethnic groups there are sometimes subsets. For instance, the prevalence of HLA-BW46 is increased in Chinese men (but not women) with Graves' disease, and the relative risk for this allele is higher in men with early onset disease (age 10–19) than in men overall. The genetic focus seems to be on antibody production rather than disease production.

SHARED HAPLOTYPES ASSOCIATED WITH AUTOIMMUNE DISEASE

The most striking set of HLA antigens that occur together as a marker for disease is HLA-A1, B8, and DRw3/DR3. The frequency of this set is increased among patients with type 1 diabetes, gluten sensitivity enteropathy, Graves' disease, dermatitis herpetiformis, chronic active hepatitis and several other diseases. For this reason, Graves' disease patients have a higher risk for developing the other autoimmune diseases associated with these markers.

While HLA genes are associated with the development of Graves' disease, they are not considered diagnostic markers. Studies indicate that the percentage of patients with Graves' disease having these genes borders on 50 percent. Clearly, there are other genes involved, particularly those governing the TSH receptor and those influencing immunoglobulin production as well as the immune response.

CTL GENES

Recently, another gene associated with the immune response, the cytotoxic lymphocyte CTLA-4, was found to be related to disease susceptibility in both Graves' disease and Graves' ophthalmopathy, especially in males. Its role appears to be associated with the second signal needed to invoke a progressive immune response provided by one of the adhesion molecules that exist on the antigen presenting cell. One of the most important adhesion molecules is B7. CTLA4 recognizes and interacts with the subset B7.2, giving a negative signal.

Environmental Triggers Associated with Graves' Disease

There is not one specific cause of Graves' disease other than the immune system defect. There is also no evidence that the thyroid gland or its protein antigens are inherently abnormal. The process that leads to disordered immunity involves a variety of factors allowing self-reactivity to occur. Very low levels of self-reactivity are normally present in most everyone. In Graves' disease, self-reactivity is accelerated due to a combination of genetic and environmental factors. There's general agreement that several different factors contribute to an individual's immune dysfunction rather than one trigger. Several triggers have been identified and others have been suspected of contributing to the development of Graves' disease. The major risk factor for Graves' disease is female sex and this is partially due to the modulation of the autoimmune response by estrogen.

Known triggers include cigarette smoke; stress; low selenium levels; infectious agents; exposure to seasonal and food allergens; sex steroids, particularly estrogens; excess dietary iodine; iodine contrast dyes; lithium; amiodarone and other medications with high amounts of iodine; interferon-alpha; interferon-gamma; interleukin-1 alpha; interleukin-2; diethylstilbesterol (DES); and trauma, including excessive palpation of the gland and ethanol injection for the treatment of nodules.

Besides trauma or injuries to the thyroid gland, thyroid cells may also be injured by oxidative stress related to the immune system's response to low antioxidant levels (Rose et al. 2002). In addition, radioiodine ablative treatment causes the production of TSH receptor antibodies and can lead to the development of Graves' disease in patients treated for thyroid cancer and other conditions. Infectious environmental triggers include retroviruses, Epstein-Barr virus (EBV), *Yersinia enterocolitica*, *Borrelia burgdorferi*, *Helicobacter pylori*, and other enteric bacteria. Infectious agents contribute to autoimmunity by mounting an endogenous interferon-alpha response. Flares of EBV are also suspected of contributing to relapses in Graves' disease (Nagata et al. 2011).

Suspected environmental triggers include goserelin acetate, which is a gonadotropin-releasing hormone (GnRH)–agonist; various monoclonal antibodies; oral contraceptives (Prummel et al. 2004), low birth weight, radiation damage to the thyroid gland, amphetamines, the TSH receptor antigen, human parvovirus B19, and aspartame in artificial sweeteners (Roberts 2004).

Aspartame has been reported to trigger Graves' disease and worsen symptoms within several weeks to 6 months after beginning aspartame consumption. Dramatic remissions occurred within several weeks to 3 months of avoiding aspartame. On multiple rechallenges with aspartame, symptoms returned within 2 days (Roberts 2004).

Sex Steroids

Estrogens have been implicated in the development of Graves' disease because this autoimmune disorder occurs more frequently in women and rarely develops before puberty. In instances where Graves' disease emerges before puberty, males and females are at equal risk. The synthetic estrogen diethylstilbesterol (DES) has been shown to cause permanent changes in T lymphocytes and natural killer (NK) cells that contribute to autoimmunity. Endocrine disruptors may trick the body into thinking there is excess thyroid hormone by binding to receptors for thyroid hormone. Endocrine disruptors include a large number of chemicals including PCBs, dioxin and furans, all of which are related to thyroid dysfunction. Dioxin and its metabolites are known to trigger both autoimmune hypothyroidism and Graves' disease.

Furthermore, the normal suppression of T and B cells during pregnancy followed by the sudden flood of estrogen may account for the incidence of postpartum Graves' disease that occurs in 5 percent to 6 percent of women after delivery. Also, estrogen is known to affect antibody formation due to its influence over B cells. In general, circulating autoantibodies and the natural disease course tend to improve in pregnancy and worsen in the postpartum period.

Iodine, Thyroid Hormone, and Autoimmune Disease

Iodine is necessary for the production of thyroid hormone. Thyroid hormone is formed when iodine combines with the amino acid tyrosine. However, the thyroid gland can't distinguish iodine from radioiodine, and it absorbs radioiodine easily. The World Health Organization estimated in 2003 that 740 million people worldwide suffer from iodine deficiency. Iodine deficiency is particularly prevalent in undeveloped countries without access to ocean fish, kelp and sea salt or where foods that block iodine (goitrogens), such as cassava and millet, are excessively consumed.

In contrast, 57 percent of people in the developing world regularly use iodized salt and commonly receive excess amounts of an unnatural form of iodine in iodized salt. In addition, iodized salt contains aluminum, which is added to prevent caking and is recognized as foreign by the immune system. In 1956, the Swiss physician H.C.A. Vogel explained that the introduction of supplemental iodine to iodine-deficient regions has always been accompanied by a rise in the incidence of Graves' disease. The renowned immunologist Noel Rose proposes that the presence of iodine increases the autoantigenic potential of thyroglobulin, a major pathogenic antigen in the induction of autoimmune thyroid disease (Rose et al. 1999).

Iodine deficiency can lead to hypothyroidism and rarely to hyperthyroidism. Iodine excess can also lead to autoimmune hypothyroidism, but it is more likely to cause hyperthyroidism. Areas in which iodine deficiency is endemic have a high incidence of thyroid nodules and toxic multinodular goiter, whereas Graves' disease is rarely seen.

The effects of iodine excess can also be transient, such as those seen in mini-epidemics of Graves' disease caused by meat contaminated with thyroid hormone or from the use of medicines such as amiodarone, which have a high iodine content. Chronic iodine excess or deficiency can, as mentioned, trigger the immune system to produce antibodies that lead to autoimmune thyroid disease (Moore 2001, 50–54).

Stress

In 1825, Parry described a patient who fell down a set of stairs while in a wheelchair shortly before developing symptoms of Graves' disease. In addition, refugees in Nazi prison camps were reported to have a higher incidence of thyrotoxicosis than seen in the general population. A higher incidence of Graves' disease has also been found in the inhabitants of countries engaged in war. The stress associated with trauma, accidents, and neck injuries is also associated with the development of Graves' disease. Besides stressful events, a stressful lifestyle has also recently been implicated in the development and onset of Graves' disease (Ogedegbe 2001). Other specific stressors have also been reported. Aggressive weight loss programs have been reported to induce Graves' disease, and administration of thyroid hormone, sometimes given for induction of weight loss, also has been followed by mini-epidemics of Graves' disease. Many over-the-counter weight loss drugs and metabolic boosters contain thyroid hormone.

Both acute and chronic stress have been demonstrated to depress the immune system perhaps secondary to the cortisol release and disturbances in cytokine levels that accompany stress. Stress-induced immune suppression is presumed to be followed by a compensatory period of immune system hyperactivity. This could precipitate autoimmune thyroid disease, as in postpartum Graves' disease, which occurs within 12 months post-delivery or termination of pregnancy.

Superantigens and Allergens

Superantigens are potent T-cell stimulatory molecules, usually infectious particles, that bind to MHC class II molecules. Particular T cells recognize this complex of antigen particle and MHC molecule, which causes them to become activated and possibly deleted. Superantigens may be extrinsic or intrinsic, although no intrinsic superantigens have yet been detected in man. Extrinsic superantigens include a group of bacterial endotoxins (staphylococcal, streptococcal and mycoplasmal). The bacterium *Yersinia enterocolitica* has been demonstrated to mimic the TSH receptor antibody in patients with Graves' disease due to molecular mimicry between retroviral sequences and the TSH receptor. Recent studies also show an association between Graves' disease and *Helicobacter pylori,* a common cause of gastric ulcers (Bassi et al. 2010).

The idea of an allergic response being a probable Graves' disease trigger was first suggested in a Japanese study that reported elevations of immunoglobulin E (IgE) in the serum of one-third of Graves' disease patients (Sato et al.

1999). Since then, cedar pollen has been identified as the most significant environmental trigger for Graves' disease in Japan. In the United States, recurrences of allergic rhinitis from pollen allergy are associated with relapses and exacerbations of symptoms in Graves' disease patients. IgE is elevated in the allergic response to seasonal irritants and food. In addition, researchers have discovered that patients with high IgE levels are less likely to achieve remission with methimazole even after long-term treatment (Yamada et al. 2000).

Patients with higher levels of IgE have also been found to be less likely to experience a reduction in TSH receptor antibodies after treatment with anti-thyroid drugs when compared to patients without demonstrable levels of IgE. Studies have also shown a more severe disease course in individuals with high levels of IgE. In addition, when the offending allergen is withdrawn, IgE levels and thyroid antibody levels both fall. Researchers have also demonstrated a rise in TSH receptor antibodies, TPO antibodies, eosinophil counts, and pollen-specific IgE activity and relapse/exacerbation of symptoms after attacks of allergic seasonal rhinitis (Takeoka et al. 2003).

Researchers theorize that Th2 lymphocytes are stimulated by allergens and thereby secrete excess amounts of IL-13, which subsequently stimulates B cell lymphocytes to synthesize more TSH receptor antibody and IgE (Yamada et al. 2000). Thus, allergens directly lead to increased production of TSH receptor antibodies as well as immunoglobulin E. Studies of patients with Graves' disease and gluten sensitivity show that a gluten-free diet causes a reduction in both IgE and TSH receptor antibodies.

Another line of research indicating a role for allergies in Graves' disease shows increased serum levels of eosinophil-derived neurotoxin (EDN) in patients with Graves' disease. Eosinophils are white blood cells with granules that pick up the red eosin stain used in making blood smears. Blood smears are part of a complete blood count (used to evaluate red cell morphology and differentiate the number of the different white blood cell subtypes). These granules contain potent neurotoxins, which can cause symptoms when eosinophil levels increase. Eosinophil counts increase in allergic reactions and parasitic infections. Researchers in Osaka, Japan, found high levels of EDN in untreated Graves' disease patients compared to patients with Hashimoto's thyroiditis and individuals with no signs of a thyroid disorder. Levels of EDN also paralleled levels of stimulating TSH receptor antibodies (Hidaka et al. 2003).

The TSH Receptor Autoantigen

A group of international researchers (Chun et al. 2003) has proposed that the molecular structure of the target TSH receptor antigen contributes to the development of stimulating TSH receptor antibodies in Graves' disease. Research shows that TSH receptor antibodies are more likely to bind to the shed A subunits of the TSH receptor rather than to subunits attached to the receptor. Studies of the adenovirus in animals induced to develop hyperthyroidism show that this virus expresses the free A subunit, which amplifies the immune response.

Other Factors That May Contribute to Graves' Disease Development

The immune mechanisms that contribute to disease from environmental agents include: increased cell destruction or apoptosis; thyroid autoantibody production; molecular mimicry; inflammation as white blood cells invade thyroid tissue; the production of cytotoxic (destructive to cells) immune system chemicals known as cytokines, especially interleukins and interferons; the hygiene hypothesis; and heat shock proteins.

Apoptosis

Depending on the tissue they represent, the body's cells survive for specific lengths of time. The programmed cell death for individual cells is known as apoptosis. This process involves a series of programmed events, including loss of the mitochondrial membrane, chromatin condensation, cell shrinkage, and degradation of cellular components. While certain degenerative diseases are associated with an increase in apoptosis, certain cancers are associated with reduced apoptosis. Environmental agents such as ionizing radiation and toxins can induce apoptotic cell death. Certain cytokines can also act as death ligands and promote apoptotic cell death. The expression of Fas ligand in the thyroid tissue of Graves' disease patients suggests that aberrant signaling pathways in apoptosis may contribute to the development of Graves' disease.

Fetal Cell Microchimerism

Intrathyroidal fetal cell microchimerism has long been suspected of contributing to autoimmunity in Graves' disease and in scleroderma. During pregnancy, fetal and maternal cells circulate between mother and fetus. For many years it's been known that fetal cells from male infants can persist in the maternal circulation for up to 20 years. Male fetal origin cells were detected in human thyroids by identifying the male specific region of the SRY region of the Y chromosome, and were detected in 6 of 7 frozen thyroid tissue specimens from patients with Graves' disease, and one of four patients with thyroid nodules. Fetal male cells are possible candidates for modulating auto-immune thyroid disease, since they might either induce an immune response or develop a sort of graft-versus-host immune response to the mother (DeGroot 2010).

Molecular Mimicry

Bacteria that cause food poisoning have long been known to trigger autoimmune arthritis. Researchers found that immune system cells that fight bacteria may also affect those normal cells that happen to carry a protein that resembles a bacterial protein. Other so-called innocent bystander cells, which may have been stressed by radiation, environmental toxins, or the body's own stress chemicals, can also fall victim to molecular mimicry and induce an autoreactive immune response.

Endocrine Disruptors and Thyroid Health

A number of chemicals, including fluoride, can displace iodine molecules and disrupt normal endocrine function. Lithium and the halogens bromide, chloride, and fluoride are known to cause autoimmune thyroid diseases, primarily Hashimoto's thyroiditis, but also Graves' disease.

Endocrine disruptors are chemicals with the ability to react inappropriately with various cell receptors, including thyroid cell receptors. Endocrine disruptors include polychlorinated biphenyls (PCBs) and related compounds such as polybrominated diphenyl ethers (PBDEs), the fungicide ethylenebis-dithiocarbamates (EBDCs), dioxin and perchlorate. Further complicating matters, each of these compounds may have subtypes or congeners that have weaker, stronger or no disruptive endocrine actions. Recent evidence shows a clear association between Agent Orange and the development of Graves' disease. In addition, the EBDC fungicides sprayed on many plants, including root and leafy vegetables and cereal grains, have been known since the 1960s to cause goiter and inhibit iodine uptake. Perchlorate, a persistent contaminant from missile and rocket fuel, is commonly found in drinking water in the southwestern United States. Perchlorate has anti-thyroid drug properties and is a known cause of hypothyroidism as well as a rarely used treatment for hyperthyroidism.

AGENT ORANGE

Vietnam War veterans who report being exposed to Agent Orange have a markedly increased prevalence of Graves' disease, compared to those with no exposure, a new study finds. Lead investigator Ajay Varanasi, M.D., a fellow at the State University of New York, Buffalo, presented results of this research at the American Association of Clinical Endocrinologists (AACE) 19th Annual Meeting on April 27, 2010, in Boston, Massachusetts.

"Environmental factors are believed to contribute to the increased prevalence of some autoimmune diseases," Dr. Varanasi told attendees. "During the Vietnam War, nearly 20 percent of the surface of Vietnam was sprayed with Agent Orange between 1962 and 1971, mainly for deforestation and crop destruction," he further explained, adding that "much of the concern over the widespread use of Agent Orange stems from the dioxin 2,3,7,8-tetrachlordibenzo-p-dioxin, or TCDD, a contaminant in the Agent Orange production process. TCDD is a persistent toxin, lasting in the soil for decades and remaining in the body for many years. TCDD has similar properties to triiodothyronine (T3) and thyroxine (T4)."

Consequently, TCDD can interfere with thyroid function and metabolism, bind to thyroid transport proteins and induce the production of thyroid metabolizing enzymes. Dr. Varanasi and colleagues assessed the prevalence of major thyroid diagnoses in the Veterans Administration (VA) electronic medical record database for upstate New York veterans born between 1925 and 1963. They compared the frequency of diagnoses of thyroid cancer, nodules, hypothyroidism, and Graves' disease in veterans who identified themselves as being exposed to Agent Orange (n = 23,939) or not exposed to Agent Orange (n =200,109).

In both groups, the average age of veterans was approximately 62 years. Nearly all veterans in both groups were male (90 percent) and had a history of smoking (93 percent). Approximately 22 percent of both groups were African American. In the group exposed to Agent Orange, 24 percent had diabetes, whereas in the non-exposed group, nearly 14 percent did (P = .01). The VA acknowledges type 2 diabetes as a presumptive disease associated with exposure to herbicides, including Agent Orange. The researchers found no difference in the rates of thyroid nodules or cancers between the exposed and non-exposed groups. Graves' disease, however, was 3 times more prevalent in the exposed group (odds ratio [OR], 3.05; 95 percent confidence interval [CI], 2.17–4.5; P < .001). Interestingly, hypothyroidism was less common in the exposed group (OR, 0.85; 95 percent CI, 0.79–0.92; P > .001).

When conducting a retrospective review of the literature, investigators found evidence of a possible mechanism by which TCDD exposure leads to Graves' disease. Previous research has shown that TCDD binds tightly to the aryl hydrocarbon receptor (AhR), which plays a role in normal immune pathways. In particular, T helper 17 (Th17) cells express high levels of AhR. TCDD, along with endogenous AhR, has been shown to promote Th17 cell growth. High levels of Th17 cells have previously been linked to autoimmune disorders, including Graves' disease. Most studies on TCDD and thyroid function, however, have provided little and inconsistent evidence of long-term TCDD effects on the human thyroid (Varanaski et al. 2010).

Interferons, Interleukins, and Monoclonal Antibodies

The cytokines interferon and interleukin are released during the immune response, and they are also produced synthetically and used as therapeutic agents. Elevated levels of IL-17, IL-22, and IL-23 are seen in the thyroid gland and blood of patients with Graves' disease.

Numerous studies show that interferons and interleukins used in the treatment of other conditions contribute to the development of Graves' disease and also type 1 diabetes. For instance, onset or worsening of thyroid autoimmunity and thyroid dysfunction have been reported to occur during treatment with interferon-alpha for chronic hepatitis and interferon-beta for multiple sclerosis. Interferon-alpha treatment of patients with chronic hepatitis due to hepatitis C virus is associated with the development of primary hypothyroidism, Graves' hyperthyroidism, and destructive thyroiditis, and is especially prevalent in women (relative risk of 4.4), particularly in women with existing TPO antibodies.

In *Thyroid Manager*, DeGroot describes a group of 34 patients with multiple sclerosis treated with CAMPATH, a humanized monoclonal antibody, in which one-third developed Graves' disease within 6 months. In addition, patients stopping immunosuppressive treatment may have rebound development of Graves' disease. These monoclonal antibody treatments may alter the function of regulatory T cells or deviate the immune system from a TH1 to a TH2 type of response.

Heat Shock Proteins

Heat shock proteins are a class of proteins produced by heat shock and other stressful stimuli, including exposure to oxidative radicals, alcohol, plant lectins, heavy metals (mercury, bismuth, lead, etc.) anoxia and infections. Heat shock proteins are immunogenic, meaning that they induce an immune response. In fact, bacterial infection can cause antibody production and T cell response. These antibodies and T cells can go on to cross-react with self-cellular heat shock proteins leading to autoantibody production. Heat shock protein 72 is expressed in thyroid tissue from patients with Graves' disease but not in normal subjects, which suggests that Graves' disease is associated with an autoimmune response to certain specific heat shock proteins.

Immune Stimulants and Thyroid Health

Exposure to allergens, infectious agents and toxins stimulates the immune system. Over time, with chronic exposure to allergens or toxins, including aspartame and cigarette smoke, or inadequate treatment for allergies, the immune system becomes ineffective and fails to launch a normal immune response. Unable to distinguish clear threats, the immune system targets the body's own tissues and cells, triggering autoimmune thyroid disorders. For instance, because of gluten's similarity to thyroid antigens, ingestion of gluten by individuals with gluten sensitivity can stimulate the development of thyroid antibodies, which in turn triggers autoimmune thyroid disease. In these cases, a gluten-free diet can reduce levels of autoantibodies that contribute to both thyroid disease and gluten sensitivity.

Other Suspected Environmental Triggers

Several reports have related the development of Graves' disease subsequent to starvation, either voluntarily by dieting or in conditions of anorexia or involuntarily in concentration camps. Studies show that women have also reported developing Graves' disease after being on diets with severe calorie restriction or using diet pills, especially amphetamines.

Metals, including cadmium, mercury, beryllium salts, tin, titanium dioxide and silica, are capable of inducing autoimmunity. Formaldehyde, which is used in the medical laboratory to preserve tissue specimens, is associated with autoimmunity because it causes enhanced resistance to bacterial challenge. Formaldehyde is found in cigarette smoke. Both formaldehyde and cigarette smoke are highly associated with autoimmune thyroid disorders. Formaldehyde is also found in auto exhaust, smog, biomedical research, insulation, industrial processes and as a breakdown product of the artificial sweetener aspartame.

Iatrogenic Contributions

Iatrogenic refers to effects caused by medical treatments and diagnostic tests or physicians. Lithium salts, which are used for the treatment of bipolar disorder, are a known trigger for Graves' disease (Brown 2003). Iodine contrast dyes used in imaging tests and the drug amiodarone cause excess accumulations of iodine in fatty tissues that can cause transient episodes of hyperthyroidism lasting several months. Various medications and treatments can adversely affect thyroid function.

Drugs such as interferon and interleukin, used for hepatitis, malignancies, multiple sclerosis and related disorders, are also known to trigger the development of autoimmune thyroid disorders and diabetes. When Graves' disease develops in patients receiving interferon alpha therapy, anti-thyroid drugs are the treatment of choice. While treatment with interferon alpha or interleukin-2 is continued, the thyrotoxic phase can be treated with beta blockers, and if necessary, with nonsteroidal anti-inflammatory drugs (NSAIDs) or corticosteroids (Pearce et al., 2003).

Avoiding Environmental Triggers

When environmental triggers are identified and withdrawn, thyroid antibody levels fall and thyroid conditions improve. In patients with allergic rhinitis and Graves' disease, avoiding pollen and treating the allergic response causes improvement in both disorders. The level of immunoglobulin E (IgE), which is increased in allergic reactions, is higher in patients with severe Graves' disease symptoms than in people with mild or subclinical disorders.

Patients with all forms of autoimmune thyroid disease are known to have low selenium levels. Whether low selenium contributes to the condition or is caused by thyroid dysfunction is uncertain. However, recent studies show that patients with Graves' disease using selenium and the antioxidant vitamins beta carotene and vitamin C along with the anti-thyroid drug methimazole showed a better response than patients using the anti-thyroid drug methimazole alone. Patients improving from or in remission from autoimmune thyroid disease have higher selenium levels compared to their initial levels at the time of diagnosis.

In the United States, stress is considered one of the most important triggers for Graves' disease. Stress causes immune system changes that promote an ineffective or erratic immune response, increase production of inflammatory cytokines and interfere with the body's own mechanisms for preventing autoimmune disease development. While stress cannot always be avoided, an individual's reaction to stress can be mediated with yoga, meditation, a nutrient-rich diet and mild exercise.

Armed with knowledge as to what environmental triggers may be contributing to and worsening their thyroid conditions, patients can incorporate appropriate lifestyle changes into their healing program. Many patients with autoimmune thyroid disease who are troubled by fluctuating thyroid hormone levels, poor responses to replacement hormone and anti-thyroid drugs, or dramatic waxing and waning of symptoms, report major breakthroughs within six weeks after avoiding their suspected environmental triggers.

5

Coexisting Conditions in Graves' Disease and Hyperthyroidism

A number of different disorders tend to coexist in patients with Graves' disease and other hyperthyroid disorders. Most of these associated conditions, for instance rheumatoid arthritis, involve shared autoimmunity and are seen in Graves' disease. Other disorders, such as vitamin B_{12} deficiency and elevated liver enzymes, may be related to autoimmunity as well as to excess thyroid hormone, which can lead to malabsorption and nutrient deficiencies. Chapter 5 provides an overview of the conditions and syndromes associated with hyperthyroidism.

Coexisting Disorders in Autoimmune Thyroid Disease

Individuals with Hashimoto's thyroiditis, Graves' disease and related disorders have a higher risk for developing other autoimmune conditions, especially glandular disorders.

Thyroid diseases are the most common of the autoimmune disorders. Autoimmune thyroid disorders include Hashimoto's thyroiditis, Graves' disease, autoimmune atrophic thyroid failure and Hashitoxicosis.

Prevalence of Coexisting Disorders in Autoimmune Thyroid Disease

Thyroid and other common autoimmune conditions often coexist and tend to cluster in families. To determine the prevalence of these coexisting disorders, researchers in the UK (Yeung 2011) tested 3286 individuals (2791 with Graves' disease and 495 with Hashimoto's thyroiditis). These subjects completed questionnaires detailing their personal and familial history of common autoimmune disorders. The researchers found that 9.7 percent of patients with Graves' disease had a coexisting autoimmune disorder and 14.3 percent of patients with Hashimoto's thyroiditis had a coexisting disorder. Rheumatoid arthritis was the most common coexisting disorder, occurring in 3.15 percent of the Graves' disease patients and 4.24 percent of the patients with Hashimoto's thyroiditis. The relative risk of developing the following autoimmune disorders was also increased in both Graves' disease and Hashimoto's thyroiditis patients: pernicious anemia, systemic lupus erythematosus (SLE), Addison's disease, celiac disease, and vitiligo.

The reported prevalence of autoimmune thyroid disease in patients with SLE is 3.9–24 percent, and the presence of thyroid antibodies in patients with SLE is 11–51 percent (Pyne and Isenberg 2002). The researchers found that the incidence of Hashimoto's thyroiditis in SLE is 5.7 percent whereas the incidence of Graves' disease at 1.7 percent is only slightly higher than that seen in the general population.

Family clustering was seen with increased hyperthyroidism in the parents of individuals with Graves' disease and increased hypothyroidism among the parents of subjects with Hashimoto's thyroiditis. Relative risk of the other common autoimmune diseases was also increased in the parents of the subjects. The researchers concluded that it is important to screen for other autoimmune disorders if individuals with autoimmune thyroid disease present with new or nonspecific symptoms (Yeung 2011).

Coexisting Syndromes

Coexisting conditions may occur in syndromes such as multiple autoimmune syndrome (MAS), Schimdt's syndrome, and autoimmune polyglandular (polyendocrine) syndromes. Here, autoimmune thyroid disorders coexist with several other specific conditions as part of a syndrome. The thyroid disorder may occur before or after the other disorders develop. For instance, patients with Graves' disease may later develop vitiligo and Addison's disease, or they may have these disorders before developing Graves' disease.

Multiple Autoimmune Syndrome

Multiple Autoimmune Syndrome (MAS) refers to three or more coexisting autoimmune conditions. In multiple autoimmune syndrome, patients often have at least one dermatological condition, usually vitiligo or alopecia areata, an autoimmune condition that leads to hair loss. In many cases of multiple autoimmune syndrome reported in the medical literature, vitiligo is the first autoimmune disease to be diagnosed. In these cases, vitiligo is usually bilateral and symmetrical (occurring in the same places on both sides of the body). In most cases of vitiligo that occur in multiple autoimmune syndrome, an autoimmune thyroid disorder is also present.

In many cases, the presence of one autoimmune disorder helps lead to the discovery of other autoimmune conditions. For instance, in an article from the Ocular Immunology and Uveitis Foundation, a patient is reported as having ocular cicatricial pemphigoid disorder in both eyes, a history of hypothyroidisim, and difficulty in swallowing. Although studies of her esophagus were nondiagnostic, additional tests showed the presence of another autoimmune disorder, oral lichen planus. Had the patient not had evidence of autoimmune disorders, her diagnosis and subsequent treatment for lichen planus may have been missed (Tesavibul 2007).

Familial or genetic, infectious, immunologic and psychological factors have all been implicated in the development of multiple autoimmune syndrome. Cytomegalovirus infection, for instance, is shown to cause the development of multiple autoantibodies. Disorders of an autoimmune nature are known to occur with increased frequency in patients previously diagnosed with an autoimmune disease. About 25 percent of patients with autoimmune diseases have a tendency to develop additional autoimmune disorders (Mohan and Ramesh 2003).

MULTIPLE AUTOIMMUNE SYNDROME SUBTYPES

Because of the frequency of certain autoimmune disorders occurring together, MAS is often classified into 3 subtypes that correspond with the prevalence of their being associated with one another. In patients with two autoimmune diseases, this classification is helpful when signs of a third disorder emerge.

1. Type 1 MAS includes myasthenia gravis, thymoma (tumor of the thymus gland), polymyositis (inflammatory muscle disease), and giant cell myocarditis (inflammatory heart muscle disease).
2. Type 2 MAS includes Sjogren's syndrome, rheumatoid arthritis, primary biliary cirrhosis, scleroderma, and autoimmune thyroid disease (Hashimoto's thyroiditis, atrophic thyroiditis, Graves' disease).
3. Type 3 MAS groups together autoimmune thyroid disease, myasthenia gravis and/or thymoma, Sjogren's syndrome, pernicious anemia, idiopathic thrombocytopenic purpura (ITP), Addison's disease, insulin-

dependent diabetes, vitiligo, autoimmune hemolytic anemia (AIHA), systemic lupus erythematosus (SLE), and dermatitis herpetiformis. The immune system markers HLA-B8 and/or DR3 or DR5 seem to be an important factor in type 3 MAS.

Other conditions commonly found in various combinations in MAS are:

- Pemphigus and autoimmune thyroid disease in type 1 MAS;
- Chronic active hepatitis, SLE, pemphigus, bullous pemphigoid, AIHA, ITP, alopecia areata and Addison's disease in type 2 MAS;
- Acquired primary hypogonadism, hypophysitis, rheumatoid arthritis, primary biliary cirrhosis, relapsing polychondritis, multiple sclerosis, chronic active hepatitis, ulcerative colitis, and scleroderma in type 3 MAS.

Pemphigus and Related Bullous Skin Disorders. Bullous skin diseases, such as the autoimmune disorder pemphigus, are characterized by the presence of blisters or erosions of the skin and mucous membranes. In some bullous disorders such as pemphigus vulgaris, blistering is the primary disease manifestation. In other disorders, such as lichen planus, blisters occur infrequently.

Bullous skin diseases may be acquired or induced or they may be autoimmune in origin. In MAS, autoimmune bullous disorders occur. Individuals with autoimmune bullous skin disorders have autoantibodies that target distinct adhesion molecules of the epidermis and dermoepidermal basement membrane zone. These antibodies cause a loss of the targeted protein's adhesive properties, which leads, in turn, to the appearance of blisters and erosions. Like most autoimmune disorders, autoimmune bullous or vesiculobullous skin disorders are more likely to occur in women. Women of childbearing age have the highest risk for developing autoimmune bullous diseases.

The autoimmune bullous disorders include:

- Pemphigus and pemphigoid disorders
- Epidermolysis bullosa acquisita
- Dermatitis herpetiformis
- Herpes (pemphigoid) gestationis
- IGA-mediated disorders

Pemphigus disorders and pemphigoid disorders (bullous pemphigoid, cicatrical pemphigoid) are considered prototypic bullous disorders because of their well-defined autoantibody-mediated development or pathogenesis. The three pemphigus disorders target desmoglein protein, and the pemphigoid disorders target Type XVII collagen and bullous pemphigoid (BP) antigen 2, BP antigen 180, BP antigen 230, and laminin 5. The end result is a loss of the skin's architecture. In the absence of a well-organized viable skin composition, blisters and erosions form craters between the tissues cells.

Pemphigus disorders may present or worsen during pregnancy, especially in the first and second trimesters. Menstruation is reported to trigger or cause relapses of pemphigus. Other suspected risk factors for pemphigus include frequent handling of certain spices, repeated minor thermal burns, and cosmetic procedures. Bullous pemphigoid primarily affects the skin, especially the lower abdomen, groin, and flexor surfaces of the hands and feet. About 10–40 percent of patients have mucous membrane involvement. The common age of onset is 65 to 75 years.

Cicatricial pemphigoid (CP) usually targets people between ages 60–80, although it has been reported in people of all ages, including children. Several subgroups of CP have been described including antiepiligrin CP, pure ocular CP, which affects only the eyes, anti–BP antigen mucosal pemphigoid, and oral pemphigoid.

Autoimmune Polyglandular Syndromes (APS)

Polyglandular or *polyendocrine* are terms referring to multiple endocrine glands. Autoimmune polyglandular or polyendocrine syndromes (APS types 1–4) are diseases involving multiple glands and sometimes other organs. Although these syndromes were reported as long ago as 1908, the term *APS* was originally defined in 1980 by Blizzard, Maclaren and Neufeldt as involving a constellation of different autoimmune disorders, including adrenal insufficiency, Hashimoto's thyroiditis, Graves' disease, type 1 diabetes, and hypoparathyroidism.

The highest risk of APS exists in patients with autoimmune adrenal failure and individuals with a family history of polyglandular failure. Autoimmune adrenal insufficiency is a significant contributor to APS, occurring in APS types 1, 2, and 4.

Type 1 APS. Type 1 APS is commonly referred to as autoimmune polyendocrinopathy-candidiasis-ectodermal dystrophy or APECED. APECED is a rare autosomal recessive illness that classically occurs in children younger than 10 years, showing up first as a chronic condition of mucocutaneous or oral candidiasis and later progressing to hypoparathyroidism and primary adrenal insufficiency.

Type 2 APS, Schmidt's Syndrome. Type 2 APS or APS2, which is characterized by adrenal insufficiency along with one or more additional autoimmune endocrine disorders, was originally known in 1926 as Schmidt's syndrome in honor of the doctor who first described it. Although it may occur at any age, APS2 primarily occurs in middle-aged adults. Women are affected about 3 times as often as men, and the mean age of onset is 36 years. Canines are also known to develop type 2 APS. The most common second disorders include thyroid dysfunction, type 1 diabetes mellitus, autoimmune gonadal failure, and pernicious anemia. In contrast to APECED, only about 20 percent of patients with APS2 who have adrenal antibodies develop adrenal failure. Approximately half of patients with APS2 report a family history of polyglandular failure. Studies show that about half of the patients presenting with autoimmune Addison's disease go on to develop APS2.

Among patients with APS2, patients with initial conditions of diabetes are more likely to develop Addison's disease. Among patients with APS2 who have thyroid disorders, patients with Graves' disease usually develop thyroid disease before adrenal disease and patients with Hashimoto's thyroiditis usually develop Addison's disease before developing hypothyroidism.

Overall, in APS2 less than 1 percent of patients who initially present with autoimmune thyroid disease or type 1 diabetes go on to develop Addison's disease. However, patients with diabetes who begin to experience unstable or poorly controlled glucose levels should be tested for both adrenal and thyroid antibodies.

Patients with APS2 often develop other autoimmune conditions, although these disorders are less likely to occur in APS2 compared to APS1. These disorders include vitiligo, myasthenia gravis, thrombocytopenic purpura, Sjogren's syndrome, rheumatoid arthritis, alopecia, hypergonadotropic hypogonadism, pernicious anemia, atrophic gastritis, hypophysitis, and primary antiphospholipid syndrome. In some cases, development of one of these other conditions is the first indication that the patient may also have APS.

Type 2 APS tends to run in families. Among immediate family members it's not unusual to find more than one person who is affected. The HLA D3, HLA D4 and HLA A1 haplotypes are suspected of causing a genetic predisposition to this disorder.

Treatment for APS2 consists of individualized, lifelong hormone replacement therapy for the affected organs and routine monitoring of other endocrine organs since they can also become affected. Significant problems can occur if patients with a family history of APS who have one autoimmune endocrine disorder aren't tested for other endocrine disorders.

Because thyroxine replacement hormone used in hypothyroidism increases metabolism and the body's needs for cortisol, treating hypothyroidism can worsen an undiagnosed condition of adrenal insufficiency in both humans and canines. A case of Addisonian crisis precipitated by thyroxine therapy has been reported in a patient whose adrenal insufficiency had not yet been diagnosed (Graves et al. 2003).

People with type 2 APS may also develop myasthenia gravis, pure red cell aplasia, pernicious anemia, seronegative arthritis, primary biliary cirrhosis, alopecia, sarcoidosis, or immunoglobulin A deficiency (which is common in people with celiac disease). Type 2 APS can also be associated with interstitial myositis, an inflammatory muscle disorder or myopathy.

Type 3 APS. APS type 3 occurs when patients with autoimmune thyroid diseases, including Hashimoto's thyroiditis, Graves' disease, idiopathic myxedema and euthyroid Graves' disease, develop a second autoimmune condition, excluding autoimmune adrenal and parathyroid disorders. The second condition in APS3 is usually type 1 diabetes, atrophic gastritis, pernicious anemia, vitiligo, alopecia, or myasthenia gravis. Patients with APS3 may later progress to APS2 if they develop an autoimmune adrenal or parathyroid condition.

Type 4 APS. APS type 4 occurs when patients develop two or more autoimmune endocrine conditions that cannot be classified as APS types 1, 2, or 3. An example would be a patient with diabetes who develops an autoimmune growth hormone deficiency or a patient with adrenal insufficiency who develops celiac disease.

Theories regarding the development of APS include: shared autoantigens by multiple endocrine organs, an environmental agent targeting various endocrine antigens, and genetic mutations. Because there are no spontaneous animal models for APS, there is no definitive theory to explain their occurrence.

Adrenal Insufficiency and Addison's Disease

Adrenal insufficiency is a condition that occurs when the adrenal glands produce inadequate amounts of the adrenal hormones cortisol, and, sometimes, aldosterone. This condition can occur as a primary or secondary disorder, and it can have congenital or acquired origins. Primary conditions, such as Addison's disease, occur in fewer than 1 per 100,000 persons. Secondary conditions of adrenal insufficiency are more common and usually related to the use of corticosteroids. Adrenal insufficiency ranges from a subclinical or mild condition to an extreme, sometimes fatal, form, which is known as an Addisonian crisis. Most primary adrenal insufficiency is autoimmune in nature and caused by Addison's disease or as the result of infection.

Autoimmune disease accounts for about 80 percent of all cases of primary adrenal insufficiency. Most other cases result from infection (with tuberculosis, cytomegalovirus, the HIV virus, fungi, and other infectious agents), or as a complication of various metabolic and genetic disorders such as adrenal hyperplasia and adrenoleukodystrophy, or as a sequelae to certain metastatic cancers. Also, in some bleeding disorders, such as antiphospholipid syndrome or in trauma, adrenal insufficiency may result from thrombosis or hemorrhage.

Addison's disease is a condition of primary adrenal insufficiency that affects all age groups. This disease is named after the London physician Thomas Addison who first described patients affected by this disorder in 1855. At the time, the typical Addison's disease patient had adrenal insufficiency caused by infection with *Mycobacterium tuberculosis,* an organism that causes tuberculosis (TB). With the introduction of effective treatments for TB, it is now only a rare cause of Addison's disease. Today, the primary cause of Addison's disease is autoimmune destruction of the adrenal glands. Nearly 80 percent of all cases are caused by adrenal cortex autoantibodies that destroy the adrenal cortex, the adrenal gland's outer layer. The adrenal cortex produces about 50 different steroid hormones. The two most important and biologically active of these hormones are cortisol and aldosterone. In classical Addison's disease, the adrenal gland fails to produce adequate amounts of both cortisol and aldosterone.

Symptoms of adrenal insufficiency include muscle weakness, apathy, fatigue, appetite loss, weight loss, nausea, vomiting, diarrhea, abdominal pain, low blood pressure (hypotension) that worsens when standing (orthostatic hypotension), hyperpigmentation or bronzing of skin (melasma suprenale), diminished ability to conserve sodium and excrete water, depression, irritability, salt craving, low blood sugar (hypoglycemia), tetany (condition of muscle spasm caused by high phosphorus levels), diminished attention span, and numbness of the extremities due to excess potassium (hyperkalemia).

Because most androgens in the female are produced in the adrenal cortex, females with Addison's disease may have decreased genital and underarm hair. Similar to other endocrine deficiencies, most people have a few predominant symptoms and do not develop all associated symptoms.

Coexisting Disorders in Graves' Disease

Coexisting autoimmune disorders are found in 9.7 percent of patients with Graves' disease, with rheumatoid arthritis being the most frequent finding (Yeung 2011, Boelart 2010), followed by pernicious anemia and atrophic autoimmune gastritis, conditions associated with vitamin B_{12} deficiency.

Autoimmune Vitamin B_{12} Deficiency

Vitamin B_{12}, which is the common name for cobalamin, is an essential vitamin obtained from dietary sources. Vitamin B_{12} deficiency is present in 1 to 3 percent of the population, although the incidence of vitamin B_{12} deficiency rises dramatically with age. Among people older than 60 years, the incidence of cobalamin deficiency is as high as 10 to 30 percent. Cobalamin deficiency is caused by diets low in vitamin B_{12}, malabsorption syndromes, infection, and the autoimmune disorders autoimmune gastritis and pernicious anemia. Malabsorption syndromes are common in hyperthyroidism, and chronic conditions of hyperthyroidism frequently lead to deficiencies of vitamin B_{12} and other nutrients.

SYMPTOMS AND SIGNS OF VITAMIN B_{12} DEFICIENCY

A number of unrelated symptoms can occur in vitamin B_{12} deficiency. Clinical manifestations of vitamin B_{12} deficiency include:

- Hematological changes, such as megaloblastic anemia (characterized by large red blood cells), and a low production of other blood cell types, which is known as pancytopenia. Types of pancytopenia seen in vitamin B_{12} deficiency include leucopenia (low white blood cell levels), thrombocytopenia (low platelet count), and anemia.
- Neurologic changes, including paresthesias, peripheral neuropathy and combined systems disease such as demyelination (loss of protective outer sheath) of the dorsal columns of the nerve cells in the spine.
- Psychiatric changes, including irritability, personality change, mild memory impairment, dementia, depression, and psychosis.
- Cardiovascular symptoms, including a possible increased risk of heart attack and stroke.

During its absorption in the body, vitamin B_{12} binds to the protein haptocorin, found in saliva. In the duodenum, vitamin B_{12} is released from haptocorin. The free cobalamin molecules are then linked to a substance known as intrinsic factor in the proximal ileum of the intestines. In this form vitamin B_{12} enters the mucosal cells that line the intestines. Here, cobalamin is released. In its free form it binds to the protein transcobalamin, and in this form vitamin B_{12} is released into the blood circulation. Within the body's cells vitamin B_{12} is freed from transcobalamin protein and it acts as a coenzyme for the synthesis of various enzymes needed for DNA synthesis and energy production.

Pernicious Anemia

Pernicious anemia is an autoimmune disorder characterized by atrophy of the gastric mucosa, selective loss of parietal and chief cells from the gastric mucosa, and an infiltration of lymphocytes into the submucosa. Immunologically, pernicious anemia is characterized by autoantibodies to gastric parietal cells (AGPA), proton pump (H+K+ATPase), and to the cobalamin-absorbing protein intrinsic factor. Intrinsic factor is a 60 kD glycoprotein produced by the parietal cells of the stomach lining that enables the absorption of vitamin B_{12}. Two types of intrinsic factor antibodies can occur. Type I antibodies block the binding of vitamin B_{12} to intrinsic factor, thereby preventing the uptake of vitamin B_{12}. Type II intrinsic factor antibodies bind to intrinsic factor and prevent the attachment of intrinsic factor–cobalamin complex to receptors in the ileum. Both types of antibodies prevent absorption of cobalamin.

Autoimmune Gastritis

Autoimmune gastritis is also called type 1 chronic gastritis. Type 2 chronic gastritis is a similar disease caused by *Helicobacter pylori* infection. Patients with chronic *H. pylori* infection, which is a suspected trigger for Graves' disease, can go on to develop autoimmune gastritis. In autoimmune gastritis, the mucosal cells of the intestines are destroyed by autoantibodies to gastric parietal cells. Unlike pernicious anemia, autoantibodies to intrinsic factor are not present in autoimmune gastritis. However, chronic autoimmune gastritis may progress to pernicious anemia. This process may take 20 to 30 years, which suggests that autoimmune gastritis is an early phase of pernicious anemia.

In one study of patients diagnosed with autoimmune thyroid disease, about one-third of subjects were found to have atrophic body gastritis (atrophic gastritis). In addition, the presence of anemia in subjects was considered suggestive of undiagnosed gastritis (Centanni et al. 1999).

AGPA antibodies occur in about 90 percent of patents with pernicious anemia and 30 percent of first-degree relatives of patents with pernicious anemia, and they are also seen in up to 50 percent of adults and 18 percent of children with *H. pylori* infection (Kumar 2007). In addition, AGPA antibodies are seen in patients with various autoimmune endocrinopathies, including autoimmune thyroid disease, and as many as 2–8 percent of normal elderly subjects may also have AGPA antibodies. The incidence of atrophic gastritis increases with age.

A recent study from Spain shows a relationship between thyroid antibodies and autoimmune gastric disorders, with patients having the highest levels of thyroglobulin and thyroid peroxidase antibodies having the highest levels of parietal cell antibodies (PCA). PCA are seen in atrophic gastritis and pernicious anemia. The predictive value for patients with autoimmune thyroid disorders to have PCA was 20.3 percent (Garcia et al. 2010).

Hyperthyroidism and the Liver

Thyroid hormone regulates the basal metabolic rate of all cells, including hepatocytes (liver cells). In doing so, thyroid hormone affects the liver's basic function. The liver, in turn, metabolizes thyroid hormones and regulates their effects. Consequently, abnormalities in thyroid hormone levels may disturb liver function; liver disease affects thyroid hormone metabolism; and a number of systemic diseases affect both the liver and thyroid gland.

The liver produces several plasma proteins that are used to transport thyroid hormone through the body. Thyroid hormones are more than 99 percent bound to these proteins, including thyroid binding globulin, thyroxine-binding prealbumin, and albumin (Malik and Hodgson 2002). While levels of inactive thyroid hormone bound to these proteins are normally constant, levels of free hormone vary according to the transport and enzyme activity within specific tissues. Consequently, thyroid status depends on thyroxine secretion as well as the normal thyroid hormone delivery of T3 to nuclear receptors.

Liver injury caused by thyrotoxicosis is common. Increases in the liver enzymes aspartate aminotransferase (AST) and alanine aminotransferase (ALT) are seen in 27 percent and 37 percent of patients respectively, and alkaline phosphatase is elevated in 64 percent of patients (Malik and Hodgson 2002). Both liver cells and bile ducts can sustain injury in thyrotoxicosis. Jaundice is rare, although when it occurs, complications of thyrotoxicosis (cardiac failure and sepsis) or intrinsic liver disease need to be evaluated.

Autoimmune Thyroid Disease and Autoimmune Hepatitis

Autoimmune hepatitis (AIH) is, like other types of hepatitis, a disorder of liver cell inflammation. Overall, symptoms and signs of hepatitis include fatigue, enlarged liver, enlarged spleen, jaundice (a yellowing of the skin and eyes), low platelet count, fever, malaise, joint pain, nausea and vomiting. In addition, patients with AIH may have acne, puffy facial features, hirsutism (increased facial hair), obesity, pigmented abdominal striae or stretch marks, and absent or decreased menstrual periods.

In one study, German researchers studied the prevalence of other autoimmune disorders in patients with autoimmune hepatitis (Teufel et al. 2010). Autoimmune hepatitis had long been associated with the autoimmune liver disorders primary biliary cirrhosis (PBC) and primary sclerosing cholangitis (PSC), but the association with other autoimmune diseases hadn't been investigated. The results of the German study showed that 40 percent of patients with autoimmune hepatitis had other autoimmune diseases. After PBC and PSC, autoimmune thyroid disorders represented the most common autoimmune disorder to coexist with autoimmune hepatitis, occurring in 10 percent of all cases.

Gluten Sensitivity

Individuals with autoimmune thyroid disorders have an increased risk for developing gluten sensitivity enteropathy and celiac disease. Thyroid antibodies also parallel gliadin and other antibodies seen in gluten sensitivity. Individuals with both autoimmune thyroid disease and gluten sensitivity who follow a gluten-free diet for three months experience declines in both thyroid and gliadin autoantibodies.

Hyperthyroidism and Rheumatological Disorders

Arthritic symptoms frequently occur in patients with thyroid disorders, and thyroid antibodies often occur in systemic arthritic disorders. Several reasons have been proposed. Because symptoms of arthritis are common in autoimmune hypothyroidism, joint pain has long been listed as a symptom of hypothyroidism. Some researchers are questioning whether hypothyroidism is responsible for arthritic symptoms and suspect that these symptoms may be caused by other coexisting autoimmune rheumatological conditions. Another theory is that thyroid autoantibodies are responsible for rheumatologic symptoms. This is supported by the fact that antibodies to thyroid hormone are commonly seen in autoimmune rheumatological disorders.

Rheumatic Symptoms

Patients with autoimmune thyroid disorders, more often Hashimoto's thyroiditis but also Graves' disease, often have rheumatic manifestations including a mild non-erosive variety of arthritis, polyarthralgia (multiple joints affected), myalgia (muscle pain), and sicca syndrome without a true Sjogren's syndrome. In studies of children with juvenile idiopathic arthritis, thyroid disease was not found to be more common than in children without juvenile arthritis (Unsal et al. 2008).

Thyroid Autoantibodies and Antinuclear Antibodies (ANA)

Besides TSH receptor antibodies and antibodies to thyroglobulin and thyroid peroxidase, patients with autoimmune thyroid disorders may also rarely have antibodies to TSH, T4, and/or T3. These antibodies are suspected, and subsequently tested for, when laboratory results are erratic and do not correlate with symptoms or other thyroid function tests. For instance, patients with T4 antibodies will have elevated FT4 levels with normal TSH levels and no symptoms of hyperthyroidism.

Symptoms in organ-specific autoimmune diseases can overlap. For instance, overlapping autoimmune liver diseases, such as autoimmune hepatitis and primary biliary cirrhosis, can coexist. Similarly, systemic lupus can overlap with other undifferentiated connective tissue disorders. In addition, there are overlapping thyroid and rheumatological disorders that may elude a definitive diagnosis. It's suspected that patients with joint pain that occurs when thyroid hormone levels are low may be expressing latent conditions of rheumatoid arthritis or undifferentiated connective tissue disease. This theory would explain why not all patients with hypothyroidism exhibit joint pain. This theory also explains why joint pain can occur in patients with thyroid antibodies who are euthyroid.

Autoimmune Clotting Disorders

A number of disorders that affect blood clotting and renal function are associated with Graves' disease.

Antiphospholipid Syndrome (APS)

Antiphospholipid syndrome (APS) refers to a number of different phenomena including arterial and venous thrombosis (blood clotting), thrombocytopenia (decreased platelet counts), and obstetric complications such as recurrent spontaneous abortion (miscarriage). Antiphospholipid syndrome is caused by autoantibodies directed against specific proteins involved in blood coagulation, the process in which blood forms a clot. Clots are essential to staunch bleeding from wounds. However, within the body, clots can cause a number of clinical conditions, including strokes (cerebral thrombosis) and pulmonary embolisms (clots within the lungs).

The autoantibodies that cause APS, antiphospholipid antibodies, anticardiolipin antibodies, and antiprothrombin antibodies, often occur in patients with Graves' disease and are common causes of miscarriages, strokes and other thrombotic (caused by blood clots) events.

There are two types of antiphospholipid syndrome: a primary syndrome, which occurs in the absence of any other underlying disease; and a secondary syndrome, which is related to systemic lupus erythematosus (SLE), other autoimmune or neoplastic diseases, or other pathological conditions. Recent studies show that high concentrations of anticardiolipin, antiphospholipid, and antiprothrombin antibodies are also associated with recurrent miscarriages, especially at 8–12 weeks gestation. Antiprothrombin antibodies appear to have two subtypes, one which interferes with blood clotting and one which does not.

LUPUS ANTICOAGULANT

Because antiphospholipid and antiprothrombin antibodies often occur in patients with SLE, these antibodies are often referred to as lupus antico-agulant whether the patient with these antibodies has SLE or not. *Lupus anti-coagulant* was originally used as a term to describe the abnormal blood clotting often seen in approximately 30 percent of patients with systemic lupus. When doctors order blood tests for lupus anticoagulant, they are looking for the presence of antibodies that can cause hyper-coagulation syndromes rather than lupus disorders.

ANTIPHOSPHOLIPID ANTIBODIES

Antiphospholipid antibody is a term used to describe several different antiphospholipid and anticardiolipin antibodies directed against specific proteins necessary for blood clotting. Although the term *antiphospholipid antibodies* also includes antibodies to beta2-glycoprotein, prothrombin, kininogens, annexin V, protein C and protein S, these antibodies do not target phospholipids. Rather they are directed at proteins with an affinity for anionic phospholipid surfaces. Most tests for antiphospholipid antibodies do not detect prothrombin antibodies. Specific tests for prothrombin antibodies must also be ordered.

Approximately 30 percent of patients with antiphospholipid antibodies are reported to have thrombotic (involving abnormal blood clotting) events (Sabatini et al. 2007). These events primarily include deep vein thrombosis of the legs and pulmonary embolism, which represent two-thirds of all events. The other thrombotic events include cerebral arterial thrombosis, spontaneous miscarriages, fetal deaths, or fetal growth retardations.

OBSTETRICAL COMPLICATIONS

Women with antiphospholipid antibodies are especially prone to second or early third trimester fetal deaths. Lack of oxygen secondary to spiral arterial blood clots is considered to be the primary cause. Low platelet counts resulting from antiphospholipid antibodies can also result in bleeding complications during delivery. When evaluating women with recurrent miscarriage, it's impor-tant to test for both antiphospholipid and antiprothrombin antibodies.

RENAL AND OTHER COMPLICATIONS

A small number of patients with antiphospholipid syndrome develop an associated kidney disease or nephropathy caused by clots in the blood vessels that serve the kidneys. It is estimated that about 1 percent of patients with APS are diagnosed with renal complications, although the true incidence of renal complications is suspected of being higher (Fakhouri et al. 2003).

Renal complications most often occur within the first five years of the diagnosis of antiphospholipid syndrome. The renal changes in APS may also be associated with abnormalities of the central nervous system, heart, and skin, related to arterial and arteriolar thromboses (blood clots). Blood clots impair blood circulation to organs and interfere with proper organ function.

Kidney Problems in Antiphospholipid Syndrome

Kidney problems known to occur in antiphospholipid syndrome include:

- APS-associated nephropathy
- Glomerulonephritis
- Lupus neprhitis and lupus nephritis rheumatism
- Arterial hypertension
- Diffuse interstitial kidney sclerosis
- Pauci-immune vasculitis

APS-ASSOCIATED NEPHROPATHY

In APS-associated nephropathy, which is the most common extra-renal complication, thrombotic (characterized by blood clots) vascular involvement of the large and intrarenal small-sized vessels of the kidneys occurs. Symptoms vary in severity.

APS-associated nephropathy can occur as a subacute or chronic condition characterized by proteinuria (excess urine protein) and hematuria (blood in urine) with mild kidney involvement. In extreme cases, APS-associated nephropathy can progress to acute renal failure. One of the earliest markers of APS-associated nephropathy is the inhibition of glomerular filtration. This causes a reduced creatinine clearance and early elevations of the blood urea nitrogen (BUN) and creatinine levels.

When the skin, heart and central nervous system are affected, APS-associated nephropathy can result in generalized ischemic (lack of oxygen) damage to the organs. This condition, which is known as a vaso-occlusive process, may involve multiple organs. Over time, these changes can lead to progressive destruction of the kidney with focal atrophy of the kidney's cortex.

VIRAL CONNECTION

In patients with coexisting conditions of APS, systemic lupus erythe-matosus, and lupus nephritis, viral triggers have been implicated. Cytomegalo-virus (CMV) is associated with arterial damage and the development of Raynaud's phenomena, whereas infection with human parvovirus B19 has been associated with hematological changes such as severe anemia, low white blood cells (leukopenia) and platelet deficiencies (thrombocytopenia). No significant association has been made with the Epstein-Barr virus (EBV) (Kakhouri et al. 2003).

Other symptoms that often accompany APS include autoimmune hemolytic anemia, livedo reticularis, skin necrosis, dementia or neuropsychi-atric events, and a severe bleeding condition referred to as catastrophic antiphospholipid syndrome.

DIAGNOSING APS

Diagnosing antiphospholipid syndrome involves a series of different tests that detect abnormalities in blood clotting.

Tests for APS include:

- Anticardiolipin antibodies
- Antiphospholipid antibodies
- IgG and IgM antiprothrombin antibodies
- Protein C functional activity
- Protein S functional activity

Other tests that screen for other hypercoagulation syndromes include:

- DVVT test
- Factor V Leiden mutation
- MTHR mutation
- APC test

TREATMENT

Treatment for APS, when indicated, includes anticoagulant therapies such as aspirin, warfarin or heparin and corticosteroids if antiprothrombin or platelet antibodies are present.

Platelet Antibodies and Autoimmune (Idiopathic) Thrombocytopenic Purpura (ITP)

Platelets are blood components, distinct from red and white cells, which are critical for the normal clotting mechanism, particularly after vascular injury. Patients with insufficient platelets bruise easily. Slight pressure may cause tiny bruises known as petechiae. In addition, patients deficient in platelets may bleed profusely from minor injuries, especially those involving the nasal or oral areas. One of the most common causes of a low platelet count is platelet destruction by platelet antibodies. Platelet antibodies can occur in patients with Graves' disease.

Platelet antibodies are diagnosed with tests designed to detect antibodies to platelet glycoproteins as well as antibodies to HLA class I antigens (HLA-A-B). Although HLA class I antibodies do not cause thrombocytopenia, they're associated with refractoriness to platelet transfusions, a treatment used to quickly restore platelet counts.

THROMBOCYTOPENIC PURPURA

Autoimmune thrombocytopenic purpura is a disorder characterized by thrombocytopenia (reduced platelet counts) and clotting disorders. Since many drugs such as heparin and other conditions can cause thrombocytopenia, other causes are usually ruled out before the patient is tested for antiplatelet antibodies and a diagnosis of idiopathic thyrobocytopenic purpura (ITP) is made.

Coexistence with Other Glandular Disorders

Individuals with hyperthyroidism can have two disorders that contribute to their hyperthyroidism. For instance, individuals with Graves' disease can have existing conditions of thyroid nodular disease or thyroiditis.

Klinefelter's Syndrome

Klinefelter's syndrome, a form of primary hypogonadism and infertility in males, has been reported in males with Graves' disease (Jong-Suk Park et al. 2004). Klinefelter's syndrome is caused by a structural sex chromosome abnormality that results in reduced testosterone levels. According to Jong-Suk Park, individuals with Klinefelter's disease have a higher risk for systemic lupus erythematosis, rheumatoid arthritis, Sjogren's syndrome and autoimmune thyroid disorders.

Turner's Syndrome

While ovarian dysfunction has often been reported in patients with autoimmune thyroid disorders, only rarely has Turner's syndrome, a form of ovarian dysgenesis, been reported in patients with Graves' disease (Hirano 1981). Turner's syndrome is also characterized by short stature, low-set ears, webbed neck, and occasional cognitive defects.

Miscellaneous Coexisting Conditions

A number of nonglandular conditions are also seen in patients with hyperthyroidism.

Aplastic Anemia

Aplastic anemia is a clinical syndrome that results from a marked reduction in the bone marrow's production of cells. The syndrome includes deficiencies in reticulocytes and red blood cells, granulocytes, monocytes and platelets.

Italian researchers described a child with Graves' disease who later developed aplastic anemia, which was presumed to be caused by the same autoimmune process rather than by any medications. The child achieved complete remission from both Graves' disease and aplastic anemia with the use of antithyroid drugs (Das et al. 2007).

Calcification of Costal Cartilage

The costal (chest cavity) cartilage can become calcified, resulting in a condition of costochondritis, including chondral enlargement or destruction, soft tissue swelling and localized calcification. Radiologists note that there appears to be an association between heavy premature costal cartilage calcification and certain systemic conditions, such as malignancy, autoimmune disorders, chronic renal failure, and thyroid disease, particularly Graves' disease (Ontell et al. 1997).

Thyrotoxic Autoimmune Encephalopathy

A form of Hashimoto's encephalopathy, thyrotoxic autoimmune encephalopathy has been found to occur in patients with Graves' disease (Seo et al. 2003). Thyroid autoantibodies and cerebral inflammation, rather than high thyroid hormone levels, are responsible for this disorder, which responds to corticosteroids but not to anti-thyroid drugs. Untreated, encephalopathy can cause cognitive dysfunction, including dementia.

Coexisting Malignancies

Individuals with hyperthyroidism and also euthyroid Graves' disease can have autonomously functioning thyroid carcinomas (Michigishi et al. 1992). At one time, thyroid cancer in patients with thyrotoxicosis was considered to be extremely rare, but researchers have discovered this perception is incorrect. Several studies have demonstrated both an increased incidence of nodules and of thyroid cancer in patients with Graves' disease, with cancer rates varying from as low as 1 percent to as high as 9 percent of cases (Stocker and Burch 2003). Stocker and Burch explain that TSH receptor antibodies, like TSH, stimulate thyroid cell growth, including thyroid cancer cell growth. The close relationship of TSH to the stimulating TSH-R antibodies seen in Graves' disease has led to the perception that thyroid cancer occurring in the setting of Graves' disease may become more aggressive as a result of stimulation by these autoantibodies. However, as they expain, there is not universal agreement that thyroid cancer is more aggressive in patients with Graves' disease.

Maltoma (mucosa-associate lymphoid tissue lymphoma) of the thyroid gland has also been identified in patients with Graves' disease (Djrolo et al. 2000, Doi et al. 2004). In his study, Doi recommended that that an enlarged thyroid in cases of Graves' disease should be examined carefully for primary thyroid lymphoma.

A higher incidence of thyroid disease has been reported in patients with infiltrating ductal carcinoma of the breast compared to age-matched controls (Giani et al. 1996). Malignant struma ovarii has also been reported to occur in a patient with Graves' disease, with struma ovarii contributing to hyperthyroidism (Kano et al. 2000). Researchers in Copenhagen reported finding coexisting Graves' disease, sarcoidosis, sarcoid granuloma, and papillary carcinoma (Zimmermann-Belsing et al. 2000).

6

Diagnosing Hyperthyroidism
and Graves' Disease

Chapter 6 describes the blood, tissue, and imaging tests that are used to diagnose hyperthyroidism and determine its specific cause. In addition, this chapter describes the use of the pituitary hormone thyrotropin (thyroid stimulating hormone, TSH) test for evaluating thyroid function by explaining how the thyroid gland works together with the hypothalamus and pituitary gland to regulate thyroid hormone levels.

The explanation of thyroid hormone regulation by the hypothalamic-pituitary-thyroid axis leads to a discussion of individual thyroid hormones, the pituitary hormone thyrotropin, which is also known as thyroid stimulating hormone (TSH), and the recommended use of thyroid function tests. This chapter also includes a description of the thyroid and other autoantibodies seen in Graves' disease.

Clinical Picture in Hyperthyroidism

In a routine physical exam, certain abnormal results detected in a chemistry profile may suggest thyrotoxicosis. These abnormalities include decreased cholesterol, high concentrations of alkaline phosphatase (a bone and liver enzyme) and increased calcium. Symptoms and signs such as weight loss or nervousness described in earlier chapters may also suggest the presence of hyperthyroidism. When hyperthyroidism is suspected, the first blood test used as a screening tool is the pituitary hormone thyrotropin (thyroid stimulating hormone, TSH), which is described in the next section.

106

The Thyroid-Pituitary-Hypothalamic Axis

The hypothalamus, at the base of the skull, is considered the true master gland since it controls the other endocrine glands, including the pituitary gland. The hypothalamus monitors all of the body's hormone levels. When slight deviations from normal occur, the hypothalamus engages other organs to correct matters.

Normally, the pituitary gland secretes TSH in small pulses throughout the day, secreting more or less TSH as necessary to provide stable thyroid hormone levels. TSH causes follicular thyroid cells to grow and produce thyroid hormone. Without adequate TSH (due to a pituitary or hypothalamic malfunction as is seen in central hypothyroidism) the thyroid gland normally is unable to produce adequate thyroid hormone.

What Drives TSH Production?

The hypothalamus in the brain monitors our thyroid hormone levels and orders the pituitary to produce more or less thyroid hormone in an effort to ensure we always have an adequate supply of thyroid hormone. The hypothalamus accomplishes this by secreting a hormone known as thyrotropin-releasing hormone or TRH. TRH directs the pituitary gland to secrete TSH. When the hypothalamus notes a rise in thyroid hormone levels, it secretes less TRH, causing the pituitary to secrete less TSH. When the hypothalamus sees that thyroid hormone levels are falling, it releases more TRH, which raises TSH levels and, in turn, thyroid hormone levels.

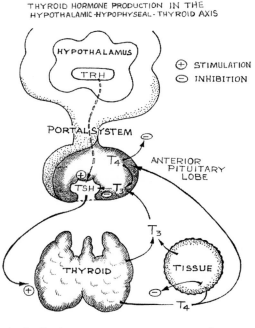

The Axis Has Its Limits

In thyroid disease, the axis normally corrects thyroid hormone levels unless the immune system takes control. For instance, in Graves' disease,

The feedback axis (courtesy Marvin G. Miller).

stimulating TSH receptor antibodies (also called thyroid-stimulating immunoglobulins or TSI) stimulate the thyroid receptor to produce more thyroid hormone. Acting in place of TSH, TSI antibodies order thyroid hormone production even when TSH falls to undetectable levels. In Graves' disease, thyroid function falls under immune system control rather than hypothalamic regulation and the regulatory axis is no longer intact.

In both hyperthyroidism and hypothyroidism, external factors disrupt the normal thyroid axis, and TSH remains abnormally low or high respectively. In hypothyroidism, damaged or defective thyroid cells are unable to produce adequate thyroid hormone. Even with a steadily rising TSH, thyroid hormone levels remain lower than the reference range. The pituitary gland regulates thyroid hormone levels by secreting more or less TSH. Consequently, low levels of TSH are seen in hyperthyroidism and high levels are seen in hypothyroidism. Usually, blood levels of TSH can be used to diagnose abnormal thyroid function.

Benefits of TSH Testing

As soon as the pituitary gland is alerted that thyroid hormone levels are changing, it adjusts secretion of TSH accordingly. Normally, TSH rises to abnormally high levels before thyroid hormone (FT4 and FT3) levels fall below the normal range. Similarly, TSH levels fall below the reference range before thyroid hormone levels rise above the normal range.

Thus, in screening for thyroid disease, the TSH test is the best early indicator of thyroid dysfunction. If the TSH level is normal, in most cases thyroid function and levels of FT4 and FT3 are usually also normal. In screening new patients, the TSH test is considered a cost-effective gold standard for evaluating thyroid function.

If the TSH result is abnormal, physicians typically order blood tests for FT4 alone or both FT4 and FT3 levels. If FT4 alone is tested and the result is normal, the FT3 level is tested. In some thyroid disorders, particularly Graves' disease and toxic multinodular goiter, T3 is released from thyroid cells at a high rate, and levels of FT3/T3 become elevated before FT4 levels rise. Because T3 is nearly 5 times as potent as T4, even a slight rise in FT3 levels can cause symptoms of hyperthyroidism requiring treatment.

In hyperthyroidism, TSH levels generally fall below .01 mu/L before thyroid hormone levels become abnormally high. In active Graves' disease, TSH is suppressed and thyroid hormone levels are elevated. In subclinical hyperthyroidism, the TSH level is low and thyroid hormone levels are normal.

Tests for thyroid antibodies are used to tell if hyperthyroidism is autoimmune, with TSI antibodies diagnostic for Graves' disease.

However, a normal TSH and the absence of TSH receptor antibodies don't exclude Graves' disease when thyroid hormone levels are elevated because TSH levels lag behind thyroid hormone levels. Although a rare occurrence, thyroid hormone levels can rise quickly in some individuals, becoming abnormally high before TSH levels fall. In very early Graves' disease, TSI antibodies can be present in the thyroid gland but haven't yet spilled out into the blood circulation, causing low TSI levels.

If T4 and T3 levels are measured, results may be elevated due to high levels of binding proteins or high levels of thyroid hormone. Although these tests aren't recommended because of interferences, some doctors use the ratio of total T3 to total T4, measuring ng/mcg (ng of T3/mcg of T4), with ratios greater than 20 suggesting Graves' disease (Bach et al. 2011, 599). Because T3 is also often synthesized in higher amounts in toxic multinodular goiter, measuring the ratio can only suggest and not confirm Graves' disease.

Levels of thyroid-binding proteins (thyroxine-binding globulin or TBG usually) or an RAI-uptake test can be used to further evaluate results when T4 and T3 levels are high despite a normal TSH and an absence of symptoms. However, tests for free T4 and free T3 (FT4 and FT4 levels) are usually used to evaluate thyroid status.

Often, conversion of T4 to T3 is impaired especially if selenium levels are low, resulting in a normal T3 and an elevated FT4 (T4 toxicosis). Occasionally, the discrepancy between T4 and T3 levels may be exaggerated, with T4 being normal and T3 alone being elevated (T3 toxicosis). In about one-third of patients with Graves' disease, T3/FT3 elevation is higher relative to the T4/FT4 elevation.

Reference Ranges

Reference values (normal ranges) and units of measurement used for a particular blood test vary depending on the analytical method used. To tell if results are abnormal, they must be compared to the range used by the testing laboratory. This range is generally listed below or to the right of the test results. Units of measurement indicate the amount of a substance present in a known volume. Results given in mcg/ml, for example, indicate how many micrograms are present in one milliliter of serum. Reference values for the following tests are listed as general guidelines.

T4 (Thyroxine) Total; Total T4; TT4

T4 is the major thyroid hormone with blood levels 10 to 20 times higher than T3. T4 is considered a prohormone needed for conversion into the more active hormone, T3. Total T4 reflects the thyroid's ability to secrete hormone in adequate concentrations. In blood, most T4 is bound (linked) to protein and unavailable to cells. T4 is thereby considered inactive. Changes in binding proteins (due to certain physiological conditions or medications) alter the total T4 concentration but rarely affect the FT4. Drugs and conditions known to increase the T4 level include: amphetamine abuse; heroin use; heparin; amiodarone; estrogen withdrawal; high doses of propranolol and occasionally prednisone (due to increased conversion of T4 into T3); iodine contrast agents used in imaging tests; acute psychosis; excess iodine; selenium deficiency (decreased conversion of T4 into T3).

Reference Range: Adults = 5.0–12.5 ug/dL or 0.8–1.5 ng/dL
    0–4 days (neonates) = 5.9–15.0 ug/dL
    21 weeks up to 20 years = 5.6–14.9 ug/dL

Interpretation: T4 levels are elevated in hyperthyroidism and when TBG and transthyretin levels are increased (in estrogen therapy, pregnancy, certain drugs). T4 is decreased in pituitary TSH deficiency, primary hypothyroidism, hypothalamic TRH deficiency, nonthyroidal illness, and when levels of TBG are decreased.

Serious illness (non-thyroidal illness) such as trauma or surgery lowers the T4 level in 25 percent of patients; consequently, in severely ill or hospitalized patients, the total T4 result may not accurately reflect thyroid status. In patients with normal TBG levels (either a normal TBG level or a normal T3-uptake test), and no evidence of coexisting non-thyroidal illness, T4 is a good index of thyroid function (NACB 2002, 8).

Free T4 (FT4, Free Thyroxine)

Free T4 or FT4 (approximately 0.03 percent of total T4) represents the active thyroxine fraction which has been cleaved from its carrier protein and is available for use by the body's tissues. FT4 levels are controlled by a negative feedback mechanism causing constant levels of FT4 regardless of the binding protein concentration. Some immunoassays may provide falsely low results due to nonspecific reactions with reagent proteins. The most accurate determinations of FT4 employ dialysis methods that remove interfering proteins.

Reference Values: Non-dialysis methods: 0.8–1.8 ng/dL for age 2 weeks to 21 years

Direct dialysis methods: 0.8–2.7 ng/dL for adults

Interpretation: FT4 levels indicate the amount of thyroxine available for use by the tissues and cells in both hypothyroidism (low levels) and hyperthyroidism (high levels). In general, a normal FT4 level indicates euthyroidism (normal thyroid function). In patients undergoing treatment for hyperthyroidism, a normal FT4 in the presence of a low TSH indicates euthyroidism. TSH and FT4 are recommended as the initial tests for evaluating patients with suspected thyroid disorders. In non-thyroidal illness, FT4 is usually normal or slightly elevated, although about 50 percent of severely ill hospitalized patients show decreased FT4 levels (NCAB 2002, 8).

Testing methods for FT4 employing standards containing free thyroxine are considered accurate, although in patients with high or low levels of TBG or other binding or interfering proteins, FT4 tests may be diagnostically accurate. When FT4 results appear erratic, the FT4 by dialysis method is available.

T3 (Triiodothyronine); Total T3

The hormone triiodothyronine (T3) is more metabolically active, but its effects are briefer. About 20 percent of T3 is produced in the thyroid gland, and 80 percent is produced by conversion from T4. The T3 level may be falsely elevated by increased binding proteins (as seen in pregnancy and in patients on estrogens). T3 is often low in sick or hospitalized patients and in patients using medications such as propranolol that inhibit the conversion of T4 into T3.

Reference Values: 94–269 ng/dL for 1–9 years

80–180 ng/dL for adults

Interpretation: Elevated total T3 levels may normally occur in pregnancy, during estrogen therapy, and in infectious hepatitis. Depressed T3 levels occur in drug therapy with dexamethasone and glucocorticoids, and in iodine deficiency. T3 values greater than 230 ng/dL are consistent with hyperthyroidism or increased binding proteins. T3 or preferably FT3 levels are necessary to assess patients suspected of having thyrotoxicosis when TSH is decreased and the FT4 value is normal. In extremely sick hospitalized patients and individuals on low carbohydrate diets, T3 is decreased and reverse T3 is increased. According to the National Academy of Clinical Biochemistry (NACB), serum T3 measurements, interpreted together with FT4, are useful to diagnose complex or unusual presentations of hyperthyroidism. For instance, in an acute recurrence or relapse in Graves' disease, the T3/FT3 tests may be elevated before TSH falls abnormally low.

Free T3 (FT3, Free Triiodothyronine)

Normally, T3 circulates as a complex in which it is tightly bound to thyroxine-binding globulin (TBG) and albumin. Only 0.3 percent of the total T3 is unbound or free, and this portion is the active form since it reacts with the body's cells. Elevations in FT3 are associated with thyrotoxicosis or excess thyroid hormone therapy. FT3 is performed by dialysis or non-dialysis methods. High protein concentrations related to pregnancy and estrogen therapy can produce falsely elevated FT3 results in direct FT3 assays. In these cases, a free T3 by dialysis is used to remove interfering proteins.

Reference Values: Adults 230–420 pg/dL or 2.3–4.2 pmol/L or 2.0–5.0 ng/L in nondialysis assays
210–440 pg/dL or 2.1–4.4 pmol/L and 200–380 pg/dL in pregnancy in tracer dialysis assays

Interpretation: When increased plasma thyroxine-binding globulin (TBG) concentration is suspected as the cause of an elevated total T3, the FT3 dialysis assay can differentiate this condition. FT3 is increased in Graves' disease, toxic multinodular goiter (TMG), T3 thyrotoxicosis, thyroid hormone resistance and in functional thyroid adenoma. FT3 is decreased in non-thyroidal illness, selenium deficiency, and conditions of hypothyroidism. In some circumstances FT3 and T3 may be superior to FT4 and T4 for monitoring patients receiving thyroid replacement therapy (Aziz 1997, 141).

Reverse T3 (rT3)

Reverse T3, a thyroid hormone considered metabolically inactive, differs from T3 in the positions of its iodine atoms. When T3 is produced, it follows either the T3 or reverse T3 pathway depending on the body's needs. Increased rT3 is produced at the expense of T3 (Aziz 1997, 146). RT3 is formed in conditions where adequate T3 is not needed and where its effects might be harmful, for instance in newborns or severe illnesses and trauma. Since the introduction of FT3 assays, reverse T3 levels are rarely ordered or needed as a clinical diagnostic test.

Reference Values: Adults: 10–24 ng/dL or 0.18–0.51 nmol/L
    1 month up to 20 years: 10–35 ng/dL
    Cord Blood: 102–342 ng/dL

Interpretation: Reverse T3 is increased in the euthyroid sick syndrome seen in many chronically ill patients; the fetus and newborn; low T3 syndrome; hyperthyroidism; in conditions of fasting, malnutrition, anorexia nervosa, and poorly controlled diabetes; mellitus, trauma, heatstroke; surgery/postsurgical recovery; and systemic illness. Reverse T3 is decreased in hypothyroidism.

Thyroid-Stimulating Hormone
(TSH, Thyrotropin)

Thyrotropin or TSH is a pituitary hormone that regulates levels of thyroid hormone in the blood. TSH is considered to be far more sensitive than FT4 in detecting changes in thyroid function, because small changes in FT4 away from the normal set-point cause large changes in TSH concentration. However, in the presence of TSH receptor antibodies, it may take many months for TSH to adequately reflect thyroid function. Consequently, low TSH levels persist. TSH receptors in the pituitary gland recognize TSH receptor antibody molecules as if they are TSH molecules. When these antibodies are present, the pituitary presumably recognizes that there is adequate TSH and halts TSH secretion.

Reference Values: 0.3–3.0 mIU/L
Note: the high end of the TSH reference range was lowered in 2003 to 3.0 although it was recommended that the upper limit be lowered to 2.5 mIU/ml (Lee 2003, 1). Worldwide, all laboratories use the same units of measurement for TSH (universal units). Therefore, this reference range is considered the same worldwide.

In screening for thyroid disorders, a TSH concentration between 0.3 and 3.0 mIU/L suggests euthyroidism, although Graves' disease patients receiving treatment are considered euthyroid as soon as their FT4 level falls within the reference range. TSH levels <0.3 mIU/L suggest a diagnosis of hyperthyroidism if FT4 and FT3 levels are abnormal, and subclinical hyperthyroidism if these levels are normal. TSH concentrations greater than 3.0 mIU/L suggest hypothyroidism. If thyroid hormone levels are normal, an elevated TSH indicates subclinical hypothyroidism.

Interpretation: In active hyperthyroidism, levels of TSH are low, often falling to <0.01 mIU/L before thyroid hormone levels rise abnormally high. In primary hypothyroidism, TSH is elevated. Typically, TSH levels lag 6–8 weeks behind thyroid hormone levels. Serum TSH concentrations begin to rise several hours before the onset of sleep, reaching maximal concentrations between 11 P.M. and 6 A.M., then declining, with the lowest concentrations occurring at 11 A.M. The diurnal variation in TSH level approximates +50 percent; consequently, time of day may influence the measured TSH concentration, although daytime TSH levels vary by less than 10 percent (Fisher 1998, 146).

TSH values decline with surgical stress, caloric restriction, and certain psychological states such as anorexia nervosa and depression. In addition, medications such as dopamine, glucocorticoids and bromocriptine cause a transient suppression of TSH.

Increased TSH Sensitivity
(S-TSH and Third-Generation Tests)

With fourth-generation TSH assays, laboratories can detect levels as low as 0.01 mIU/L. Many laboratories, however, use older methods with sensitivity levels of 0.03 mIU/L. Fourth-generation methods are recommended for monitoring T4 replacement or suppressive (used in cancer) therapy when it's important to know if TSH is being secreted or not.

THYROXINE-BINDING GLOBULIN (TBG)

TBG, a protein produced in the liver, binds both T4 and T3. Thyroid hormone molecules combine with protein in order to be transported through the blood. Because TBG accounts for 75 percent of plasma protein thyroxine-binding activity, increased levels of TBG alter total T4 and T3 concentrations. TBG levels are high at birth, peaking at about the fifth day, which accounts for the higher T4 and T3 levels seen in newborns.

Reference Values:

1–5 Days 2.2–4.2 mg/dl for Males and Females		
	Females	*Males*
1–9 years	1.5–2.7 mg/dL	2.0–2.8 mg/dl
10–19 years	1.4–3.0 mg/dl	1.4–2.6 mg/dl
20–90 years	1.7–3.6 mg/dl	for males and females

Interpretation: TBG concentration should be interpreted in conjunction with the T4 results. The T4/TBG ratio should be 0.25–0.60. Elevated ratios indicate hyperthyroidism and reduced ratios indicate hypothyroidism. Certain diseases and medications alter serum TBG levels. TBG is increased by estrogen therapy, oral contraceptive agents, tamoxifen (despite being an estrogen antagonist), pregnancy and hepatitis. TBG may be decreased in cirrhosis, in the nephrotic syndrome and by androgens including anabolic steroids. The non-steroidal anti-inflammatory drugs fenclofenac, mefenamic acid, aspirin and salicylate compete with T4 for binding to TBG, with effects depending on the total drug concentration. Therapeutic doses of salicylate lower serum T4 by 40 percent and T3 by 30 percent.

THYROGLOBULIN (HTG)

Thyroglobulin is a large molecular weight protein produced by the thyroid gland. Normally hTG is found only in the thyroid gland, where it stores thyroid hormone. Thyroglobulin is released in increased amounts in certain conditions, particularly thyroid cancers, and in hyperthyroidism.

Reference Values:
<59.4 ng/ml in patients with normal thyroids
<5 ng/ml in patients without thyroid glands

Interpretation: The serum thyroglobulin level reflects physical damage or inflammation of the thyroid gland as well as the magnitude of TSH stimulation. All forms of TSH-dependent hyperthyroidism, including Graves' disease, toxic nodular goiter and thyroiditis, cause elevated serum thyroglobulin. The main uses of thyroglobulin levels are for postoperative monitoring of patients with thyroid cancers, differential diagnosis of hyperthyroidism due to exogenous causes (with excess replacement thyroid, thyroglobulin levels are low), and for determining hypothyroidism in infants if there is any functional thyroid tissue present. Thyroglobulin autoantibodies interfere in most testing methods for thyroglobulin. Therefore, antithyroglobulin antibodies are measured in all samples submitted for thyroglobulin assays.

T3 UPTAKE (TBG ASSESSMENT)

The T3 uptake test is rarely used to assess the protein-binding capacity of thyroxine (T4). Fluctuations in TBG concentrations lead to changes in T4 and T3 levels. The test is based on the ability of TBG to bind with T3 tracer and provides an indirect measurement of TBG. With new methods available to measure FT4 and FT3, the T3 uptake, which can be used with a T4 level to calculate an index (FTI, FT7, FT4 index) to approximate how much FT4 is present, is considered an obsolete test.

Reference Values:
26 percent to 40 percent uptake

Interpretation: The T3 uptake test is increased in hyperthyroidism, renal failure and malnutrition and decreased in hypothyroidism, pregnancy and acute hepatitis.

Thyroid Autoantibodies

Tests for thyroglobulin and TPO autoantibodies, which are seen in Hashimoto's thyroiditis and Graves' disease, are used to confirm or rule out autoimmune thyroid disease (AITD). However, tests for stimulating TSH receptor antibodies (TSI, stimulating TRAb) are used to confirm Graves' disease. The absence of TSI, however, does not exclude a diagnosis of Graves' disease since these antibodies may form circulating immune complexes (CICs) and thereby escape detection. These antibodies may also be present in the thyroid gland but haven't yet been released into the blood circulation. Most patients with AITD have a combination of thyroid antibodies. Serbian researchers studied the possibility of autoantibody-negative Graves' disease in 255 newly diagnosed patients. In this patient group, 20 percent of patients had tested negative for TSH receptor antibodies. Further studies showed that only 234 of these patients had Graves' disease. The misdiagnosed patients were found to have conditions of either autonomous hyperthyroidism (Plummer's disease), painless thyroiditis, or euthyroid Graves' disease. The researchers concluded that TSH receptor autoantibody-negative Graves' disease is extremely rare (Paunkovic and Paunkovic 2006).

TPO antibodies are seen in 90 percent of patients with Hashimoto's thyroiditis and in 70 percent of patients with Graves' disease. With standard tests TSI antibodies are seen in 80 percent of patients with Graves' disease. However, when tests for total TSH receptor antibodies (TBII) and thyroid growth immunoglobulins (TGI) are also tested in Graves' disease patients, test positivity increases to 95 percent and 90 percent, respectively (Leavelle 1997, 504–05). Sensitivity in TSI testing is also increased in laboratories that use the Thyretain laboratory method for TSI. Thyretain is the only FDA-approved TSI test. It was introduced by Diagnostic Hybrids in August 2009.

TSH (Thyrotropin) Receptor Antibodies (TRAb)

Three types of TSH receptor antibodies exist: stimulating (TSI), blocking, and binding TRAb. In active Graves' disease, TSI antibodies cause hyperthyroidism, although most patients have a combination of these antibodies with TSI predominating. TSI acts as an agonist, mimicking TSH and causing excess thyroid hormone production. TSI are diagnostic for Graves' disease and also Hashitoxicosis. In Hashitoxicosis, patients primarily have hypothyroidism but also have TSI antibodies, which cause transient symptoms of thyrotoxicosis.

TSH receptor antibodies react with the TSH receptor found on cells of the thyroid gland, pituitary gland, lymphocyte, kidney, brain, bone, adipose tissue, and thymus gland (Davies et al. 2005, 1976.) The TSH receptor is the major autoantigen in Graves' disease. Studies suggest that cleavage of the receptor can lead to the shedding of some of the extracellular A subunits. These subunits react with TSH receptor antibodies in human blood to break peripheral tolerance and induce the development of Graves' disease (Rocchi 2005, 11). In addition, TRAb show functional heterogeneity, which explains why some people with lower TSI levels have more severe symptoms than individuals with higher levels.

Effects of TSH Receptor Antibodies on TSH Levels

For many years, researchers have known that TSH levels remain suppressed in patients with Graves' disease. This was thought to be partially caused because the normal pituitary-thyroid-hypothalamic axis was disrupted by immune system dysfunction. In 2001 Leon Brokken and his colleagues in the Netherlands discovered that the TSH receptors in the pituitary gland recognize both TSH and TSH receptor antibodies but presumably cannot differentiate between the two. Recognizing the antibodies as if adequate TSH remained in the blood circulation, the pituitary halted its release of TSH into the circulation. Consequently, one of the reasons for the persistently low TSH levels in euthyroid Graves' disease patients was explained (Brokken et al. 2001, Brokken et al. 2003, Utiger 2003).

Thyroid-Stimulating Immunoglobulins (TSI, Stimulating TRAb)

TSIs react with the TSH receptor on thyroid cells in place of TSH, stimulating thyroid cells to grow and produce/release excess thyroid hormone. According to Specialty Laboratories, TSI antibodies are present in 95 percent of Graves' disease patients (Aziz 1997, 149) with higher levels often seen in individuals with large goiters, severe exophthalamos, pretibial myxedema and patients treated with radioiodine ablation. However, due to difficulties in interpretation of results, patients may be mistakenly told that their results are negative. TSI are increased in Graves' disease, Hashitoxicosis and transient neonatal thyrotoxicosis (passively transferred via the maternal circulation). TSI antibodies are also often seen in low titers in subacute thyroiditis. The TSI level is also used in pregnancy to detect the presence of TSI, which can pass into the fetal circulation.

Reference Range: <125 percent activity

TSI Result Interpretation

Most tests for TSI measure the change in thyroid hormone concentration in a culture of hamster thyroid cells after the addition of a patient's serum. The change is measured as a percent activity. At 125 percent activity, most patients will have symptoms of hyperthyroidism. Because blocking TRAb can block the activity of TSI, and there is variability in the potency of TSI, patients with lower TSI levels can have symptoms. TSI levels in the normal population are usually <2 percent activity. Patients with a TSI of 90 percent activity are presumed to have Graves' disease but are often told their results are negative because the results are below the cutoff. Patients with hyperthyroidism should keep copies of all test results and examine results carefully.

BLOCKING TRAB

TSH receptor–blocking antibodies (TRBAb, TSBAb) in patients with Graves' disease usually causes no symptoms, but when they predominate, they may cause hypothyroidism, especially after treatment when TSI levels decline and blocking antibodies appear (Henry, 1991, 824). Blocking TRAb inhibit TSH-generated cAMP in thyroid cells, causing hypothyroidism. In some laboratories, total TRAb is measured and compared to the TSI assay to determine if blocking TRAb are present. Discrepancies (low TSI, high TRAb) are usually due to the presence of blocking TRAb. High levels of blocking TRAb occur in atrophic thyroiditis and severe hypothyroidism, but atrophic thyroiditis may occur in the absence of blocking antibodies. Blocking antibodies are seen in 59 percent of patients with nongoitrous autoimmune thyroiditis and 10 percent of patients with goitrous autoimmune thyroiditis (Aziz 1997, 149).

Reference Range: = <10 percent inhibition

Indications: Increased in atrophic thyroiditis, Hashimoto's thyroiditis, and transient congenital hypothyroidism.

THYROTROPIN RECEPTOR–BINDING INHIBITORY ANTIBODIES (TRAB, BINDING TYPE, TBII)

TBIIs interfere with the binding of TSH to the TSH receptor and are commonly seen in atrophic (condition where thyroid cells atrophy, leading to hypothyroidism) rather than goitrous thyroiditis. Assays for binding TRAb frequently reflect the presence of either or both the stimulatory and inhibitory immunoglobulin classes since both types bind to the TSH receptor. Thus, in some assays, a measure of TBII includes a measurement of TSI.

Reference Range:
TRAb, binding type = <10 percent inhibition
10 percent to 100 percent inhibition in Graves' disease

Indications: Increased in Graves' disease, atrophic thyroiditis, postpartum autoimmune thyroid disease, neonatal Graves' disease and transient neonatal hypothyroidism.

Other Thyroid Autoantibodies Seen in Graves' Disease

The thyroid autoantibodies most frequently seen in Graves' disease, besides TRAb, are antibodies to thyroglobulin and thyroid peroxidase, and thyroid growth–stimulating immunoglobulins (TGI). Antibodies to T4, T3 and TSH occasionally exist in patients with AITD, but they're rarely tested unless results for T4, T3 or TSH appear to be falsely elevated. Using sensitive assays, about 25 percent of women and 10 percent of men in the general population have autoantibodies to thyroid peroxidase (TPO) or thyroglobulin, and these antibodies are also seen in thyroiditis, making them a less specific indicator (McLachlan and Rappaport 1996, 483).

In addition, antibodies also exist to megalin (the thyroid cell TG receptor) and to the thyroidal sodium/iodide symporter. In addition, antibodies reacting to components of eye muscle and fibroblasts are present in sera of patients with Graves' ophthalmopathy. The immune reactivity in Graves' disease includes development of antibodies to these antigens, cell-mediated immune responses due to lymphocyte reactivity, development of circulating antigen/antibody complexes, and the release of various cytokines capable of perpetuating and modulating the immune response.

Thyroid Growth–Stimulating Immunoglobulins (TGI)

Autoantibodies with the ability to increase DNA synthesis in thyrocytes (thyroid epithelial cells that produce thyroid hormone) are termed thyroid growth–stimulating immunoglobulins (TGI). TGI are seen in patients with Graves' disease, autoimmune thyroiditis and nonspecific goiter. When Graves' disease patients are tested for both TGI and TSI, nearly 100 percent of patients are positive for one or the other antibody (Fisher 1998, 199).

Reference Range <130 percent of basal activity

Interpretation: Used in the diagnosis of Graves' disease when TSI is negative and for differential diagnosis of goiter. Increased in Graves' disease, autoimmune thyroiditis and nonspecific goiter.

Thyroglobulin Antibodies, Antithyroglobulin Antibodies (TgAb, ATG, ATA)

Antithyroglobulin antibodies were the first autoantibodies to be discovered. TgAb are seen in most patients with Hashimoto's thyroiditis and in lower titers in 50 percent of patients with Graves' disease. The prevalence of TgAb in normal women is 18 percent, with higher frequencies in older women (Fisher 1998, 169). In men the prevalence is much lower (3 to 6 percent). In all cases the prevalence of TgAb increases with age (Aziz 1996, 150–51).

Reference Range = <2 IU/ml

Indications: Indicated for confirmation of autoimmune thyroid disease, pre-screening before thyroglobulin assay. The test may be used to distinguish Graves' disease from toxic multinodular goiter. Increased in Hashimoto's thyroiditis, Graves' disease and postpartum thyroiditis.

Thyroid Peroxidase (TPO) Antibodies (Previously Known as Anti-Microsomal Antibodies)

The thyroid microsomal antigen is a component of the carrier vesicles within thyroid follicular cells in which newly synthesized thyroglobulin is transferred to the follicular lumen for storage. The primary autoantigen (element eliciting an autoimmune response) in the microsomal particle is the enzyme thyroid peroxidase. Consequently, thyroid peroxidase antibodies (TPO Ab) are a more sensitive determinant of the microsomal particle of thyroid cells and are considered as markers of thyroid inflammation. In the laboratory, TPO Ab have replaced anti-microsomal antibodies. TPO Ab are present in the serum of almost all patients with Hashimoto's thyroiditis and 57 to 88 percent of patients with Graves' disease. Low-level TPO titers are also found in 10 to 13 percent of normal women and 3 percent of normal men (Aziz 1996, 150–51).

Reference Range = <2.0 Iu/ml

Interpretation: Indicated for confirmation of autoimmune thyroid disease.
Elevated in Hashimoto's thyroiditis, primary hypothyroidism, Graves' disease and postpartum thyroiditis.

Laboratory Test Interferences

Certain drugs directly interfere with thyroid function because they cause changes in the absorption of thyroid hormone in the body or in the body's ability to convert T4 into T3. Drugs that affect levels of binding proteins or lead to the production of anti-human (heterophile) antibodies can also interfere with tests for thyroid function and thyroid antibodies. Medications and other substances can cause markedly different results when blood samples are obtained shortly after ingestion of the interfering substance. An excellent resource on drugs that affect thyroid hormone levels can be found at http://www.ncbi.nlm.nih.gov/pmc/articles/PMC1070767/ (accessed December 10, 2012). Thyroid hormone and TSH levels can also be falsely elevated by antibodies to T3, T4, and TSH, heterophile antibodies, and rheumatoid factor (Despres and Grant 1998). For instance, it's been found that patients with recurrences of Epstein-Barr virus (EBV) infection can have transient production of T3 autoantibodies that cause transient elevations of T3/FT3 test results (Shimon et al. 2003). Antibodies to T3, T4, and TSH are more common in thyroid disease patients, with a prevalence as high as 10 percent (Despres and Grant 1998).

Abnormal thyroid function test results aren't always related to abnormal thyroid function. Besides interferences from medicines, the non-thyroidal sick state causes suppressed hormone levels. In evaluating laboratory results, the effects of interfering medications (along with the time of last dose and dietary influences) as well as the patient's condition and symptoms must be taken into consideration. The following medications and conditions can influence thyroid laboratory tests.

- Medications affecting liver function (acetaminophen, vitamin A derivatives) accelerate T4 metabolism causing disproportionately high levels of T3.
- Anticonvulsants: Both phenobarbital and phenytoin (Dilantin) inhibit TSH secretion in rats. At concentrations above the therapeutic range, phenytoin inhibits T4 binding to TBG and induces accelerated T4 metabolism with increased conversion to T3. The net result is a 15–20 percent lowering of T4 and FT4. Phenytoin interferes with binding of T3 to pituitary receptors. Carbamazepine (Tegretol) has similar effects (Bayer 1991, 1–11).
- Dopamine (L-dopa), dopamine agonists, and bromocriptine produce a prompt, transient suppression of TSH secretion and radioiodine uptake. In patients with true hyperthyroidism, thyrotropin levels are often undetectable. By increasing dopamine levels for 1–3 weeks, amphetamines also suppress TSH (Dong 2000, 102).

- Glucocorticoids, particularly in "stress" doses, inhibit TSH secretion acutely, decrease serum TBG and impair the conversion of T4 to T3. The net effects are a low T4 and a slightly decreased FT4, a low or very low T3, and a low TSH. In patients with primary hypothyroidism, TSH may be suppressed into the normal range, confusing diagnosis.
- Androgens, including anabolic steroids, decrease TBG levels in the blood, thereby lowering T4 and T3 while leaving FT3 and FT4 unaffected.
- Estrogens, tamoxifen, methadone, octreotide, amphetamines, and heroin increase the level of TBG and its binding in the blood, increasing T4 and T3 while leaving FT3 and FT4 unaffected (Henry 1991, 119–20).
- Beta adrenergic receptor antagonists (propranolol, metoprolol) and calcium channel blocker drugs inhibit the conversion of T4 to T3, resulting in decreased T3 and FT3.
- Iron, aluminum and calcium may prevent the complete absorption of T4 if ingested within two hours of a therapeutic dose. Lithium decreases levels of both T4 and T3.
- The nonsteroidal anti-inflammatory drugs (NSAIDs) fenclofenac, diclofenac, mefenamic acid, aspirin and furosemide compete with T4 for binding to TBG to a degree depending on doses. Therapeutic doses of salicylate (aspirin) lower serum total T4 by 40 percent and serum T3 by 30 percent. Naproxen lowers serum T3, but not T4, while TSH isn't altered. NSAIDs and free fatty acids have been shown to displace T3 from binding to nuclear receptors, diminishing the effects of T3 (Henry 1991, 315–20).
- Amiodarone contains 37 percent iodine. Thus, some effects occur while the drug slowly metabolizes. Amiodarone impedes the conversion of T4 to T3 with resulting decreases in T3 and rT3. Because metabolism is lowered, levels of T4 and FT4 are increased.
- Sertaline (Zoloft) is associated with elevated TSH levels in patients on thyroxine, indicating a decrease in the effectiveness of their thyroxine replacement hormone.
- A transient elevation of FT4 occurs in acute psychosis, estrogen withdrawal, iodine administration, the onset of T4 therapy (until levels stabilize), gallbladder contrast agents, initial response to high altitude exposure and selenium deficiency due to decreased peripheral conversion of T4.

Non-Thyroidal Autoantibodies in Graves' Disease

Individuals with Graves' disease often have other autoantibodies even in the absence of other autoimmune disorders. Autoantibodies seen in Graves' disease include parietal antibodies, antinuclear antibodies (ANA), DNA antibodies, pituitary antibodies, acetylcholine receptor antibodies, gliadin antibodies, liver membrane antibodies, and antibodies to the adrenal steroidogenic enzymes and ovarian components of the pituitary.

ANA antibodies may occur as a result of therapy with anti-thyroid drugs and beta adrenergic blocking agents such as propranolol in a condition known as drug-related lupus (DRL). DRL usually occurs within 4 months of drug use, although it can occur at any time and resolves when the offending drug is withdrawn.

Genetic Markers

Although Graves' disease has an association with several HLA antigens, these markers are not routinely tested and do not aid in diagnosis. Genetic tests are rarely used to help diagnose conditions of thyroid hormone resistance and familial dysalbuminemic hyperthyroxinemia when diagnosis is difficult.

Biopsy Tests

Thyroid biopsies are used to evaluate nodules in individuals with autonomously functioning nodules and toxic multinodular goiter. Thyroid nodules can also be present in patients with Graves' disease or thyroiditis. Because 20 percent of patients with thyroid cancer have been found to have thyroglobulin antibodies (Check 2007), an evaluation of nodules is especially important in thyroid patients.

A study of Graves' disease patients showed an increased incidence of both nodules and thyroid cancer, with cancer rates varying from 1 to 9 percent (Stocker and Burch 2003). In their article, Stocker and Burch also report that the aggressiveness of thyroid cancer in Graves' disease patients is a controversial subject, although it's generally thought that stimulating TSH receptor antibodies, like TSH, stimulate the growth of thyroid cancer cells. Other studies show an incidence of thyroid cancer (6.2 percent) and nodules (17–27 percent) in Graves' disease patients, with nodules more common in women and in iodine-deficient areas (Mishra and Mishra 2001). In Graves' disease patients treated with anti-thyroid drugs or radioiodine, more than 50 percent of the nodules disappeared or decreased in size during post-treatment follow-up (Carnell 1998). However, the incidence of papillary, and occasionally follicular, thyroid cancer after radioiodine ablation is increased (Greenspan 1997, 250).

The evaluation of FNA specimens in Graves' disease patients with nodules can pose diagnostic difficulties because the cytomorphologic changes in Graves' disease may mimic nuclear features of papillary thyroid carcinoma (Dabbs 2004). Dabbs reports that nodules from patients who have had radioiodine ablation are even more difficult to assess because they may have significant atypical cells. Changes typical of papillary cancer such as prominent nuclear elongation and pale powdery chromatin with intranuclear grooves must be carefully evaluated for a differential diagnosis.

In the general U.S. population, the prevalence of thyroid nodules is on the rise, occurring in 3–7 percent of the population (Abad 2009) although autopsy studies show a 50 percent prevalence of nonpalpable nodules in patients without a history of thyroid disease, calling the occurrence of nonpalpable thyroid nodules an epidemic (Abad 2009).

Fine Needle Aspiration (FNA) Thyroid Biopsy

Biopsies are used in conjunction with imaging tests to determine the type of thyroid nodule present. The tissue make-up of nodules is studied by aspirating a small tissue sample, which is studied microscopically. Results are reported as benign, malignant, suspicious (indeterminate) or nondiagnostic. Nondiagnostic means that the sample was unsatisfactory and might contain foam cells, cyst fluid or blood. Most often (70 percent of the time) results are benign (Abad 2009) and nodular goiter is the most frequent lesion encountered in FNA (Auger 2003). Benign nodules include colloid nodules (most common), macrofollicular adenoma, lymphocytic thyroiditis, granulomatous thyroiditis, hyperplastic nodule, colloid cyst, and simple cyst. Nodules are considered toxic when they produce excessive amounts of thyroid hormone, causing thyrotoxicosis.

The Afirma Thyroid FNA Analysis

Physicians using the Afirma Thyroid FNA Analysis may be able to reduce the amount of inconclusive results that typically result from manual FNA evaluations. In the case of inconclusive FNA results (15–30 percent of results), patients must consult with their physicians to decide if surgical removal of nodules is needed. The Afirma test, with increased sensitivity, helps make diagnosis more certain by studying the cells for genetic changes that confirm thyroid cancers. More information on the Afirma analysis is available through Veracyte at www.veracyte.com/afirma.

Imaging Tests

With increased TSI testing sensitivity, the RAI-uptake (RAI-U) test is no longer routinely used to identify Graves' disease as the cause of hyperthyroidism and it is no longer recommended (Bahn et al. 2011, 598). RAI-uptake is more often used to differentiate thyroiditis from Graves' disease when antibody test results are ambiguous. Ultrasonography is frequently used to determine thyroid volume or size or to detect nodules and to rule out toxic multinodular goiter as the cause of hyperthyroidism.

Radioiodine Uptake Scan (RAI-U)

The radioiodine uptake (RAI-U) test is the only direct test of thyroid function because it measures the thyroid gland's ability to absorb iodine. Laboratory tests are indirect, measuring hormones that may be affected by pituitary function. However, the uptake is increased in most types of hyperthyroidism with the exception of iodine ingestion and thyroiditis. Therefore, it can suggest but not confirm Graves' disease. The accompanying scan shows a diffuse pattern and identifies nodules or other growths that cause increased absorption.

RAI-U usually employs the radioisotope I123 as a tag for I-127, the body's stable form of iodine. RAI-U reflects the thyroid gland's clearance of iodine. This test is not relied on as much as previously because of improved laboratory tests. The diagnostic accuracy of the RAI-U does not approach that of measuring TSH plus FT4 or FT3 levels to determine hyperthyroidism, followed by a TSI determination to confirm Graves' disease (Larsen et al. 1998, 315–20, 438).

The major advantage of RAI-U over antibody testing is that it can be performed locally, generating faster results. Also, RAI-U has value in excluding thyrotoxicosis not caused by conditions of a hyper-functioning thyroid such as ectopic thyroid tissue, or iodine-induced thyrotoxicosis. The major disadvantage of the RAI-U is that patients must ingest radioiodine, which increases the body's cumulative exposure to radiation, and radioiodine can occasionally worsen symptoms of hyperthyroidism. In addition, because of dietary changes (iodine subsidization, processed foods) that have led to an increased iodine intake, the normal or reference range for the RAI-U test among the U.S. population has significantly increased since RAI-U first came into use, making it a less significant indicator than in the past.

RAI-U Principle

The principle of the radioiodine uptake scan is simple. External X or gamma irradiation is capable of uniformly penetrating the entire thyroid gland within seconds to minutes following a given dose. Just as the thyroid takes up iodine, it takes up radioiodine without recognizing the difference. Radioiodine particles are absorbed and incorporated into the thyroid follicle. Here they remain while undergoing radioactive decay.

Localized in the gland, the distribution of radiation from radioiodine particles depends on the type and energy of the emissions, the follicle size and the distribution of iodine within the follicle. The mean range of particles in the thyroid is variable. It's much shorter for non-beta emitters such as I123 than for beta emitters such as I-131, I-132 and I-133.

RAI-U PROCEDURE

The procedure involves the oral administration of radioiodine, usually I-123 taken in a drink or as a capsule. The residual radioiodine is later measured using imaging tests. RAI-U measures the amount of iodine taken up by the thyroid in a given length of time varying from 2 to 24 hours. The RAI-U is dependent on the activity of the thyroid's iodine trapping mechanism, the rate of organic binding of iodine within the gland, and the rate of iodine release.

In a hyperthyroid patient with a minimal endogenous iodine intake and a fast turnover rate, the RAI-U measured at an earlier time is usually elevated, although at 24 hours it may fall within the normal range. Thus an earlier time, generally six hours, is recommended for the uptake measurement. A high concentration of dietary iodine will interfere with the uptake of radioiodine. If the scan is to be performed within four hours of the dose, rather than at 24 hours, the patient is advised to fast. Any medications containing iodine or anti-thyroid agents and imaging test contrast agents can interfere with this test. RAI-U is contraindicated in patients who are pregnant or breast-feeding. While I-123 has a shorter half-life than I-131, patients are advised to avoid close contact with small children.

REFERENCE RAI-U RANGE

The normal or reference RAI-U range varies in different geographical regions. Reference ranges are given for the time interval between dose and scan, which is usually 24 hours. Normal ranges using I-123 are usually about 2–12 percent at two hours, 5–15 percent at six hours, and 8–35 percent at 24 hours. RAI-U is increased in most conditions of hyperthyroidism, iodine deficiency, pregnancy, hydatidiform mole, recovery phase of subacute thyroiditis, rebound after TSH suppression or following withdrawal of strong solution of potassium iodine or anti-thyroid drugs if TSH is elevated, therapeutic lithium, chronic thyroiditis if TSH elevated and inborn errors of thyroid hormone synthesis.

RAI-U can also be increased in disorders in which iodine accumulation is normal but hormone secretion is impaired, such as in patients with abnormal thyroglobulin synthesis. RAI-U is also increased in calorie restriction, soybean ingestion since it binds thyroxine in the gut, nephrotic syndrome, and chronic diarrheal states.

RAI-U is decreased in primary and central hypothyroidism, status post-thyroidectomy, post-radioiodine ablation, thyroid hormone administration, destructive or active phase of subacute thyroiditis, postpartum or sporadic lymphocytic (painless) thyroiditis, iodine excess and the ingestion of thion-amides, sulfonamides, perchlorate, thiocyanate, amiodarone, glucocorticoid therapy and salicylates at levels greater than 5 grams per day. Drugs having minor effects include phenybutazone, resorcinol and sulfonylureas.

INTERFERENCES

Exposure to excess iodine is the most common cause of a decreased RAI-U. Special offenders are organic iodinated dyes used as X-ray contrast media and the heart medication amiodarone. Depending on the contrast dye used, the RAI-U may be falsely suppressed for up to several months. A single large dose of iodide can depress the test for several days, and chronic iodide ingestion may affect the results for many weeks. Because its high iodine content is stored in fat, amiodarone may interfere with test results for as long as several months.

RAI-U and Scan in Graves' Disease

Most patients with hyperthyroidism caused by Graves' disease have an elevated RAI-U. However, in elderly patients, the RAI-U is less likely to show elevated levels. RAI-U in subacute, silent or postpartum thyroiditis and exoge-nous thyroid administration is usually low, and in subclinical hyperthyroidism the uptake may be normal. In severe thyrotoxicosis, Graves' disease patients may very rarely take up and dissipate their oral dose of radioiodine so quickly that the uptake is decreased by the time the residual radioiodine is measured.

The accompanying scintiscan is used to determine the absorbed radioio-dine's pattern of distribution. In Graves' disease this distribution appears dif-fusely (predominantly even distribution of radioiodine) scattered and the gland enlarged. In patients with nodules as the cause of their hyperthyroidism, hot nodules will take up more radioiodine than surrounding tissue and cold nodules will take up less. However, the thyroid doesn't function as a single homogeneous unit. Radioautographic studies reveal variations among different areas of the gland and in different follicles. In fact, there may be iodine pools in the thyroid gland that are cleared at different rates, also causing discrepant test results.

Radioiodine Concerns

According to Dr. John Gofman, a physician and doctor of nuclear and physical chemistry, radioiodines that deliver beta particles provide the same effects as external X-rays, provided the same quantity of ionizing radiation energy is delivered to a specific tissue or organ when administered at a comparable age. While evaluating the effects of ionizing radiation on chromosomes for the Atomic Energy Commission, Dr. Gofman found that because cell division proceeds slowly in the thyroid, the effects of ionizing radiation may take more than 30 years to emerge. This is particularly true, he reports, for adults exposed to low doses at low dose rates (Gofman 1991, 20–45).

Because of the ability of the thyroid gland to concentrate up to 12 grams of radioiodine, it is said to be uniquely susceptible to the biologic effects of radioiodine exposure. Results may vary, from no discernible clinical effects to metabolically important processes such as acute radiation thyroiditis and to the induction of both benign and malignant neoplasms. Furthermore, there are no available long-term studies of irradiated populations or their progeny followed to the completion of their lifespans.

RADIOISOTOPES

Although I-123 is most often used for the RAI-U, some radiologists use I-131 for this test despite its longer half-life and greater toxicity. Technetium-99m is also used for diagnostic studies of thyroid structure because its emissions are favorable, and the pertechnetate material utilized in this procedure is readily available from a generator system rather than from the nuclear waste materials used for radioiodine. The half-life of technetium-99m is six hours and it doesn't produce beta emissions. Although the material is actively trapped in the thyroid much like iodine, it doesn't undergo organification and the total body radiation dose is much less than that of radioiodine (Bach et al. 2011, 599). A technetium pertechnetate thyroid scan has the ability to differentiate between Graves' disease or nodular thyroid disease since it provides better anatomical definition.

Ultrasonography

Ultrasonography is based on the principle that body tissues have a property called acoustic impedance. Sound waves entering tissue can be either transmitted through the tissue or reflected (echoed). The ease of distinguishing cystic from solid lesions in tissue is based on the different properties of acoustic impedance. For example, tissue that is calcified has a much higher impedance than other tissue. Ultrasound is very sensitive in its ability to detect thyroid lesions and in distinguishing solid lesions from simple and complex cysts. However, ultrasonography is unable to distinguish between malignant and benign lesions.

In Graves' disease, the thyroid is usually enlarged. Its echo pattern is inhomogeneous and normal to low in intensity compared to normal glands, which have a more uniform echo texture. Using color flow Doppler equipment, the intense vascularity of the thyroid in Graves' disease can be easily demonstrated. This technique also offers an ideal measurement of thyroid volume, which indicates size. The intensity of the flow pattern, however, is not correlated to disease severity. Since a diminishment of thyroid volume is one of the first indicators of response to therapy in Graves' disease, ultrasonography is sometimes used during the course of antithyroid drug therapy to monitor treatment response.

Computed Tomography

Rarely, computed tomography (CT) is used to help determine the cause of hyperthyroidism. CT in hyperthyroidism is usually used to study orbital changes in patients with eye changes. In the thyroid gland, differences as small as 0.5 percent in the density of soft tissues can be determined using CT. Easily visualized because of its high iodine content, the thyroid can be viewed as a three-dimensional image in relation to the trachea, esophagus and surrounding structures. The radiation dose used is relatively small and there is minimal exposure to other areas of the body.

The procedure requires the patient to remain supine with his neck hyperextended. This position provides elevation of the thyroid in the neck and prevents interferences from the shoulders. A frontal scan is taken to locate the landmarks of the neck. Scanning then begins at the level of the vocal cords. During each scan, which takes one to three seconds, the patient is directed not to swallow.

In Graves' disease, CT demonstrates thyroid enlargement with homogeneous density. Total iodine content is increased, but the iodine concentration is decreased, which results in a decreased CT density, with results usually measuring 50 percent to 70 percent of the normal value.

Magnetic Resonance Imaging (MRI)

MRI is rarely used to diagnose Graves' disease and like CT is more likely to be used when patients complain of pain or hoarseness. MRI is a noninvasive technique of imaging tissues based on their magnetic properties. Improvements in soft tissue contrast permit superior definition of many anatomic structures of the neck in multiple planes with thinner sections, higher resolution, and shorter scanning times. Limitations include sensitivity to physiologic tissue that affects imaging quality and the inability of MRI to identify calcification as readily as CT.

In Graves' disease, the thyroid is enlarged, occasionally lobulated, with a slightly heterogeneous, diffusely increased signal on both T1 and T2 weighted images. The intensity on T2 weighted images often exceeds that of fat. The thyroid to muscle signal ratio is linearly related to both the serum thyroxine (T4) concentration and the 24 hour radioiodine uptake scan. Following radioiodine ablation, the signal ratio falls proportionately in response to changes in the serum T4 and radioactive iodine uptake. Changes may reflect differences in tissue water content, thyroglobulin content, blood flow or vascularity of the thyroid.

7

Conventional Treatment
Options for Hyperthyroidism

The three major conventional therapies used for hyperthyroidism have remained the same for more than 60 years. However, a survey of 2011 current practice trends for treating Graves' disease in North America shows that anti-thyroid drug therapies are used more often, and the use of radioiodine has declined (Burch et al. 2011). This was also confirmed in another study of pre-scriptions used for anti-thyroid drugs in the U.S. (Emiliano et al. 2010). In addition to this dramatic change, several new therapies are under investigation. Chapter 7 describes available conventional therapies, the reasons for the increased popularity of anti-thyroid drugs, research studies, and the recommended guidelines for treating conditions of hyperthyroidism.

The Treatment Survey

More than two decades have passed since members from the American Thyroid Association (ATA), European Thyroid Association, and Japan Thyroid Association were surveyed on management practices for patients with hyperthyroidism due to Graves' disease. Twenty years ago, radioiodine ablation was used most often in the United States, infrequently in Europe, and rarely in Japan. In Europe and Japan, most patients were treated with anti-thyroid drugs.

In the 2011 survey conducted by Henry Burch, Kenneth Burman and David Cooper, U.S. and international members of the ATA, The Endocrine Society (TES), and the American Association of Clinical Endocrinologists (AACE) were sought to document current practices in the management of Graves' disease to evaluate differences in treatment practices (Burch et al.

2012). The researchers also compared these results to both those documented in earlier surveys and to practice recommendations made in the 2011 ATA/ American Association of Clinical Endocrinologists (AACE) hyperthyroidism practice guidelines (Bahn et al. 2011). Results: A total of 730 respondents participated in the survey. The preferred mode of therapy in uncomplicated Graves' disease was antithyroid drugs (ATDs) by 53.9 percent of respondents, radioactive iodine (RAI) therapy by 45.0 percent, and thyroid surgery in 0.7 percent Compared with 1991, fewer U.S. (59.7 percent vs. 69 percent) and European (13.3 percent vs. 25 percent) respondents would use RAI therapy. Methimazole and carbimazole were the preferred ATDs, with only 2.7 percent of respondents selecting propylthiouracil. Patients with Graves' ophthalmopathy were treated with ATDs (62.9 percent) or surgery (18.5 percent) and less frequently with RAI plus corticosteroids (16.9 percent) or RAI alone (1.9 percent).

The researchers concluded that striking changes have occurred in Graves' disease management over the past two decades, with a shift away from RAI and toward ATDs in patients with uncomplicated Graves' disease. Apparent international differences persist but should be interpreted with caution. For instance, the use of RAI slightly increased in Asia, where it had been used infrequently in the past, although the use of RAI in Asia is still significantly less than in other parts of the world. Current practices also diverge in some areas from recently published guidelines, particularly in regard to ATD dosing.

Prescribing Practices Study

In 2010, David Cooper and his team at Johns Hopkins Medical School began a study of ATD prescribing habits in the United States. The results showed that between 1991 and 2008, methimazole became the most frequently prescribed ATD. Prior to this study, PTU accounted for two-thirds of all prescriptions. Between 1991 and 2008 there was a 19 percent increase in PTU (from 348,000 to 415,000 prescriptions annually) and a 9-fold (800 percent) increase in methimazole (from 158,000 to 1.36 million prescriptions annually). Methimazole's popularity compared to PTU is related to its superior side effect profile, greater efficacy in severely hyperthyroid patients, and its longer mode of action. In addition, in the 1990s, methimazole became available as a generic, causing it to be more affordable than in the past. PTU, which now has a black box warning due to its potential to cause liver problems, is generally reserved for patients who are pregnant, allergic to methimazole and in possibly life-threatening conditions of thyroid storm (Emiliano et al. 2010).

Reasons for the Change

Changes rendered by provisions of the Health Insurance Portability and Accountability Act (HIPAA) of 1996 gave patients access to their own laboratory results and thereby empowered patients. Typically, physicians explain laboratory results before giving copies of the results to patients, but in some states and when direct access testing is used, patients receive results directly, a situation currently under scrutiny (O'Reilly 2011).

HIPAA also mandates that the diagnosis should be explained, and treatment options, along with their pros and cons, should be discussed. The 2011 ATA guidelines state: "Once the diagnosis has been made, the treating physician and patient should discuss each of the treatment options, including the logistics, benefits, expected speed of recovery, drawbacks, potential side effects, and cost (Bahn et al. 2011, 600). This is a far cry from the situation in the past where patients were told they had hyperthyroidism and scheduled to have RAI ablation, often before the cause of hyperthyroidism was confirmed. In addition, with medical information widely available on the Internet, patients are able to research their own conditions and therapies, with more patients asking for anti-thyroid drugs. Environmental concerns have also led to dissatisfaction with radioiodine as a treatment.

Treatment Considerations

Many factors influence treatment choice, including the cause of hyperthyroidism, the presence and size of nodules, coexisting conditions, symptoms and their severity, access to medical facilities, age, and general health. The likelihood of remission also factors in, with spontaneous remission likely in milder conditions of thyrotoxicosis.

Spontaneous Remission

Although spontaneous remission is reported to occur in 30–40 percent of patients with Graves' disease (Graves' disease, Encyclopaedia Britannica, http://www.britannica.com/EBchecked/topic/242366/Graves-disease, accessed October 1, 2012), most doctors feel that because serious complications might arise, all patients should be treated aggressively. In other cases of hyperthyroidism such as following iodine ingestion or thyroiditis, spontaneous remission is part of the disease course, and treatment is typically withheld. Consequently, some doctors advise that hyperthyroid patients with mild symptoms be monitored before starting treatment since for them spontaneous remission is likely.

Multiple Treatment Considerations

Patients do not necessarily use one treatment exclusively and many patients move spontaneously from one thyroid disorder to another. An important consideration is that with aggressive therapies, there's no way to restore destroyed thyroid tissue, whereas with medical therapies, the medications can be stopped or the dose adjusted if unwelcome symptoms occur. In addition, if symptoms recur after a patient achieves remission with ATDs, a different treatment may be recommended. However, if the previous treatment had worked reasonably well, it is usually used again and reasons for the relapse are investigated.

Conventional Treatment Options

There is no one specific cure for hyperthyroidism although, regardless of the cause, treatment has traditionally focused on (1) destroying the thyroid gland, using radioiodine ablation or thyroidectomy surgery and putting a quick halt to hyperthyroidism by reducing the amount of functional thyroid tissue that can produce thyroid hormone; or (2) using ATDs, and occasionally dietary interventions, to limit the amount of thyroid hormone that can be produced. ATDs are also known to mildly suppress the immune system, which helps reduce production of thyroid antibodies. In Graves' disease, TSI antibodies are the cause of hyperthyroidism.

In some cases of hyperthyroidism, such as conditions related to TSH excess (pituitary tumors) or HCG hormone, thyroid hormone levels are often watched but not treated. Alternately, the primary cause of the hyperthyroidism is treated, which affects thyroid function. For instance, many patients with latent infections have persistent conditions of Graves' disease that are treated with antibiotic or antiviral therapies. These protocols are described in Chapter 8.

The major conventional treatments for hyperthyroidism are described in the following sections. One or more of these treatments are used in all cases of chronic hyperthyroidism. The sections on therapies are followed by a description of treatment protocols used for the less common causes of hyperthyroidism. While most doctors do not offer nutritional guidance, diet plays an important role in the development of many hyperthyroid conditions, and nutrient deficiencies are responsible for many symptoms. While some doctors advise patients on diet, most do not. Therefore, dietary influences are described in Chapter 8 with complementary medicine.

Antithyroid Drugs and Goitrogens

Antithyroid drugs (ATDs) are goitrogens. Goitrogens are chemical compounds that have the ability to lower thyroid hormone levels. The earliest description of goitrogenic activity is credited to Chesney, who in 1928 observed that rabbits fed a cabbage diet developed hyperplastic thyroid glands devoid of colloid. The body temperature of the rabbits varied, and adding iodine to the rabbits' diets reversed their conditions. This was the first clue that foods could contain phytochemicals with goitrogenic properties (Goodman and Gilman 1955, 1544). This description also illustrated the individual response to goitrogenic therapies.

Other foods of the genus *Brassica* were also found to be goitrogens, and the active goitrogenic chemical was identified as acetonitrile. Interest in this topic waned until 1942 when Richter and Clisby discovered that thiourea in *Brassica* seeds had even greater goitrogenic properties than acetonitrile. In 1943, Astwood began to investigate thiourea. He ultimately discovered that all goitrogens prevent the synthesis of thyroid hormone.

GOITROGEN EFFECTS

Astwood found that goitrogens as a whole act to deplete the thyroid gland of hormone, to lower the concentration of circulating hormone, to decrease basal oxygen consumption, and to cause compensatory stimulation of TSH secretion by the pituitary gland, which results in thyroid hyperplasia. Foreshadowing the use of block-and-replace therapy, Astwood found that when he added iodine to a goitrogen simultaneously, the animals were prevented from developing thyroid hyperplasia and a decline in oxygen consumption. This showed that goitrogens do not block the peripheral actions of thyroid hormone on tissues and that the morphological changes in the thyroid gland depend on compensatory hyperactivity of the anterior pituitary related to a rise in TSH (Goodman and Gilman 1955, 1544–45). In other words, at the right dose, goitrogens lower thyroid hormone levels without necessarily causing hypothyroidism.

THIOUREA DERIVATIVES AND OTHER IONS

These early studies quickly led to the development of chemicals with goitrogenic properties for their use as anti-thyroid drugs. Most of the studied plant and synthetic compounds possessed the thioureylene radical. Studies showed that after goitrogen withdrawal, the thyroid gland gradually regained its ability to produce thyroid hormone and store thyroxine in its colloid. The researchers also found that the cytological change that occurs in the pituitary as a result of goitrogens is similar to that which follows thyroidectomy, although the effect with goitrogens is temporary. Goitrogens are readily absorbed from the gastrointestinal tract and are distributed to all body tissues. About 60 percent of an administered dose is destroyed in the body with the remainder appearing in the urine for 24 hours (Goodman and Gilman 1955, 1550–51).

Although several anti-thyroid drugs were developed in the 1940s, the anti-thyroid drugs that remain in use in the United States include the thionamides propylthiouracil (PTU) and methimazole. Aniline derivatives such as sulfonamides and polyhydric phenols such as resorcinol are also ATDs, but they are rarely used. Other compounds with antithyroid properties include strong solutions of potassium iodide, lithium, thiouracil derivatives, oral cholecystographic agents, amiodarone, and iodide transport (ionic) inhibitors.

In Great Britain and Europe, carbimazole (Neo-Mercazole), a derivative of methimazole, is used. Carbimazole is metabolized to methimazole, which accounts for its antithyroid effect. Thus, the effects of carbimazole and methimazole are identical.

EFFECTS ON AUTOIMMUNITY

Patients treated with ATDs experience a decrease in their TSI levels. This immunosuppressive action occurs within the thyroid, the site of ATD concentration. ATDs also cause a decrease in thyroid antigen expression in thyroid cells and reduce the amount of prostaglandins and cytokines released by thyroid cells. These phenomena cause a subsequent impairment or relaxation of the autoimmune response.

ATDs also inhibit the generation of oxygen radicals in T and B lymphocyte cells and in antigen-presenting cells. This may contribute to the decline seen in TSI levels of patients using ATDs. Also, patients prepared before surgery with ATDs demonstrate thyroid glands that are depleted of lymphocytes compared to control patients.

TIMEFRAME FOR EFFECTIVENESS

ATDs are very effective in reducing thyroid hormone levels and controlling the symptoms of hyperthyroidism. However, the effects aren't immediate. Newly diagnosed patients have large stores of thyroid hormone within their thyroid colloid. It takes 4–6 weeks for this hormone to dissipate. Consequently, higher starting ATD doses are used. At about 4–6 weeks, the FT4 level falls within the normal range, symptoms are reduced, and the drug dose is lowered. At this time only enough of the drug is needed to reduce the production of new thyroid hormone. The lowest dose needed to keep the FT4 level near the high end of the range is used, with the dose lowered over time (Moses 2012).

MEDICATIONS AND DOSAGE ADJUSTMENT

The 2011 ATA guidelines note that methimazole be used in virtually every patient who chooses antithyroid drug therapy for Graves' disease, except during the first trimester of pregnancy when PTU is preferred; in the treatment of thyroid storm; and in patients with minor reactions to methimazole who refuse RAI or surgery (Bahn 2011, 603).

Individuals vary in their susceptibility to and their requirements for goitrogens. Therefore, dosage must be determined by the response of the patient (Goodman and Gilman 1955, 1532). Once improvement is observed, the dosage is often substantially reduced in an effort to maintain a normal metabolic state. The TSH level may remain low for many months, and a low TSH during treatment is not a sign of hyperthyroidism. Patients on ATDs are considered euthyroid when their FT4 falls into the reference range.

Occasionally, however, patients are prescribed a hefty dose of ATDs and told to return for a follow-up visit in two or three months. This may lead to marked hypothyroidism. Patient response can be so variable that the initial use of ATDs requires constant vigilance on the part of the patient and the doctor. Most doctors order thyroid labs four to six weeks after the start of anti-thyroid drug treatment.

SIDE EFFECTS

Although their actions are similar, methimazole and PTU do not have the same chemical structures. For this reason, cross-reactivity between the drugs is uncommon, and side effects that occur with one ATD usually do not occur when the other ATD is used. The most common reaction is a mild, occasionally purpuric, urticarial papular rash that subsides spontaneously (Goodman and Gilman 2006, 1529). Minor skin reactions (rash, hives, urticaria) occur in up to 5 percent of patients using ATDs (Bahn et al. 2011, 604). These symptoms may be managed with concurrent antihistamine therapy without stopping the ATD. Joint pain, hair loss, and weight gain have been reported to occur with ATD use but are mainly observed when high doses of ATDs are used and thyroid hormone levels fall too low for the body's needs, causing symptoms of hypothyroidism.

Both PTU (0.44 percent incidence) and to a lesser extent methimazole (0.12 percent) may cause agranulocytosis (Goodman and Gilman 2006, 1528). Agranulocytosis is a critical decrease in segmented neutrophilic white blood cells. Agranulocytosis associated with methimazole is more likely to be dose-related. Signs of infection such as sore throat or fever should be reported promptly, especially during the first 4 weeks of therapy.

About 50 percent of patients using PTU develop anti-neutrophilic cytoplasmic antibodies (ANCA), which is associated with the development of vasculitis. ANCA and vasculitis are rarely seen in patients using methimazole (Goodman and Gilman 2005, 1529).

Because agranulocytosis develops abruptly, patients are not routinely monitored with CBC tests for agranulocytosis after starting treatment unless symptoms occur. However, the ATA guidelines recommend that patients have CBC and liver function tests at the time of diagnosis (Bahn 2011, 603). Many physicians also repeat these tests 4–6 weeks after starting treatment. The ATA guidelines also recommend that patients on PTU be assessed for liver function when they experience itching, rash, jaundice, pale stools, dark urine, joint pain, abdominal pain or bloating, anorexia, nausea or fatigue (Bahn et al. 2011, 604). Because hyperthyroidism can also cause abnormal liver function tests, results should be compared to those taken at baseline.

Transient elevations of liver enzyme (transaminase levels) are commonly seen in up to one-third of patients using ATDs. Up to 4 percent of patients taking PTU can have significant elevations (threefold above the upper limit of the reference range) with a lower prevalence seen in patients using MMI (Bahn et al. 2011).

PTU can cause fulminant hepatic necrosis that may be fatal. This finding has led to a black box warning. Methimazole can rarely affect the liver with symptoms more likely to occur in the biliary than hepatocellular system.

GOITER CHANGES

In one-third to one-half of patients undergoing ATD treatment, the thyroid gland decreases in size. In the remaining patients, the thyroid may remain unchanged or it may become enlarged, which is usually due to ATD doses that are too high, causing hypothyroidism. An increase in goiter size may rarely be due to a naturally occurring progression of the disease, in which case the dosage of ATDs must be increased. This can be differentiated with FT4 and FT3 levels. The serum TSH level is not helpful at this time as it may not yet reflect the changes in thyroid hormone and may remain subnormal or suppressed for many months after the T4 and T3 levels have changed.

REMISSION AND TREATMENT FAILURE

Remission rates in Graves' disease vary, with permanent remission rates higher in Europe and Asia than in the United States. Although nonadherence is considered the primary reason for patients not achieving permanent remission, treatment failure can also occur in patients with other conditions such as sarcoidosis of the thyroid gland. It's important to verify that remission has occurred with TSI tests or by weaning meds slowly to see if TSH is still secreted normally in patients on very low ATD doses.

Propylthiouracil

Discovered five years before methimazole, propylthiouracil (PTU) was once the ATD of choice. However, in 2010 PTU was associated with a higher incidence of liver damage and now has a black box warning. In the 2011 treatment survey, among 704 respondents indicating a preferred treatment, 83.5 percent would select methimazole, 13.8 percent carbimazole, and 2.7 percent PTU. In contrast, a 1990 ATA survey indicates that 73 percent of physicians would choose PTU as their preferred medical treatment.

Advantages of PTU include its shorter plasma half-life (75 minutes), staying in the blood circulation only 2–3 hours, and thereby lowering thyroid hormone levels faster. For this reason, PTU is often used in the emergency room setting for treating thyroid storm. In addition, although both PTU and methimazole cross the placenta and are found in breast milk, PTU does so to a lesser degree and is the drug of choice during the first trimester of pregnancy. PTU also partially inhibits the conversion of T4 into T3, reducing FT3 levels in patients with T3 toxicosis. PTU's metabolism is also not affected by kidney or liver disease. The usual starting dose for PTU is 300 mg using doses of 100 mg every 8 hours.

PTU should be discontinued if liver transaminase enzyme levels (either elevated at onset of therapy, found incidentally or measured because of symptoms) reach 2–3 times the upper limit of normal and fail to improve within 1 week with repeat testing. After discontinuing the drug, liver function tests should be monitored weekly until there is evidence of resolution. If resolution is not evident, prompt referral to a gastroenterologist or hepatologist is warranted. Except in cases of severe PTU-induced hepatotoxicity, MMI can be used to control the thyrotoxicosis without ill effects (Bahn et al. 2011, 604).

Methimazole (Tapazole; MMI; Active Metabolite of Carbimazole)

Methimazole (MMI) has a half-life of 4–6 hours and is said to be 10–50 times as potent as PTU, although its effects are not as consistent. Peak serum concentrations occur 1–2 hours after ingestion. The intrathyroidal metabolism of methimazole is slow, with drug concentrations measured 17–20 hours after ingestion similar to those measured 3–6 hours after ingestion. A dose as low as 0.5 mg may have an effect, but a dose of 1.0–1.5 mg is needed if effects are to last for 24 hours. The usual starting dose for methimazole is 20 mg per day with maintenance doses ranging from 2.5 to 10 mg, and lower doses used when weaning off medication. Methimazole can be given once daily because of its longer half-life and its long duration of action. However, blood levels remain more stable when methimazole is taken in 2–3 divided doses (Goodman and Gilman 2006, 1527–30). Doses for methimazole and carbimazole are the same because carbimazole is completely metabolized to methimazole (Abraham et al. 2005). Drug metabolism is not affected by renal (kidney) disease, although it is prolonged in patients with hepatic (liver) disease. Methimazole also offers protection against Graves' ophthalmopathy. Precautions regarding the use of methimazole in pregnancy are included in Chapter 9.

Block-and-Replace Protocol

In the block-and-replace protocol, a small dose of thyroxine is given in conjunction with an ATD. The rationale in adding thyroxine is to prevent the patient from becoming hypothyroid while thyroid hormone production is reduced. The advantage is that the gland is kept at rest while optimal FT4 and FT3 levels are maintained. This protocol initially requires frequent monitoring with blood tests, but once blood levels are stable, repeat labs can be performed every 3 months. In the United States, controversy surrounds this protocol, and a data analysis of comparison studies shows similar remission rates for titration dosing (ATD alone, reducing the dose over time) and block-and-replace protocols (Abraham et al. 2005). Data analysis showed a higher dropout rate for the subjects using block-and-replace.

THE ORIGINAL PROTOCOL

Originating in Japan, where it yielded remission rates as high as 96 percent (Yamamoto et al. 1983), the block-and replace-protocol hasn't yet met with the same success in the United States, where remission rates vary considerably. The markedly higher remission rates reported in the early Japanese studies appear to be directly related to the use of tangible guidelines such as T3 suppression tests tor TSI levels to determine when remission has taken place. Initially, patients were given 300 to 450 mg daily of PTU or 30 to 45 mg of MMI until they became euthyroid. Then 1.0 ug/kg of body weight of T3 was added to the regimen.

At 6-month intervals, the patients were given a 20-minute RAI-U scan (T3 suppression test). When uptake results reached 10 percent, or 10 percent to 15 percent on 2 consecutive readings, the drugs were discontinued (normal RAI-U is about 25 percent). The time for suppression to occur ranged between 12 and 111 months with a mean of 4 years. The patients were then monitored at 6-month intervals for thyroid hormone levels. Of the patients who eventually relapsed, most of them had achieved early remissions (within 1 or 2 years). No patients who went into remission after 40 months of treatment had relapses (Yamamoto 1983).

Once treatment begins, thyroid function tests including levels of FT4 and FT3 should be performed every 2–4 months. Once euthyroidism is established, patients should be monitored at 4- to 6-month intervals. Treatment response is associated with a decrease in goiter size. If the goiter increases, hypothyroidism has probably occurred, although lab tests may be necessary to distinguish hypothyroidism from hyperthyroidism caused by the natural progression of the disease. Since hypothyroidism may have adverse effects on preexisting Graves' opthalmopathy, it's important that the treatment is frequently monitored.

While both drugs are gradually reduced as remission nears, in one popular protocol, the ATD dose is reduced and patients remain on thyroid replacement hormone alone for one year or longer. Because 20 percent of Graves' disease patients spontaneously move into hypothyroidism (which, similar to the course in hyperthyroidism, can run its course and resolve), some patients remain on replacement hormone indefinitely. Block-and-replace protocols are helpful for patients who show a strong goitrogenic response to very low doses of ATDs and become hypothyroid easily when titration therapy is used.

A Minimum ATD Maintenance Dose

Japanese researchers used a minimum maintenance dose of 5 mg MMI every other day to keep patients euthyroid for 6 months before stopping ATDs completely. Their study resulted in a remission rate of 81 percent (Kashiwai et al. 2003). Using the lowest dose needed to keep FT4 near the recommended high end of the range, many patients are kept on doses as low as 1.25 mg methimazole before stopping meds.

In a related study, researchers found that TSH levels are inversely proportional to TSI levels. They discovered that patients who are able to secrete TSH on a minimal ATD dose can be considered in remission. They concluded that the TSH level may be more reflective of the circulating TSI concentration than is thyroid gland function. It's important when using this model that patients be on a minimal ATD dose or TSH may be a reflection of too high of an ATD dose (Kabadi and Premachandra 2007).

Discontinuing ATD Treatment

Debate surrounds the duration of ATD therapy (both titration and the block-and-replace protocols), and with the normal variability seen in Graves' disease, an absolute time frame can't be established. What's important is confirming that remission has occurred before stopping medications. Writing in the *New England Journal of Medicine*, David Cooper, M.D., reports that "treatment with ATDs for 12–18 months is the usual practice, but some patients opt for long-term antithyroid drugs treatment (years or even decades) and there is no theoretical reason why a patient whose disease is well controlled with a small dose of antithyroid drug could not continue antithyroid drug therapy indefinitely." (Cooper 2005).

It's not uncommon for patients, especially younger patients, to have transient symptoms of hyperthyroidism during the first 6 months after the withdrawal of antithyroid drugs. Japanese researchers recommend that physicians follow these patients with laboratory tests for at least one month unless they have unbearable symptoms or complications before resuming ATDs (Kubota et al. 2004).

Higher remission rates are associated with low antibody titers, small goiters, initial T3 toxicosis, milder symptoms and older patients since they usually have milder symptoms. One study (described in Chapter 8) reports higher remission rates using ATDs in conjunction with traditional Chinese medicine. The longer the course of therapy, the more likely it is to see a reduction in antibody titers. Thus, most physicians feel therapy should be continued for at least 12 months.

Surgery (Thyroidectomy)

While surgery in the United States is recommended in only 20 percent of Graves' disease cases (Burch et al. 2012), its prevalence has increased in the past two decades while the use of radioiodine has declined. Surgery is recommended for patients with large goiters showing signs of compression, when large nonfunctioning photopenic, or hypofunctioning nodules are present, in patients with coexisting hyperparathyroidism requiring surgery, females planning pregnancy in less than 6 months, and patients having suspicious thyroid nodules or multinodular goiters (Bahn et al. 2011). Because of its rapid effects, surgery is also sometimes recommended for patients with very large goiters and severe thyrotoxicosis since there is a higher failure rate with radioiodine in these individuals.

Factors indicating that surgery isn't a good option include substantial comorbidity (high surgical risk) such as cardiopulmonary disease, end-stage cancer, or other debilitating disorders. Pregnancy is a relative contraindication in which surgery should be used only when rapid control of hyperthyroidism is needed and ATDs can't be used. Thyroidectomy should also be avoided in the first and third trimesters of pregnancy because of the possibility of birth defects from anesthetic agents, increased risk of fetal loss in the first trimester, and increased risk of preterm labor in the third.

Before deciding on surgery, patients should have an initial trial with ATDs to lower thyroid hormone levels and determine their normal disease course. They should also consult with more than one surgeon and determine the type of surgery that would be most beneficial. Having access to advanced imaging studies, today's surgeons can study the thyroid's anatomy and density beforehand, and they can predetermine the thyroid gland's relationship to the parathyroid glands and other adjacent structures. Also, fine precision surgical tools facilitate identification of the laryngeal nerves. The current success of thyroidectomies can also be attributed to the implementation of pretreatment protocols that render the patient euthyroid before surgery and prepare the tissue to facilitate cutting.

PRETREATMENT

Before surgery, the patient's thyroid hormone levels are lowered with ATDs (takes about six weeks for euthyroidism), with ATDs continued until the day of surgery. Strong iodine solution (three drops of Lugol's solution or five drops SSKI used twice daily) is also given for 7–10 days before surgery to prepare the tissue. Iodine makes the thyroid tissue less vascular (firmer), which facilitates surgery. Patients who are allergic to ATDs or noncompliant can be treated with iopanoic acid, dexamethasone and propranolol for 5–7 days prior to surgery. These drugs are discontinued before surgery.

SURGICAL PROCEDURE OPTIONS

Thyroidectomy procedures include subtotal, near-total, or total thyroidectomy. The most commonly used procedure is the bilateral subtotal thyroidectomy in which 1–2 grams of thyroid tissue is left on both sides. This is also considered the safest procedure. Debate surrounds the amount of tissue that should be removed, with most surgeons leaving 2–3 grams of tissue on either side of the neck.

Alternately, the surgeon may perform a procedure known as a Hartley-Dunhill procedure in which a total lobectomy is performed on one side and a subtotal thyroidectomy is performed on the other side, leaving about 4–5 grams of thyroid tissue. In patients with coexisting eye disease, total thyroidectomy is recommended because it is associated with a decreased level of stimulating TSH receptor antibodies. However, unless the immune system heals, it can continue to produce TSI antibodies, and eye symptoms can worsen. In addition, some patients without evidence of eye changes can develop clinically significant Graves' ophthalmopathy years after surgery. While most TSH receptors (the antigenic prompt for TSI) are located within the thyroid gland, they're also present in other organs.

ADVANTAGES AND DISADVANTAGES OF SURGERY

Surgery offers a prompt reduction of symptoms with a decreased incidence of severe hypothyroidism when compared to radioiodine therapy. In addition, surgery typically requires fewer outpatient visits than ATDs do, and the surgeon is able to detect and remove an existing thyroid carcinoma during surgery if one happens to be present.

ADVERSE EFFECTS AND COMPLICATIONS

Disadvantages include the rare possibility (approximately 1 percent) of recurrent laryngeal nerve injury that can result in permanent vocal cord injury, and hypoparathyroidism (transient in 13 percent of patients and permanent in 1 percent) (Schwartz 1999, 1673). The earliest symptoms of hypoparathyroidism, which may appear from 1 to 7 days after surgery, include anxiety and depression, followed by heightened neuromuscular excitability and spasm. Usually, hypoparathyroidism is transient and can be treated with calcium, although at the onset it is impossible to predict if the condition is temporary or permanent. Following surgery, the patient's serum calcium level is temporarily decreased and the phosphorus level increased. This decrease in blood calcium level (hypocalcemia) is independent of hypoparathyroidism and thought to be caused by the bone's retention of calcium. It is frequently accompanied by a transient rise in the serum alkaline phosphatase level.

Mortality from thyroid surgery is rare. Bleeding onto the operative site, the most serious postoperative complication, can rapidly cause death by asphyxia. Also, if the laryngeal nerve is damaged bilaterally, the airway can be obstructed, requiring an emergency tracheostomy.

Permanent hypothyroidism occurs in 4–40 percent of surgical patients (Schwartz 1999, 1673). Long-term studies indicate that the incidence of developing hypothyroidism after surgery in Graves' disease patients increases over time, which may be due to the natural progression of the disease with the process possibly being accelerated by the surgical destruction of thyroid tissue. This is similar to the cumulative incidence of hypothyroidism over time seen after radioiodine treatment, but it's not as severe. The incidence of hypothyroidism appears to be related to the amount of thyroid tissue left.

Radioiodine Ablation

In the United States, the use of radioiodine ablation for hyperthyroidism is waning. Radioiodine therapy is primarily used in patients resistant to ATD treatment. Radioiodine is contraindicated in women who are pregnant or breast-feeding or who plan on becoming pregnant. Other relative contraindications include progressive ophthalmopathy, large, dense thyroid glands, and the presence of isolated nodules. In Europe, radioiodine is used infrequently, and rarely on women younger than 40 years. Although radioiodine is frequently recommended for elderly patients, some physicians feel that the increased risk of thyroid storm in the elderly puts them at too much risk (Burger 1995, 530–31).

How Radioiodine Works

The thyroid gland absorbs radioiodine, a form of ionizing radiation, in a manner similar to its absorption of iodine. Ionizing radiation includes particulate radiation (mainly alpha and beta particles) and electromagnetic radiation (including gamma and X-rays), which have extremely high frequency and short wavelengths. Radioiodine releases alpha and beta particles and gamma rays and each has its own rate of decay.

Iodine in its natural state has a molecular weight of 127. The radioisotopes of iodine in current use are produced by irradiation in nuclear reactors, cyclotron-charged particle irradiation, or in a process that separates them from nuclear fission products. Ionizing radiation is emitted when radioactive isotopes decay. Ionizing radiation disrupts the atoms and molecules of the tissues through which it passes. Because living tissue is composed of atoms joined into molecules, it is vulnerable to ionizing radiation. The molecular disruptions caused by irradiation produce ions and free radicals that can cause further biochemical damage, including cell death, reproductive effects and cancer.

The Question of Linear Energy Transfer

As radiation impinges on matter and bombards ions, it releases energy in a process called linear energy transfer (LET). Estimation of the cumulative dose over time is known as dosimetry and the absorbed dose is defined as the energy absorbed per unit mass in joules per kilogram (gray or Gy; 1 Gy = 1 joule/kg of tissue) or in ergs per gram (rad).

Radiation kills cells by damaging their DNA, although DNA is not the only target. Although it was originally thought that effects of radiation were proportional to dose, the National Research Council lists several deviations from this rule, including the type of tissue targeted, the growth stage of the cells, cell sensitivity and the dose rate. Recent studies indicate that the energy transfer of radioisotopes may not be linear. Despite popular and universal application for a half century, this concept has yet to be validated or disproved. In studies of cell damage from Nagasaki bomb survivors, a purely cubic model, not a linear model, was found to fit the data best (Burger 1995, 528).

Radioiodine was first produced in 1937, and by 1950 when I-131 was made available, it evolved as a standard treatment for hyperthyroidism. Initially, the use of radioiodine was limited because of the controversy surrounding radiation, already under criticism for being indiscriminately used in treating acne, thymus enlargement, tonsillitis, hemangioma (birthmark) and pertussis (whooping cough).

When radioiodine was being considered as a treatment for hyperthyroidism in the mid–1950s, physicians became alarmed by the results of a 1950 study in which 10 of 28 patients with thyroid cancer had undergone previous irradiation. Subsequent studies showed an increased tumor risk with low doses of irradiation.

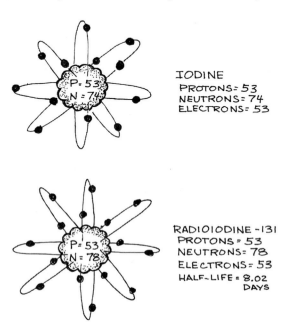

IODINE
PROTONS= 53
NEUTRONS= 74
ELECTRONS= 53

RADIOIODINE –131
PROTONS = 53
NEUTRONS= 78
ELECTRONS= 53
HALF–LIFE = 8.02
DAYS

Iodine and radioiodine molecules (courtesy Marvin G. Miller).

However, the Cooperative Thyrotoxicosis Therapy Study, comparing surgery, antithyroid drugs and radioiodine ablation for post-treatment cancer deaths, which was conducted at 26 institutions and involved thousands of patients, concluded that radioiodine is a safe treatment for hyperthyroidism. With publication of these results, radioiodine wended its way to the center stage of the treatment arena in the U.S. However, the debate regarding the safety of radiation continues to this day and is discussed later in this chapter.

BIOLOGICAL EFFECTS OF RADIOIODINE

When radioiodine is localized in the thyroid gland, its distribution depends on the type of radiation and the energy of the emissions, with 73 percent to 96 percent of the total radiation dose from radioiodines attributed to particulate irradiations. The mean particle range is highly variable, although it is known to be longer for beta emitters such as I-131. Although I-131 emits both gamma and beta irradiation, beta particles are responsible for the destruction seen in thyroid cells. Since their path length exceeds the diameter of thyroid cells, thyroid cells are irradiated even if they haven't trapped radioiodine. However, in patients with large, dense thyroid glands, the rays may be unable to fully penetrate the cells, inhibiting complete ablation.

Determining an optimal ablative dose is difficult because of individual sensitivity and the varying size of the individual thyroid follicles. At the usual ablative doses, follicular cells are destroyed and the biological effects are primarily on thyroid function. Following ablation, radioiodine particles lodge in the thyroid follicle and remain while undergoing radioactive decay. The effective half-life of I-131 ranges from 2 to 8 days, with a mean of 5.5 days.

Half-life denotes the time for the original dose to be reduced by 50 percent. The amount remaining will be further reduced by 50 percent every 5.5 days. For radioiodine, usually 8 to 10 half-life cycles are required for the entire dose to be reduced (44 to 55 days). However, the actual time for radioiodine to leave the body depends on the dose. Since atoms are being reduced in the process, with an initial dose of 1 trillion atoms, when reduced by half each 5.5 days, it will take considerable time for the total RAI dose to be reduced.

Because the rate of cell division in the normal thyroid is quite slow, sublethal radiation effects such as the development of both benign and malignant neoplasms may take many years to become clinically apparent, especially at low doses. When higher doses are used, most of the thyroid tissue is destroyed and the incidence of neoplasms is lower. To date, no irradiated population has been adequately studied through its life span. What studies have been done focus on mortality.

CELLULAR DAMAGE FROM RADIOIODINE

Dr. Joseph Gong, a cell biologist at the State University of New York at Buffalo, has studied the effects of ionizing radiation for the Atomic Energy Commission for many years. His lifelong passion has been to quantify these effects. Cellular effects of radiation, he has found, include a prolonged increase of red cell precursors known as normoblasts in the bone marrow and the presence of a subpopulation of erythrocyte (red cells) with transferrin (involved in iron uptake) receptors. By measuring the percentage of erythrocytes with transferrin receptors present in a blood sample, Dr. Gong can assess radiation injury. Dr. Gong has studied the effects of external radiation on humans and is able to measure the lifelong cumulative effects (Gong 1999, 713). The effects in people with hyperthyroidism have never been studied.

CHROMOSOMAL DAMAGE

Although several studies have shown distinct leukocyte (white blood cell) chromosomal abnormalities in patients treated with radioiodine, the clinical importance is unclear. However, the whole body is exposed to radiation following radioiodine therapy. The Nuclear Regulatory Commission reports that a whole-body dose as low as 0.1 Gy or 10 rad in 100,000 persons would cause 800 additional deaths from cancer (Beir 1990).

Gonadal irradiation is of particular concern because radioiodine is ultimately excreted in the urinary bladder. The estimated gonadal dose is thought to be similar to that of other common radiographic procedures such as barium enema and intravenous pyelography. One recent study showed that ionizing radiation is carcinogenic even without hitting the cell nucleus, an event that was previously thought necessary for mutations. Study results indicate that genetic damage at low-dose radiation exposures is likely to be more significant than previously thought. Apparently, irradiation of the cytoplasm by alpha particles creates highly reactive free radicals that migrate to the cell nucleus and mutate the DNA (Conway 1999).

RAI PRETREATMENT

Because radioiodine can cause a temporary increase in thyroid hormone levels, some physicians lower their patient's thyroid hormone levels with ATDs before ablation. However, pretreated patients often require a larger RAI dose. For this reason, it's recommended that patients stop ATDs for 3–5 days before ablation to allow adequate uptake of radioiodine by the thyroid. The ATDs are then restarted 3–7 days later, and generally tapered over 4–6 weeks as thyroid function normalizes (Bahn et al. 2011, 601).

RADIOIODINE PROCEDURE AND MODE OF ACTION

Patients are advised to avoid ingesting excess iodine for two weeks prior to ablation, and iodine contrast dyes are to be avoided. Excess iodine may interfere with the body's uptake of radioiodine. Strong iodine solution (SSKI) should not be used for the first three days after radioiodine treatment. However, it may be started on the fourth day to relieve symptoms of thyrotoxicosis until thyroid hormone levels fall.

Radioiodine treatment is usually administered in the form of a drink of I-131 commonly referred to as a radioactive cocktail. Taken orally, I-131 is dissolved in water or swallowed as a capsule. I-131 is rapidly absorbed and quickly concentrated, oxidized and organified by thyroid follicular cells. There is no general agreement on what constitutes an optimal dose. The methods of calculating the dose are controversial, although most systems consider the RAI-U results and the size and density of the thyroid.

Radioiodine therapy is generally designed to deliver 5,000 to 10,000 rads to the thyroid tissue. This can usually be achieved by a dose of approximately 7.5 mCi. Many clinics have settled on an arbitrary dose calculated to result in the delivery of 185 to 222 Mbq (5 to 7 mCi) of I-131 to the thyroid gland 24 hours after administration. The standard dose has also been listed as 5.9 Mbq (160 uCi) per gram of estimated gland weight, which leads to a higher incidence of hypothyroidism. Thus, some physicians using this method administer prophylactic doses of thyroxine.

RADIATION SAFETY

Radiologists are required to explain the biological risks, including the increased risk for Graves' ophthalmopathy, to the patient before RAI is administered. The consent form the patient must sign follows guidelines directed by the Nuclear Regulatory Commission and is designed to ensure that the patient has been informed of other available treatment options, the progression to hypothyroidism that occurs, and other potential risks.

Following ablation, the patient is instructed to avoid intimate contact, including kissing, for at least 3–4 days. Because the thyroid glands of infants and young children are most susceptible to radiation, patients are instructed to avoid carrying infants on the shoulder and to avoid hugging children where thyroid-to-thyroid contact might occur. Since radioiodine is excreted via the urine, the toilet should be flushed 2 to 3 times after use, and the hands should be thoroughly washed. Pregnancy is not advised for 6 to 12 months after ablation. Some of the guidelines recommended by the Nuclear Regulatory Commission include:

- Use private toilet facilities, if possible, and flush twice after each use.
- Bathe daily and wash hands frequently.
- Drink a normal amount of fluids.
- Use disposable eating utensils or wash utensils separately from others.
- Sleep alone and avoid prolonged intimate contact for 3 or 4 days.
- Launder linens, towels, and clothes daily at home, separately. No special cleaning of the washing machine is required between loads.
- Do not prepare food for others that requires prolonged handling with bare hands.
- Avoid becoming pregnant for 6–12 months after treatment.
- Many facilities require a pregnancy test within 24 hours prior to RAI in women of childbearing age who have not had a surgical procedure to prevent pregnancy.

Patients who need to travel immediately after radioactive iodine treatment are advised to carry a letter of explanation from their physician. Radiation detection devices used at airports and federal buildings may be sensitive to the radiation levels present in patients up to 3 months following treatment with I-131. Depending on the amount of radioactivity administered during your treatment, your endocrinologist or radiation safety officer may recommend continued precautions for up to several weeks after treatment. The Society of Nuclear Medicine has prepared a list of guidelines that is available at http://interactive.snm.org/index.cfm?PageID=11031 (accessed December 1, 2012).

ADVANTAGES, DISADVANTAGES AND LONG-TERM RISKS OF RAI

The advantages of radioiodine ablation are that it is quickly administered, generally effective, relatively inexpensive and initially painless. It requires few office visits until hypothyroidism develops. The disadvantages are that it invariably causes permanent hypothyroidism, and it may affect other organs such as the salivary glands, the gastric glands, the parathyroid glands, the pancreas and the gonads. Difficulties in determining an optimal dose and misinterpreted laboratory results (the persistent suppression of TSH causing some doctors to think the patient is still hyperthyroid) cause many patients to have a second ablation. In addition RAI is known to significantly induce or exacerbate Graves' ophthalmopathy and pretibial myxedema. By stimulating the immune system, RAI can also lead to the development of other autoimmune disorders.

Worsening of Graves' ophthalmopathy is reported to not occur immediately in patients using corticosteroids with RAI. However, Graves' ophthalmopathy is associated with TSI antibodies, and these antibodies can remain elevated for many years after RAI. It's not unusual for patients to develop Graves' ophthalmopathy many years after RAI.

Controversy also surrounds the cancer risk associated with radioiodine. Although most mortality studies report that radioiodine causes no increased deaths from cancer, a recent study in the British medical journal *Lancet* involving 7,417 patients treated between 1950 and 1991 in Birmingham, United Kingdom, indicates that although the overall risk of cancer is low, there is a significant increase in cancers of the thyroid and small bowel following radioiodine ablation. The authors of this study suggest that the increased relative risk for these cancers indicates a need for long-term vigilance in those receiving radioiodine (Franklyn et al. 1999).

Another provocative study of roughly the same United Kingdom cohort reports that among hyperthyroid patients treated with radioiodine, mortality from all causes and mortality due to thyroid disease, cardiovascular and cerebrovascular disease (stroke) and fracture are increased. The highest incidence of mortality occurred in the first year following treatment and was observed primarily in women. The overall risk was confined to patients who were older than 49 at the time of treatment. The overall risk of fracture was confined to patients who were older than 59 at the time of treatment, which put them in the age range typically associated with increased fracture at the time of the study. Mortality from all causes increased with increasing cumulative doses of radioiodine (Franklyn 1998). Although this study has been criticized, with critics saying that the causes of death were related to age more than to RAI, many patients criticize the fact that there are no studies indicating the incidence of cancer apart from cases listing cancer as the cause of death.

A report of the Cooperative Thyrotoxicosis Therapy Follow-up Study Group indicates that radioiodine does not increase total cancer deaths, although it poses a significantly increased risk of death from thyroid cancer. Thyroid cancer risk is reported to possibly be a result of the original thyroid disease, although this increased risk is not seen in patients treated with ATDs or surgery (Ron et al. 1998).

In 2010, researchers reviewed the data on 18,156 hospitalized Graves' disease patients and found an increased risk of thyroid and parathyroid tumors in the first 2 years following RAI. Cancer sites with observed excess included the mouth and breast (Shu et al. 2010). In a study of 10,552 Swedish patients with hyperthyroidism treated with radioiodine, researchers found a significant increase in cancer mortality, especially in cancers of the digestive and respiratory systems (Metso et al. 2007). In another study, Jane Franklyn and her colleagues found cardiovascular disease mortality increased in patients with hyperthyroidism after radioiodine therapy, but not in patients with overt hypothyroidism who are treated with T4 (Franklyn et al. 2005).

RADIATION THYROIDITIS AND HYPOPARATHYROIDISM

Radiation thyroiditis develops within the first few weeks of treatment and may lead to an exacerbation of symptoms resulting in serious consequences including thyroid storm related to the release of stored hormone from ruptured thyroid follicles. Milder side effects include sore throat and pain on swallowing, which are associated with thyroidal inflammation and tenderness. On the cellular level, side effects include thyroid epithelial cell swelling and necrosis, disruption of follicular cells, edema and infiltration with leukocytes. After this acute phase, the thyroid gland is marred by fibrosis, vascular narrowing and lymphocytic infiltration. These changes are associated with a reduction in thyroid volume, which reflects thyroid damage.

In hyperthyroidism, radioiodine reduces symptoms by destroying thyroid tissue, preferentially the active follicular cells. Biological effects of I-131 include impaired replication of intact follicular cells, atrophy, fibrosis and a chronic inflammatory response that may ultimately result in permanent thyroid failure (Chiovatae et al. 1988). The parathyroid glands are exposed to radiation and parathyroid reserve may also be diminished in some patients.

HYPOTHYROIDISM

Permanent hypothyroidism occurs in nearly everyone who has RAI. Although the incidence of hypothyroidism is greatest during the first two years following treatment, 25 to 50 percent of patients become hypothyroid within the first year. The incidence increases at a rate of approximately 5 percent with each successive year with nearly all patients becoming hypothyroid within 10 years (Greenspan 1997, 226).

The sudden onset of hypothyroidism in a previously thyrotoxic patient may result in severe muscle cramps, especially in large muscle groups such as the trapezius or latissimus dorsi or the proximal muscles of the extremities. Psychiatric symptoms, including psychosis, may also develop when thyroid hormone levels fall quickly. The development of hypothyroidism and thyroid failure are related to thyroid cell destruction and also the increasingly high titers of stimulating TSH receptor antibodies seen following ablation.

RELAPSE FOLLOWING RADIOIODINE

Relapse following radioiodine is most often seen in patients having larger pretreatment thyroid volumes that I-131 rays can't fully penetrate. Relapse is also associated with the volume of the thyroid tissue remaining after treatment with larger volumes associated with relapse, except in the case of transient enlargement due to the inflammatory response. Often, when patients are told treatment wasn't successful, they have a low TSH level, which is expected and not a sign of persistent hyperthyroidism. Post-RAI, thyroid status is based on thyroid hormone levels. Usually, euthyroidism and goiter shrinkage are evident within 6–8 weeks after radioiodine therapy. Hypothyroidism can occur within weeks to many months after treatment.

Ionic Transport Inhibitors and Dexamethasone

Ionic inhibitors are substances that interfere with the thyroid's ability to concentrate iodide into iodine. These substances are monovalent hydrated ions that resemble iodine. Thus, they are able to displace it, inhibiting thyroid hormone synthesis.

One of the first ionic inhibitors discovered is the heart medication thiocyanate. Its natural ability to block thyroid hormone synthesis led researchers to develop compounds with similar modes of action. Some of the goitrogen plant compounds metabolize into thiocyanate after ingestion.

Perchlorate is 10 times as active as thiocyanate. Years ago, perchlorate was routinely used to treat hyperthyroidism using doses of 2 to 3 grams. At such excessive doses, perchlorate was found to cause aplastic anemia, which can be fatal. Since early 1990, perchlorate treatment has seen a revival using lower doses, 750 mg (0.75 grams). Perchlorate is used to treat the thyrotoxicosis of Graves' disease and also amiodarone-induced hyperthyroidism. Perchlorate is present in concentrations of up to 1.0 percent in many fertilizers and as an atmospheric by-product of solid fuel propellant used in rockets, missiles and fireworks. These environmental sources of perchlorate are suspected of causing hypothyroidism in children.

Other ionic inhibitors include lithium, which is used in the treatment of bipolar disorder, fluoride, bromide, chlorine and iodinated radiographic contrast agents such as sodium iopanoate and sodium ipodate. Lithium is sometimes used in severe thyrotoxicosis in place of strong iodine solution in patients who are allergic to iodine. Lithium carbonate inhibits thyroid hormone secretion with the advantage that it doesn't interfere with radioiodine uptake. Lithium is generally used at a dose of 300 to 450 mg given every 8 hours resulting in a serum concentration of 1 mEq/L, which has a therapeutic range of 0.5 to 1.5 mEq/L. The fluoride compound fluoborate is considered as effective as perchlorate.

Although they are still occasionally used, contrast agents have side effects that make them undesirable treatment agents for long-term use. Ipodate used in doses of 1 gram daily causes a prompt reduction of serum T4 and T3 in hyperthyroid patients. The effects of ipodate include iodine release and inhibition of T4's conversion to T3. As with strong iodine solution, withdrawal of ipodate may result in an exacerbation of symptoms.

Dexamethasone administered as a 2 mg dose every 6 hours inhibits thyroid hormone secretion and the peripheral conversion of T4 to T3. Dexamethasone also has an immunosuppressive effect and is sometimes used along with beta adrenergic blocking agents and strong iodine solution to provide rapid relief in cases of thyroid storm.

The major advantage of these compounds is that they do not generally produce hypothyroidism, yet they effectively relieve symptoms of thyrotoxicosis. The disadvantage is the frequency of recurrence if they are not used until the hyperthyroid disorder runs its course.

Beta Adrenergic Blocking Agents (Beta Blockers)

Beta blockers are used as an adjuvant therapy to relieve symptoms of thyrotoxicosis that result from excessive catecholamine stimulation, primarily cardiac symptoms and anxiety. The major effects of beta blockers are on the cardiovascular system (slowing the heart and decreasing its contractions). Beta blockers decrease tremulousness, palpitations, tachycardia, excessive sweating, heat intolerance, nervousness, anxiety, eyelid retraction and the Graves' stare, but they do not normalize the metabolic rate. Beta blockers also reduce blood pressure in hypertensive patients but have no effect in patients with normal blood pressure. Beta blockers are usually used early in therapy and stopped when thyroid hormone levels fall back into the reference range.

PROPRANOLOL AND RELATED DRUGS

Propranolol is the drug usually prescribed (except in patients with bronchial disorders, chronic obstructive pulmonary disease or asthma since propranolol aggravates bronchospasm) because it has a slight diminishing effect on the conversion of T4 to T3. The dose initially prescribed is 20 to 40 mg of propranolol to be taken up to four times daily or 50 to 100 mg of atenolol or metoprolol, which can be taken once daily due to its longer half-life. For patients with severe symptoms, propranolol or esmolol can be given intravenously. For patients with congestive heart failure, beta blockers should be avoided. For patients with asthma, cardioselective beta blockers, such as atenolol and metoprolol, are used.

Many patients with mild to moderate symptoms are instructed to take the medications as needed (without exceeding the maximum dose) with the precaution that beta blockers can cause sluggishness at high doses in some patients. As the patient moves toward euthyroidism, the dosage is generally decreased, and discontinued when the patient becomes euthyroid. After continuous long-term treatment, beta adrenergic antagonists should not be discontinued abruptly, as this can exacerbate angina and pose a risk of sudden death. Increased sensitivity to catecholamine stimulation may persist for one week. Therefore, when taken regularly, the drug should be tapered and withdrawn slowly.

SIDE EFFECTS AND PRECAUTIONS

Side effects of beta blockers include decreased plasma potassium, decreased intraocular pressure, light-headedness, depression, lassitude, weakness, fatigue, visual disturbances, vivid dreams, an acute reversible syndrome characterized by disorientation for time and place, short term memory loss, nausea, vomiting, thrombocytopenic purpura, agranulocytosis and rare occurrences of drug-related lupus.

Beta blockers may mask symptoms of thyrotoxicosis, and an abrupt withdrawal of the drug may be followed by an exacerbation of hyperthyroid symptoms, including the potential progression to thyroid storm. While beta blockers are often used as the sole therapy in patients with mild or subclinical hyperthyroidism, they are not recommended as the sole pretreatment agent before surgery since abrupt withdrawal is associated with thyroid storm.

Lugol's Solution, Saturated Solution Potassium Iodine (SSKI)

Before the discovery of radioiodine, saturated solutions of potassium iodine (SSKI, Lugol's) were used to treat hyperthyroidism. SSKI contains more iodine (6 mg/day or more) than could be obtained through diet (U.S. diet provides 300–700 mcg iodine). Once the only medical treatment available for hyperthyroidism, SSKI is primarily used today to quickly lower thyroid hormone levels in thyroid storm or as a therapeutic option mainly used by naturopaths. SSKI inhibits the release of thyroid hormone from the thyroid gland and it also causes a transient inhibition of thyroid hormone synthesis known as the Wolff-Chaikoff effect.

Because the body has a natural regulatory mechanism or form of autoregulation known as the "escape from the Wolff-Chaikoff effect," the effects of SSKI are naturally limited to 12 days, preventing hypothyroidism from developing. Autoregulation is a protective measure influenced by levels of iodine and thyroid hormone. The body's autoregulatory mechanism causes an escape from this inhibition, thereby preventing blood levels of thyroid hormone from becoming critically low and causing goiter or hypothyroidism. The protocol for using SSKI therapy in hyperthyroidism must be managed by a skilled practitioner experienced in titrating the dose appropriately to ensure a constant lowering of thyroid hormone levels.

Specific Conditions of Hyperthyroidism and Their Treatments

While most conditions of hyperthyroidism can be treated with any of the treatments, certain treatments are highly recommended for specific disorders, and in some cases, specific treatments are used.

Percutaneous Ethanol Injection (PEI) for Nodules

Injections of ethanol can be administered directly to toxic thyroid nodules, cysts and large nontoxic thyroid nodules. PEI has been shown to be an effective therapy for reducing thyroid volume in specific areas of thyroid tissue. In hyperthyroid patients, anti-thyroid drugs are initially used to restore euthyroidism.

Ultrasound-Guided Laser Thermal Ablation (LTA) for Nodules

Percutaneous laser thermal ablation is used to reduce both hyperfunctioning and compressive nodules. The safety and usefulness of LTA, which has previously been used to ablate tumors, has been proven effective by Italian researchers (Spiezia et al. 2007). The researchers used color and power Doppler ultrasonography to guide the ablation, and the effects of LTA on thyroid nodules were monitored by ultrasound during the procedure. The researchers concluded that PEI under ultrasonographic guidance is an effective and safe treatment of benign hot and cold thyroid nodules, causing shrinkage of thyroid nodules, normalization of thyroid function in hyperfunctioning nodules, and improvement of patient's compliance.

Levothyroxine Suppressive Therapy for Nodules

Benign toxic nodules are often treated with levothyroxine in an effort to lower TSH levels. TSH causes thyroid cells to grow and produce hormone. By raising thyroid hormone levels to or slightly above the FT4 reference range, TSH is suppressed and unable to cause cell growth or thyroid hormone production. However, the efficacy of levothyroxine on reducing the size of thyroid nodules is still controversial. The American Thyroid Association (ATA) does not recommend routine use of this procedure because of side effects of the therapy (enhanced coagulation), questionable effectiveness of its long-term use, and regrowth after cessation of the therapy. However, data from multiple randomized control trials and meta-analyses suggest that levothyroxine suppression therapy may result in decrease of nodule size in regions of the world with borderline low iodine intake (Demir et al. 2009).

Treatment of Resistance to Thyroid Hormone

Resistance to thyroid hormone (RTH) is a dominantly inherited condition of impaired tissue responsiveness to thyroid hormone that can cause hypothyroidism, hyperthyroidism of variable severity and, occasionally, symptoms of simultaneous thyroid hormone deficiency and excess. Nearly all cases of RTH are caused by mutations in the thyroid hormone receptor beta gene. The mutant thyroid hormone receptor molecules have either reduced affinity for T3 or impaired interaction with one of the cofactors involved in the mediation of thyroid hormone action.

Treatment for hyperthyroidism in this condition consists of anti-thyroid drugs to normalize thyroid hormone and beta blockers to reduce symptoms. Researchers say it is reasonable to expect specific treatments in the near distant future. One suggestion would be selection of an oocyte that doesn't have the mutation from the affected mother that could be used in in vitro fertilization (Weiss and Refetoff 1999).

Treatment in TSH Receptor Mutations, Familial Kopp

In order to achieve a permanent cure for hyperthyroidism in individuals with TSH receptor mutations, it is necessary to destroy all thyroid tissue, either by thyroidectomy followed by radioiodine therapy or radiotherapy alone. In younger patients, temporary therapy with thionamides can be considered. Because the condition may not be readily recognized and confused with Graves' disease, patients treated with thionamides or insufficient amounts of radioiodine have frequent relapses.

Treatment Outcome Studies

While these studies primarily include patients with Graves' disease, the outcomes of treatment are applicable for other patients with hyperthyroid disorders.

In one Swedish study involving 174 Graves' disease patients, younger patients (20 to 34 years) were treated with their choice of surgery or ATDs in conjunction with thyroxine (block-and-replace approach), while older patients were given the added option of radioiodine ablation. Two years after treatment, most patients recommended their treatment to others. In patients with Graves' ophthalmopathy, 20 percent reported that the eye problems were much more troublesome than the thyroid problems. The costs of treatment, with surgery being most expensive, were not as significantly different when relapses were taken into consideration (Ljunggren et al. 1998).

In another study conducted in Chile over a period of 30 years, Graves' patients treated with surgery, PTU or radioiodine were compared to determine the efficacy of achieving euthyroidism. Surgery resulted in euthyroidism in 70.2 percent of patients. Radioiodine ablation accounted for the highest rate of hypothyroidism (72.1 percent) regardless of the ablative dose used. PTU used alone achieved remission in only 26.4 percent of patients. However, when PTU was combined with T4, the success rose to 62.5 percent. In the block-and-replace protocol designed by Yamamoto described earlier in this chapter, which is guided by RAI uptake suppression tests, 87.5 percent of patients achieved long-standing euthyroidism. The authors of this study recommend using anti-thyroid drugs as a first approach and assessing the RAI-U or TRAb levels after six months. If improvement is seen, T4 is added to the regimen. If there is no improvement at this time, it's recommended that radioiodine or surgery be used (Pineda et al. 1998).

Treatments Under Investigation

Arterial Embolization

Thyroid arterial embolization is a procedure in which the arteries leading to the thyroid gland are blocked. This interferes with the thyroid gland's ability to produce thyroid hormone. Embolization techniques are approved in the United States for parathyroid gland and hepatic surgeries.

At this writing, there are no American physicians certified to perform thyroid arterial embolization, although they are available in Canada, Asia and Europe. Thyroid arterial embolization is used in patients with severe hyperthyroidism who cannot tolerate or who prefer not to use conventional treatment methods (radioiodine ablation, thyroidectomy, or anti-thyroid drugs). Arterial embolization is also used in patients whose severe hyperthyroidism puts them at risk for surgery or ablation (Xiao et al. 2002).

The Novel Molecule

National Institutes of Health (NIH) researchers are investigating the cause of Graves' disease and looking for therapies aimed at stopping the disease process. The novel molecule making headlines is a small-molecule antagonist that directly inhibits or prevents TSI antibodies from activating the TSH receptor. When TSI activates the TSH receptor on thyroid cells, the cells are ordered to produce excess thyroid hormone. Blocked by the novel molecule, TSI doesn't cause hyperthyroidism. TSI also contributes to the development of Graves' ophthalmopathy (thyroid eye disease) when these antibodies activate TSH receptors on orbital cells; and they contribute to pretibial myxedema when they activate the TSH receptor on dermal cells. This novel antagonist molecule offers great promises for these disorders as well.

In this study, Dr. Marvin Gershengorn and Susanne Neumann and their teams at the Clinical Endocrinology Branch of the National Institute of Diabetes and Digestive and Kidney Diseases and National Institutes of Health Chemical Genomics Centers at the National Institutes of Health (NIH) have isolated this molecule and they've shown that it inhibits receptor signaling. This was demonstrated in four patients with active Graves' disease using in vitro systems.

The researchers have investigated several analogs of the small-molecule antagonist and are currently working with the best molecule for human study. In this model system, NCGC00229600 inhibited both basal and TSH-stimulated cAMP production although TSH binding was not affected. The small-molecule antagonist has not yet been studied in clinical trials. Further research in patients with both Graves' disease and Graves' ophthalmopathy is expected to begin in the near future. A small molecule capable of stimulating the TSH receptor has already been tested in animal trials (Neumann et al. 2011).

Therapeutic Peptides

Researchers are developing antagonistic peptides that interfere with the action of TSH receptor antibodies as well as peptides that bind to TSH receptor antibodies, preventing them from reacting with the TSH receptor (Park et al. 1999).

8

Complementary and Alternative Treatments for Hyperthyroidism

In recent years the use of alternative medicine in treating hyperthyroidism has become more widespread, both as a complementary therapy used with conventional medicine and as the sole therapeutic agent. Dietary changes, supplements, herbal medicines, psychosocial stress relief, homeopathy, and energy therapies are some of the most popular therapies. Alternative therapies for hyperthyroidism are generally part of a wellness protocol aimed at lowering thyroid hormone levels and healing the underlying causes.

Alternative Medicine's Treatment Goals

Alternative and allopathic medicine have identical goals for treating hyperthyroidism. They both aim to reduce the amount of thyroid hormone available to the body's cells. Some alternative therapies, particularly herbal medicine, have anti-thyroid properties and have a similar mode of action to the ATDs. Similar to ATDs, alternative treatments differ from aggressive conventional therapies for hyperthyroidism in that they promote the body's own natural healing ability.

Alternative Healing Philosophy

Alternative medicine is shaped by Western cultural context as well as Eastern tradition, and it employs a variety of options, varying between the simplicity of attending a weekly yoga class to a more detailed life plan that

160

completely adheres to holistic guidelines. Alternative medicine recognizes that each of us has an inherently unique physical and psychological profile or constitution resulting from predisposed hereditary, social and environmental factors. Also, one's inherent life force is taken into consideration.

This vital life force is called chi or qi in China, and kundalini in ancient India. For optimal health, this vital force must be in balance, and its flow must not be blocked. Its polar opposites are the yin and yang of traditional Chinese medicine, the kyo and jitsu of Japanese shiatsu, and the Ayurvedic doshas. Holistic medicine focuses on correcting these imbalances and allowing the free flow of energy. Thus, five patients with similar symptoms would likely all be prescribed different treatments tailored to their unique constitution and flow of vital energy.

Dietary Influences

Diet plays an important role in both the development and treatment of hyperthyroidism. Thyroid hormone is produced when iodine and tyrosine molecules combine. Diets high in iodine can cause hyperthyroidism, a fact that the makers of Hill's pet food considered when they developed a cat food low in iodine (Hill's y/d) for use as a treatment in feline hyperthyroidism. Several small studies show the product lowers thyroid hormone levels, but it's not certain how successful this product will be due to taste concerns, adherence, and other factors. See http://www.askavetquestion.com/yd.php (accessed December 12, 2012).

Besides the question of iodine, food allergens can trigger or worsen Graves' disease by stimulating the immune system. Patients with both gluten sensitivity and an autoimmune thyroid disorder show increases in both gliadin and thyroid antibodies when they eat gluten and a reduction in antibodies and symptoms when they refrain (see also Chapter 2). Food dyes, aspartame, and other chemicals can also stimulate the immune system causing a similar increase in thyroid antibodies. Overall, improvement is seen when hyperthyroid patients follow gluten-free diets and avoid processed foods.

The Role of Iodine

Although iodine is of particular importance in hyperthyroidism, its role in the general population is variable. A study on the short-term ingestion of kelp shows that iodine excess can cause either hypothyroidism or hyperthyroidism in patients genetically predisposed to thyroid disease, although the effect is minimal in normal subjects (Clark et al. 2003). This confirms previous research showing that iodine is a trigger for autoimmune thyroid disease, both hypothyroidism and hyperthyroidism.

Strong solutions of saturated potassium iodide (SSKI, Lugol's), doses much higher than provided by diet, inhibit the production of thyroid hormone and the release of thyroid hormone from the gland and are used as a treatment for hyperthyroidism (see Chapter 8). Excess iodine also causes some hyperthyroid patients to have an unnatural desire for prolonged sleep, although this tendency may be caused by calcium deficiency more than iodine excess (Vogel 1991, 155–65).

The daily requirement for iodine is 75–150 mcg daily. Iodine in amounts greater than 150 mcg daily can trigger the development of Graves' disease in genetically predisposed individuals. Alternately, patients with autoimmune thyroiditis or who have been treated with radioiodine ablation are particularly sensitive to the anti-thyroid effects of iodide and experience a worsening of hypothyroidism with excess dietary iodine.

Iodine Excess and Deficiency

As mentioned, excess dietary iodine can increase or decrease hormone synthesis depending on a person's iodine status, thyroid status and individual sensitivity. Excess iodine can cause goiter as well as rashes, asthma and acne. Considering that iodine is present not only in food but in many vitamin and mineral supplements, kelp extracts, and certain drugs used for respiratory (iodinated glycerol compounds) and heart problems (amiodarone), it's not difficult to unintentionally ingest excess iodine.

Iodine deficiency can lead to hypothyroidism, and it's associated with a higher incidence of toxic multinodular goiter. Geographical areas such as Greece where iodine deficiency is prevalent are associated with milder conditions of Graves' disease.

Goitrogens

Goitrogens are foods with phytochemicals that lower thyroid hormone levels (see Chapter 8). Adding 1 to 1.5 cups daily can be as effective as a low dose of anti-thyroid drugs. Goitrogens include: cabbage, kale, kohlrabi, rutabaga, Brussels sprouts, turnips, cauliflower, rape, mustard greens and other members of the Brassica family; the cyanoglucosides, which include cassava, maize, bamboo shoots, sweet potatoes and lima beans; and the non–Brassica cruciferae with goitrogenic properties, which include horseradish, cress and radish. Levels of goitrogens are highest in the seeds of these plants. Other goitrogens include peanuts, soy, sweet potatoes, millet, peaches, and members of the mint family, including mint, borage, basil, oregano, marjoram, oregano, mustard greens, pears, almonds and spinach, lemon balm, rosemary, lavender and hyssop.

Effects of Soy on Iodine Absorption

Soybean extracts also have goitrogenic properties. Soy lowers thyroid hormone levels by decreasing the amount of iodine that is absorbed from the intestine. In the 1950s, soy protein was found to cause goiter and iodine deficiency in infants fed soy formula. The problem was corrected by supplementing soy formula. Recent research suggests that a problem with soy still exists. Soy isoflavones inhibit thyroid peroxidase, an enzyme essential for the body's synthesis and metabolism of thyroid hormone. Unfermented products such as tofu, soymilk, texturized soy protein, and soy protein isolate are reported to pose the most risk (Osborne 1999).

Diet in Hyperthyroidism

Most general dietary recommendations for hyperthyroidism involve a predominantly whole foods diet with adequate but not excess protein. Substances to be avoided include excess dietary iodine, sugar, dairy products, processed foods, hot spicy foods, and gluten if gluten sensitivity is present or suspected. Because of the many nutrient deficiencies associated with hyperthyroidism, high-nutrient foods should be selected.

A Macrobiotic Approach

William Duffy, in his English version of *You Are All Sanpaku* by George Oshawa, includes Graves' disease in the sixth stage or phase of diseases caused by an imbalance of yin and yang. Disorders in the sixth stage are a long time in the making, he writes, but improvement can be seen almost immediately by following a dietary regimen based on macrobiotic principles. For optimal results in severe cases, he recommends a protocol known as Regimen Number 7, which allows only unrefined cereals.

His prescription for healing includes avoiding sugar (including fruit and fruit juices), limiting liquids and animal products (including dairy products), avoiding nightshade vegetables, avoiding all processed or imported foods, and avoiding spices, coffee and teas. Fish, shellfish, and wild game are permitted. He recommends that one's daily diet include 60 percent to 70 percent unrefined grains or cereals and 20 percent to 25 percent baked or cooked vegetables, and that food be chewed 50 times (Duffy 1965).

Nutrient Deficiencies

In hyperthyroidism, the body's cells consume increased oxygen, depleting nutrient supplies. The increased bowel motility seen along with conditions of gluten sensitivity contributes to malabsorption of nutrients, especially oil-soluble vitamins and B vitamins. Specific nutrient deficiencies cause new symptoms and aggravate others.

Vitamin A

Deficiencies of vitamin A may cause diminished adaptation to darkness in some patients (night blindness). Both thyroxine (thyroid hormone) and vitamin A share the transport protein transthyretin, or TTR (protein that transports hormones within the body). Excess thyroid hormone binds to most of the TTR, preventing vitamin A's absorption and its conversion from carotene. Vitamin A and vitamin B_2 (riboflavin) are essential for proper thyroid function.

Coenzyme Q10 (CoQ10)

Coenzyme Q10 (CoQ10), which is also known as ubiquinone, is a naturally occurring nutrient present in the mitochondria in each cell of the body. First identified by researchers at the University of Wisconsin in 1957, CoQ10 is important for energy metabolism. In addition, CoQ10 has antioxidant and anti-inflammatory properties and acts as a cofactor in that it enhances the effectiveness of other vitamins, particularly B vitamins. Coenzyme Q10 is depleted in hyperthyroidism, and a deficiency of CoQ10 is responsible for the characteristic muscle weakness that occurs in this disorder.

Low levels of CoQ10 are associated with many diseases, including chronic pulmonary diseases, cardiovascular diseases including congestive heart failure, migraine disorders, muscular dystrophies, hypertension, diabetes, some cancers and autoimmune diseases and Parkinson's disease. However, of all the diseases studied, the lowest blood levels of CoQ10 have been found in people with hyperthyroidism, including autoimmune hyperthyroidism (Graves' disease). Studies suggest the low levels of CoQ10 in hyperthyroidism cause a defect in cellular energy transport (Mancinie et al. 2006). Most studies show that supplements containing 30–60 mg used once daily are necessary for the maintenance of optimal CoQ10 levels. In subjects with hyperthyroidism or who take statin drugs, doses of 100 mg daily may be needed.

Vitamin D and Calcium

Disturbances in vitamin D and calcium metabolism are also seen in hyperthyroidism, with levels of 25 OH vitamin D often markedly decreased. Normally, once peak bone mass (primarily under genetic control) is achieved, the bone mass remains stable for years, although resorption and formation are constantly occurring. In resorption, osteoclast cells cause bone to break down. In bone formation, osteoblasts form bone. Thyroid hormones directly stimulate bone resorption, resulting in hypercalcemia (elevated serum calcium) as calcium is released from bone. This condition is reversed when thyroid balance is restored. Severe hypercalcemia may cause vomiting, anorexia, polyuria and occasionally impairment of renal function.

Parathyroid Hormone and Vitamin D

Parathyroid hormone (PTH) and vitamin D work together to ensure adequate blood calcium levels. Calcium regulates the release of PTH from the parathyroid glands. Hypercalcemia causes decreased PTH secretion or transient hypoparathyroidism. Vitamin D supplementation counteracts the rapid calcium excretion, restoring normal calcium levels. Vitamin C and K levels (needed for bone matrix synthesis) must also be adequate.

The resultant low PTH levels interfere with the body's conversion of vitamin D (which is dependent on adequate PTH). Diminished intestinal absorption of vitamin D results in increased urinary calcium loss. A slight increase in thyroid hormone levels can initiate this process, which can ultimately result in osteoporosis.

Vitamins C, E and B

Deficiencies of both vitamins C and E cause thyroid cell hyperplasia (increase in cell number due to excessive cell proliferation), raising thyroid hormone levels. Changes in lipid metabolism and malabsorption of fat-soluble vitamins cause vitamin E deficiencies. A combination of vitamin E and C deficiencies may cause hyperthyroidism.

Thyroid hormones regulate the conversion of dietary riboflavin (vitamin B_2) into its two active flavin coenzymes. Enzyme activity is increased by thyroid hormones. Consequently, vitamin B_2 reserves are diminished in thyrotoxicosis and vitamin B_2 deficiency may contribute to Graves' ophthalmopathy. Vitamin B_2 also regulates reproductive organs, and deficiencies can cause reproductive problems.

Vitamin B_{12} and vitamin B_3 (niacin) cannot be properly absorbed unless the thyroid is functioning properly. B_{12} deficiency can cause mental illness, neuralgia and other neurological disorders. Niacin is needed for the proper metabolism of carbohydrates, proteins and fat. Serum concentrations of vitamin B_{12} and folic acid are often low in thyrotoxicosis. However, the cause may also be related to a concurrent autoimmune condition, such as autoimmune atrophic gastritis or pernicious anemia. Thiamine (vitamin B_1) deficiency, recognized as a cause of high output cardiac failure, occurs in thyrotoxicosis since vast quantities of B_1 are depleted.

Bone Loss in Hyperthyroidism

Hyperthyroidism generally causes increased excretion of calcium and phosphorus and demineralization of bone. These changes may result in conditions of weak, soft or brittle bone such as osteitis fibrosa, osteomalacia or osteoporosis. As hyperthyroidism is treated, bone changes generally resolve, especially in premenopausal women.

In young individuals, normal bone formation usually compensates for bone loss. In children, hyperthyroidism is associated with increased skeletal growth, and hypothyroidism is associated with reduced growth. Thyroid hormones are critical for cartilage growth and differentiation and they enhance the response to growth hormone. The risk of developing secondary osteoporosis is greatest in postmenopausal women.

Iodine, Magnesium, Copper, Manganese, Zinc, and Selenium

Minerals utilized in the production and metabolism of thyroid hormone include manganese, iron, phosphorus, calcium, magnesium, sulfur, zinc, copper and selenium. Proper iodine absorption requires adequate magnesium. High levels of zinc are associated with hyperthyroidism. Of particular importance is the balance between zinc and copper, which is normally 8:1. This balance is essential for proper functioning of the hypothalamic-pituitary-thyroid axis that regulates thyroid levels in the blood, and for thyroid hormone production and metabolism. As zinc levels rise, copper levels become low relative to zinc, upsetting the critical balance.

Adequate selenium (at doses of 200 to 400 mcg) is critical for the body's conversion of T4 to T3 and for the production of the deiodinase enzymes needed to convert T4 into T3. It's important not to exceed 400 mcg selenium daily. High concentrations of selenium, like iodine, are reported to decrease thyroid hormone synthesis, and toxicity occurs at doses greater than 800 mcg. Low selenium levels lead to the production of thyroid antibodies, whereas supplemental selenium has been found to lower thyroid peroxidase (TPO) antibody levels (Gartner et al. 2002).

Calcitonin, a thyroid hormone produced by C cells in the thyroid gland, promotes anabolism by regulating calcium's role in forming bone tissue. In hypercalcemia, which is common in hyperthyroidism, the thyroid gland secretes excess calcitonin. Calcitonin increases the activity of the bone-producing cells known as osteoblasts and reduces activity of the osteoclasts, which break down bone. Calcitonin reduces serum calcium levels by promoting calcium absorption and bone development. The function of calcitonin is directly opposite that of PTH.

Essential Fatty Acids

Essential fatty acids (EFAs) are not produced in the body. They must be derived from diet. Hyperthyroidism causes EFA deficiencies. Both the thyroid gland and the brain require sufficient EFAs to function properly. EFA deficiencies may cause cardiovascular and circulatory abnormalities, acne, eczema, failure of wounds to heal, mental deterioration, fatty liver and atrophy of exocrine glands. Essential fatty acids, including omega-3, omega-6, and omega-9 fatty acids, are found in varying types and quantities in evening primrose oil, marine fish oil, borage oil and flaxseed oil. Omega-3 is especially deficient in hyperthyroidism.

Low-Dose Naltrexone (LDN)

Used in low doses, the opiate antagonist naltrexone is found to improve immune function by boosting endorphin circulation. Consequently, the effects are similar to those seen in acupuncture. The use of LDN in treating patients with multiple sclerosis (MS) was first proposed in the mid–1980s by Dr. Bernard Bihari, a New York City neurologist. In his clinical practice, the Harvard-educated Bihari found that a low dose of naltrexone (1.5 to 4.5 mg daily) taken at bedtime offered benefits to patients with MS and other autoimmune conditions including Graves' disease, Graves' ophthalmopathy, and rheumatoid arthritis.

Since then, additional studies performed at Penn State and a number of anecdotal reports have confirmed Bihari's findings and demonstrated the effectiveness of naltrexone for Crohn's disease, Parkinson's disease and other conditions. The effects of naltrexone are also thought to be attributed to the removal of the regulatory effects on the immune system exerted by endogenous opioid peptides, which could activate Th2 and suppress Th1 cytokines (Moore and Wilkinson 2009, 29–44).

LDN has become a popular adjuvant treatment in Graves' disease and is frequently used in patients using anti-thyroid drug therapy. Although clinical trials are lacking, patients overwhelmingly report beneficial effects, especially on eye symptoms.

Origins of Alternative Therapies Used for Hyperthyroidism

Opinions on the cause and treatment of disease may differ depending on the background of the herbalist or practitioner. Chinese medicine generally blames environmental factors as the cause of disease and aims to restore balances of yin and yang, whereas Ayurvedic medicine credits digestive problems for most diseases related to qi imbalance.

Yin and yang refer to the opposing polarities, such as hot and cold, which govern man as well as the universe. Yin and yang relationships are apparent in the relationship of the sympathetic to the parasympathetic divisions of the autonomous nervous system. Overactivity of the sympathetic nervous system results in excess yang ailments. Overactivity of the parasympathetic system produces excess yin disorders.

Herbal Medicine

The healing effects of plants have been known for as long as records of civilization exist. Folk medicine records from cultures as diverse as Indian, Chinese, Arabic, Tibetan, Russian, European and Native American describe identical healing effects for thousands of different herbs and plant parts. From a crude system of trial and error passed down through the ages, herbal medicine has evolved into several well-documented *materia medicas*. Currently, there are five well-defined branches of herbalism: European, Asian-Arabic, Chinese, Indian (Ayurvedic) and Russian.

Adverse Effects and Precautions

While recognizing the efficacy of herbal medicine, most botanical researchers do, however, advise caution, fearing that many consumers do not realize the potency of herbs. Critics deride the lack of regulations currently guiding the herbal industry in the United States. Numerous studies have shown a significant variance in the quantity of active phytochemical substances present in herbal samples manufactured by different laboratories.

Standardized Preparations and Safety Issues

In Germany, where about 70 percent of physicians routinely prescribe herbs, herbal preparations are standardized. Capsules listed as standardized (compared by chemical analysis to known or standard concentrations) and said to contain 40 mg of an active substance or extract derived from a given herb can be trusted to contain that amount.

In 1978 the Federal Health Agency in Germany (now known as the Federal Institute for Drugs and Medical Devices) established an expert committee known as Commission E to study the safety and efficacy of herbal preparations. Each herb that is evaluated is subsequently presented in a monograph that includes positive and negative assessments based on chemical analysis, clinical trials, toxicology studies and a number of other stringent guidelines.

In buying herbs it is best to look for standardized extracts unless your practitioner advises that the whole plant or certain plant parts such as the roots are to be used. Different plant parts such as roots and leaves often contain one or more different active ingredients. Their effects may be unrelated or they may work synergistically.

Note: Dosages listed for the following herbs refer to the dried herbs (drugs), generally listed in grams (g), and not to the amounts in concentrated extracts unless specifically indicated. Some herbs listed below lower both TSH and thyroxine. This may confuse hyperthyroid patients (whose TSH levels are already low). However, with a lower level TSH, less TSH can bind to the TSH receptor and cause thyroid hormone production. Consequently, thyroid hormone levels fall. As the FT4 and FT3 levels approach normal, TSH levels eventually rise (unless TSH receptor antibodies are present) although it may take several months for this to be reflected in blood levels. However, some herbs can be dangerous in hyperthyroidism and it's important to investigate herbs that are prescribed.

HARMFUL HERBS

The German Commission E, in its extensive government-sponsored study of the safety and efficacy of herbs, lists kelp, sargassum and bladderwack as posing risk in individuals with hyperthyroidism (they have an iodine content >150 mcg). Iodine in excess of 150 mcg, according to the commission's herbal monographs, can aggravate or induce hyperthyroidism in susceptible individuals (Blumenthal 1998).

Dr. Vogel, writing in *The Nature Doctor*, reports that in some instances the body's natural iodine balance is disrupted by artificial iodine, particularly that found in iodized salt. He reports that iodized salt, with its unnatural composition, may cause palpitations in susceptible individuals, although sea salt doesn't have this effect (Vogel 1991, 156).

Kelp (Laminaria Hyperborea, Laminaria). Kelp should be avoided in hyperthyroidism unless it's used as a homeopathic preparation. However, naturopaths often report that hyperthyroidism and hypothyroidism are similar disorders of thyroid imbalance. Based on this premise, some alternative healers infer that both disorders can be rectified with preparations of kelp or sargassum (seaweed), or other iodine rich herbs such as fucus (bladderwack). However, excess iodine is potentially dangerous for patients with hyperthyroidism, and many patients have experienced an exacerbation of symptoms when using tonics containing kelp or iodine.

Herbs Approved for Hyperthyroidism

A number of different herbs have been proven effective in hyperthyroidism because of their abilities to reduce thyroid hormone levels, reduce symptoms, and reduce thyroid antibodies. Herbs should be used under the direction of an experienced practitioner who can monitor thyroid function tests and ensure that herbs with anti-thyroid properties are not stopped abruptly. Most practitioners use tonics containing several complementary herbs. The patent tonic Thyrosoothe contains Lycopus, Melissa, and Leonurus. It is widely used for hyperthyroidism and available at many health food stores and through Amazon.com. Herbs used in hyperthyroidism include the following:

Lactuca virosa (wild lettuce, prickly lettuce, lettuce opium, green endive, acrid lettuce, lactucarium). The medicinal parts of Lactuca are the dried latex (milky plant contents) and the leaves.
> EFFECTS: Analgesic and spasmolytic (reduces spasms or convulsions). Also reported to act as a tranquilizer or narcotic.
> USES: Used to treat whooping cough, bronchial catarrh, asthma and urinary tract diseases. In Graves' disease, lactuca is used for its muscle-relaxing effects.
> CONTRAINDICATIONS: Used only under medical supervision.
> PRECAUTIONS: Drug has a potential for causing allergic reactions.
> DOSAGE: As an alcohol extract used only under medical supervision.

Leonurus cardiaca (motherwort, lion's tail, lion's ear, throw-wort). The medicinal parts are the fresh above ground parts collected during the flowering season.
> EFFECTS: Mildly negatively chronotropic (tempering reproductive hormones), hypotonic (decreasing muscle tension), sedative.
> USES: Cardiac insufficiency, arrhythmia, nervous heart complaints, thyroid hyperfunction, flatulence.
> CONTRAINDICATIONS: None at recommended therapeutic dosage.

PRECAUTIONS: None at recommended therapeutic dosage.

DOSAGE: 4.5 g of herb comminuted for infusions and other oral preparations.

Lithospermum ruderale* or *L. officinale. The medicinal parts are the dried roots, flowers, leaves and seeds that contain lithospermic acid and rosmarinic acid. A freeze-dried extract is often used.

EFFECTS: Lithospermum has antithyrotropic (inhibits thyroid hormone production and release) and antigonadotrophic (inhibits release of gonadotrophin sex hormones). Reported to also inhibit TSH secretion. *L. officinale* is also reported to inhibit the peripheral conversion of T4 to T3.

USES: Mild thyroid hyperfunction.

CONTRAINDICATIONS: Lithospermum should not be used in hypothyroidism or in instances of thyroid enlargement not related to thyroid dysfunction.

PRECAUTIONS: To be used under the guidance of a naturopathic practitioner.

DOSAGE: Prescribed on an individual basis; usually sold as a tonic also containing *Lycopus virginicus, Melissa officinalis,* and occasionally *Thymus serpyllum.*

Lycopus virginicus, Lycopus europaeus (bugleweed, lycopi herba, gypsywort). Lycopus consists of the fresh or dried above-ground plant parts as well as their preparations.

EFFECTS: Lycopus has antigonadotropic and antithyrotropic effects, inhibiting the peripheral conversion of T4 to T3. It also decreases levels of the pituitary hormone prolactin, which induces lactation, and it has a mild diuretic effect. It is also reported to inhibit TSH release, and is one of the most common herbal treatments for hyperthyroidism, reducing symptoms of chest tightness, palpitations, and tremor.

USES: Mild to moderate thyroid hyperfunction with disturbances of the vegetative nervous system; breast pain or tenderness.

CONTRAINDICATIONS: Lycopus should not be used in hypothyroidism or in instances of thyroid enlargement not related to thyroid dysfunction. There should not be any simultaneous administration of thyroid hormone preparations.

PRECAUTIONS: No known hazards or side effects at recommended therapeutic dosage.

Enlargement of the thyroid gland is possible at very high doses of Lycopus (similar to other anti-thyroid agents, hypothyroidism can result from high doses). Because of its strong anti-thyroid effects, sudden discontinuation of Lycopus can lead to exacerbation of symptoms.

DOSAGE: 1 to 2 g (about 1 teaspoon) of dried herb for teas or as an ethanol extract equivalent to 20 mg of drug used 3 times daily. The German Commission E notes that each patient has his own individual optimal level of thyroid hormone. Only rough estimations of dosage are possible for thyroid disorders, in which age and weight must be considered.

Melissa officinalis (lemon balm, sweet mary, dropsy plant, honey plant, cure-all, bee balm, balm mint, sweet balm, garden balm). Melissa contains the fresh or dried leaf as well as its preparations.

EFFECTS: sedative, carminative (releases excess gas from the colon).

USES: Nervous sleeping disorders and agitation, gastrointestinal complaints; memory enhancer; inhibits TSH. In folk medicine, decoctions of the flowering shoots are used for nervous complaints, lower abdominal disorders, gastric complaints, hysteria and melancholia, bronchial catarrh, palpitations, vomiting, migraine and hypertension.

CONTRAINDICATIONS: None known.

PRECAUTIONS: None at recommended therapeutic dosage.

DOSAGE: 1.5–4.5 g of herb prepared as a tea, up to 8 or 10 g of the drug daily.

Passiflora incarnata (passion flower, granadilla, maypop, passion vine). The medicinal parts of passiflora are the dried herb and the fresh aerial parts.

EFFECTS: Sedative.

USES: Nervousness, insomnia, nervous agitation, nervous gastrointestinal complaints.

In folk medicine, use for depressive states such as hysteria, agitation and insomnia.

CONTRAINDICATIONS: None at recommended therapeutic dosages.

PRECAUTIONS: None at recommended therapeutic dosages.

DOSAGE: 4 to 8 g of the drug used as infusion taken two to three times daily and half an hour before bedtime.

Scutellaria lateriflora (skullcap, American skullcap, greater skullcap, blue pimpernel, helmet flower, hoodwort, mad-dog weed, madweed, Quaker bonnet). The medicinal part of Scutellaria is the pulverized herb of the 3- to 4-year-old aerial plant, which is harvested in June. Active compounds include scutellarin, a flavonoid glycoside, and iridoids.

EFFECTS: Sedative, antispasmodic, hypotensive, anti-inflammatory.

USES: Hysteria, seizure disorders, chorea, and other nervous disorders; reduces nervous tension while revitalizing the nervous system

CONTRAINDICATIONS: None at recommended therapeutic dosages.

DOSAGE: 1 to 2 g capsules up to three times daily; often used with passion flower

Silybum marianum and Silibinin (milk thistle, Marian thistle). The medicinal parts of milk thistle are ripe seeds or extracts.

EFFECTS: hepatic (liver) aid; alters the structure of hepatocytes (liver cells) in a way that prevents penetration of poison into the interior of the cell. Also stimulates liver cell regeneration. Silymarin is a collective name for a mixture of active phytochemicals and flavonoids present in milk thistle. Silibinin strongly inhibits leukotriene production, making it an effective inflammatory agent.

USES: Used as a tonic for functional disorders of the liver and gallbladder. In traditional Chinese medicine, detoxifying the liver has a healing effect on the eyes, making milk thistle a valuable treatment for Graves' ophthalmopathy. Beneficial for liver symptoms associated with autoimmune disease.

CONTRAINDICATIONS: None at recommended dosages.

PRECAUTIONS: None at designated therapeutic dosages. Reports of nausea when taken on an empty stomach.

DOSAGE: 12 to 15 g of the drug or an equivalent of 200 to 400 mg of Silymarin extract or a combination extract with 150 mg Silymarin and 600 mg Silibinin.

Valeriana officinalis (valerian, garden valerian, amantilla, heliotrope, vandal root). The medicinal parts of valerian are the carefully dried underground parts including roots.

EFFECTS: Sedative, sleep inducer, spasmolytic, muscle relaxant.

USES: Nervousness, insomnia, restlessness, sleeping disorders due to nervous conditions, mental strain, lack of concentration, excitability, stress, headache, neurasthenia, epilepsy, hysteria, nervous cardiopathy, menstrual related agitation, nervous stomach cramps, angst.

CONTRAINDICATION: Not to be used for extended periods.

PRECAUTIONS: None at recommended therapeutic dosage; occasional gastrointestinal and allergic complaints. Long-term use can cause headache, restlessness and cardiac disorders.

DOSAGE: 2–10 g of the drug or 1 to 2 mg (1000 to 2,000 mcg) of 0.1 percent standardized extract of valerenic acid.

Traditional Chinese Medicine

Traditional Chinese medicine (TCM) is a disciplined science with a formulary of treatments intended for use under the guidance of a doctor of Chinese medicine or an herbalist/acupuncturist. Diagnosis involves an intricate process involving an examination of the entire body, especially the tongue. The exam includes visual inspection, listening and smelling, palpation and inquiry. Diseases that are manifested as imbalances in the body's energy system are classified according to their internal or external origin.

Internal causes of disease in TCM include emotions and lifestyle, whereas external causes include seasons, and climactic conditions known as the Six Excesses — wind, cold, summer heat, dampness, dryness and fire. Treatment is based on a system of polar opposites with cooling treatment (yin) used to rebalance symptoms of hot disease (yang). Symptoms are important, but they are always subsidiary to energy healing. A TCM practitioner will never contradict the laws of energetic medicine. Instead, he will likely devise a treatment method that works symptomatically through the laws of energy medicine that promote balance of the Five Elements and also yin and yang. The Five Elements are a comprehensive template that organizes all natural phenomena into five master groups or patterns in nature: Wood, Fire, Earth, Metal, and Water. Each of the elements include sub-categories, for instance a season, a direction, climate, stage of growth and development, internal organ, body tissue, emotion, aspect of the soul, taste, color, or sound.

Treatment

Treatment involves a combination of dietary changes, massage, herbal preparations, animal ingredients and acupuncture intended to redistribute opposing forces of qi. If the body's energy is balanced, it's less likely that disease can take hold. Chinese herbs are not intended to work alone but as a protocol including one or more of the other elements listed. The primary goal is restoration of the body's energy known as qi. After TCM treatment is underway, the patient typically develops symptoms of detoxification that would be considered signs of illness under other circumstances. The symptoms, called discharge, occur in three stages and are signs that the body is ridding itself of excesses.

TCM as a Complementary Agent during ATD Therapy

In one study, integrationist researchers used TCM of RQNY (replenishing qi and nourishing yin) to complement a small dose of Tapazole in an integrative treatment effort directed at treating Graves' disease. The study, conducted at the Institute of Integration of Traditional and Western Medicine in Shanghai, involved two groups of 42 patients, monitored over a period of 18 to 24 months. Results indicate that combination therapy with TCM was much more effective than the use of Tapazole therapy alone (Zha 1997).

Chinese Herbal Medicine

In Chinese medicine, herbs may be ground and bound with honey and rolled into pills or pellets. Alternately, herbs may be pulverized into a powder that is dissolved in hot water or as a brewed soup and consumed like a tea. In general, herbs are taken on an empty stomach once daily upon rising, and no food is consumed for one half hour afterward.

Chinese herbs may be classified as inferior (or medicinal) for use in cases where disease has already taken hold. An example is coptis or Chinese goldenseal. Inferior herbs are generally used for infections and inflammation and are taken for short periods. General or preventive herbs such as bupleurum are used to prevent and heal disease that is already present. Superior or promotional herbs are called tonics and may be taken without consulting a herbalist. They can be generally taken over long time periods.

TCM typically involves combinations rather than individual herbs. Although most tonics contain a number of different herbs, only a minute quantity of each herb may be present. Customized TCM preparations using concentrated extracts of each ingredient are reported to be highly effective and are available for a variety of different conditions. Patent remedies with low doses of several different ingredients are also available and widely available in Chinese import stores such as Pearl River in New York City. Customized remedies for hyperthyroidism are prescribed on an individual basis and may include the following preparations:

Ch'ai hu kuei kan chiang t'ang

INDICATIONS: for yin individuals; treats disorders rooted in the chest such as heart palpitations, tightness, hot and cold flashes and insomnia. For heart disease, endocarditis, valvular disease.

Ch'ai hu ch'ia lung ku mu li t'ang

INDICATIONS: for yang individuals, treats tachycardia, seizure disorders, discharges excess energy (chi), hysteria, insomnia, inability to concentrate, benefits the nervous and glandular systems.

Long dan xie gan wan

INDICATIONS: for yang individuals, treats tachycardia and other symptoms of hyperthyroidism.

Tian wang bu xin wan35 (heart-yin tonic)

INDICATIONS: for yang individuals, treats tachycardia, benefits the nervous and glandular systems. Individual ingredients include Radix Rehmanniae Glutinosae, Radix Ginseng, Tuber Asparagi, Chochinchinesis, Tuber Ophiopoponis Japanici, Radix Srophulariaee, Ningponensis, Radix Salvaiae Miltiorrhizae, Selerotium Poriac Cocos, Radix Polygalae Tennuifoliae, Radix Schisandrae Chinsensis, Semen Biotae, Orientalis, Semen Zizyphi Sponosae, Radix Platycodi Grandiflori.

Jiaogulan (xianco)

INDICATIONS: helps the body adapt to stress, lowers blood pressure, prevents heart disease, acts as an adaptogen strengthening the immune system, nourishes the adrenal glands and raises energy levels. Jiaogulan also helps patients using radiation therapies maintain the immune system cells needed to protect against infection. The dose is reported to be 20 mg taken three times daily.

Immunomodulators

An overactive immune system characterizes Graves' disease. This doesn't mean that the immune system is overly effective. In fact, the immune system in Graves' disease is weak and no longer effective. Causes of weakness include exposure to chemicals, overuse of antibiotics, chronic infections, chronic stress, and uncontrolled allergies. Unable to launch an appropriate immune response, a weakened immune system responds erratically, targeting the body's own cellular proteins as if they were foreign antigens. This immune overactivity leads to autoimmunity, hypersensitivity reactions, additional allergies, and inflammation. Sustained periods of hyperimmunity may lead to immune exhaustion and collapse. Immunomodulators are substances that correct or balance the immune system, strengthening (not stimulating) weak immune systems and boosting sluggish immune systems. The goal of therapy in using immunomodulators is to restore immune system health, which helps limit autoantibody production and reduces autoimmune symptoms.

Immunomodulators also offer protection from stress-induced immune system depression (for example the immune system depression seen after strenuous exercise). Also, immunomodulators lower the production of pro-inflammatory substances as well as the stress hormone cortisol. The best known immunomodulators are plant sterols and sterolins derived from plant fats such as beta sitosterol. Although fruits and vegetables are natural sources, their sterols are leached out by cooking water or, when frozen, destroyed by enzymes during the thawing process. Besides sterols, several other substances including in the following sections have the properties of immunomodulators.

Plant Sterols/Sterolins

DOSAGE: 20 mg capsule of the product which is sold commercially under the name Sterinol may be taken three times daily on an empty stomach. Sterols are also in ingredient of the Polynesian plant *Morinda citrifolia* (noni, nonu, nono). Sterols are contraindicated for individuals who have had tissue or organ transplants. Patients on insulin therapy may experience changes and should have their insulin levels monitored while taking sterols.

Reishi mushroom extract (*Ganderma lucidum, Ganodera)*

DOSAGE: Sold as tablets, liquid tonic or as a tea with dosage information accompanying product. Reishi shows significant anti-inflammatory effects, protects the liver and diminishes allergic responses.

German chamomile (*Matricaria recutita*)

DOSAGE: 3 g of dried herb taken as an infusion of tea. May be used four to five times daily between meals. Alternately, 6 to 8 500 mg capsules may be used. Unlike other forms of chamomile, German chamomile rarely causes allergies. German chamomile tea bags are reported to be effective in reducing swelling when used as compresses over the eyelids. Briefly steep the bags in warm water, cool slightly and place the moist bags over closed eyes for 15 minutes. Note: Only chamomile or black tea should be used.

Flower pollen extract (Cernitil and Prostaphil Patent Preparations)

DOSAGE: 240 mg of the water soluble extract or 12 mg of the oil soluble extract in capsule or tablet form.

Oral Tolerance

Oral tolerance is classically defined as the suppression of immune responses to antigens that have been administered previously by the oral route.

Multiple mechanisms of tolerance are induced by the administration of oral antigens, and this suppresses the autoimmune response. Although oral tolerance is the focus of research at many leading research institutions, its origins lie in alternative medicine. Naturopaths use various forms of oral tolerance, including organotherapy, a form of homeopathy.

The basic concept is that the immune reaction that occurs in the gut causes T lymphocyte cells to either adapt or be destroyed. In the absence of autoreactive T cells, the immune system remains tolerant of the body's own proteins. In cases of autoimmunity, a small amount of a similar protein (from another species) that is ingested renders T cells inactive and stimulates the production of regulatory T cells. The regulatory T cells, in turn, release cytokines that dampen killer T cells and curb inflammation. Oral tolerance holds more promise in autoimmune diseases in which T cells (due to their release of cytokines), rather than autoantibodies, cause damage.

In addition to oral tolerance, nasal tolerance has also been shown to be effective in suppressing inflammatory conditions with the advantage of a lower dose requirement. Oral and nasal tolerance have been found to suppress several animal models of autoimmune diseases including experimental allergic encephalomyelitis (EAE), uveitis, thyroiditis, myasthenia, arthritis and diabetes in the nonobese diabetic (NOD) mouse, plus non-autoimmune diseases such as asthma, atherosclerosis, colitis and stroke. Oral tolerance has been tested in human autoimmune diseases including multiple sclerosis, rheumatoid arthritis, uveitis and diabetes and in allergy. Positive results have been observed in phase II trials, and new trials for arthritis, multiple sclerosis and diabetes are under way (Faria and Weiner 2006).

Homeopathic Preparations

Homeopathy involves treating the patient with highly diluted natural remedies that, if given in larger doses, would cause the particular symptom that is being treated. For instance, a dilute preparation of nux vomica, a substance traditionally used to induce vomiting, is used to prevent motion sickness.

Healing Principle

Homeopathy works with and not against nature, using minute dilutions of a substance that is prepared into powders and tablets, granules spun and pressed into sugar, or liquids suspended in a 10 percent or 20 percent ethanol solution taken as drops. Dry or pelleted homeopathic preparations should be rolled gently from their container onto a dry tongue, and in general, food or liquids should not be ingested for 30 minutes before and after the dose. The preparation should be allowed to dissolve on the tongue, not swallowed or chewed. Liquid preparations are dissolved into water and sipped slowly. In severe disorders, substances may be prescribed to be initially taken every two hours followed by a tapering of dosage.

Dosing

Most homeopathic preparations result from 1:100 dilutions, and each 1:100 dilution is described as having a dose of C. A substance diluted 1:100 six consecutive times is listed as a dose of 6 C. The more dilute the substance, the more powerful or potentized the effect is reported to be.

Diagnostic Applications

A remarkable contribution of homeopathy is its diagnostic approach. Homeopathic practitioners study the patient as a whole, analyzing the trivial complaints and seemingly innocent personality traits that make individuals unique. These traits are represented as constitutional types and are related to a particular element deficiency. Remedies, depending on their dosage, are often listed as effective for several seemingly unrelated conditions.

Individualized Treatment

In hyperthyroidism the uniqueness of each patient is fully appreciated and treatment is prescribed accordingly. The constitutional drug or the one apt to be most beneficial is one that most effectively treats the patient as a total sum of individual strengths and weaknesses, mentally, emotionally and physically.

The most beneficial homeopathic preparations used for hyperthyroidism address the rage at being held down or overlooked, which is considered by some to be the primary cause, which is consistent with theories relating to chakra imbalances. *Natrum muriaticum* is most often recommended. Combined with herbs and acupuncture, full effects should be seen in four weeks. Substances which may be prescribed for hyperthyroidism include the following preparations.

Arnica montana for bruising, eyestrain, black eyes, fever (arnica gel or cream applied to eyelids is beneficial for eye swelling and pain. Not to be used on broken skin).

Calcarea phosphoricum for difficulty concentrating, discontentment, bone and teeth pain, weakness and fatigue after illness.

Coffea for insomnia, toothache.

Fucus vesiculosus, a derivative of sea kelp, used for goiter, exophthalmos, tachycardia and tremor.

Iodum for symptoms of hyperthyroidism; people needing this have an obsessive desire to keep compulsively busy due to the persistent frightening thoughts they get when forced to remain still.

Kelpasan (1x–6x potency) for thyroid dysfunction.

Lycopodium for nervousness and sleeplessness, alopecia.

Natrum muriaticum for vasomotor disturbances such as the irregular pulse and palpitations of Graves' disease, eczema, acne, and skin blemishes, especially when accompanied by dry mucous membranes.

Pulsatilla for hot flushes disturbing sleep, tendency toward weepiness, fondness for sweets, little thirst.

Sepia (one of the sea remedies) for restlessness related to the menstrual cycle, impatience, menopausal complaints, candidiasis, irritable at home while extroverted with company.

Spongia tosta for palpitations and cardiac tremor.

Thyroidinium — See following section on organotherapy.

Organotherapy

Organotherapy is a newly emerging branch of homeopathy especially suited for the treatment of organ-specific diseases. The homeopathic substances used in organotherapy are derived from the corresponding organs of animals. For instance, thyroid tissue is available in an organotherapy pellet called *thyroidinum*. In conditions of autoimmune hyperthyroidism, *epiphysinum*, which is derived from the pineal gland, is used to heal the immune system.

According to organotherapy researchers, besides strengthening and balancing the affected organs, organotherapy provides a source of animal antigens. Following the principles of oral tolerance therapy described earlier in this chapter, these animal antigens react with their target autoantibodies, for instance thyroid antibodies in autoimmune thyroid disorders, preventing the autoimmune reaction that causes autoimmune disease. Furthermore, the damaged organ or tissue, which is spared from participating in the autoimmune reaction, is allowed to restore itself and heal.

The potencies for organotherapy include:

Potency 4C of an organ remedy used to stimulate organ function

Potency 7C of an organ remedy to regulate organ function

Potency 9C of an organ remedy to suppress function of the targeted organ

Potency 200K is considered optimal for regulating organ function

Potency 9C or lower of a hormone remedy is used to stimulate hormone action

Potency 12C of a hormone remedy is used to regulate hormone action

Potency 15C or higher of a hormone remedy suppresses hormone function (Bhatti 2010).

Ayurveda

Ayurveda is a 5,000-year-old medical discipline with roots in ancient India, traditionally practiced by 20 percent of the world's population. Recently adopted in the West, it focuses on treating imbalances of the body's doshas: Vata, Pitta, and Kapha.

Imbalances of doshas are seen as constitutional types with characteristic symptoms of the dominant dosha. These imbalances contribute to disease. The goal of Ayurveda is to balance one's doshas with the environment. For instance, to pacify Pitta, which is characteristically quick and hot, cooling foods such as green salads might be prescribed.

According to Ayurveda, the life energy force known as Prana flows through the body by the force of Vata, which regulates movement. Vata is divided into five parts that regulate different bodily systems. Prana Vata regulates the nervous system, for instance, while Udana Vata regulates cognition, speech and memory. Imbalances may block energy flow. Drugs in Ayurvedic medicine are not used to tranquilize but to strengthen the nerves. In Ayurvedic medicine, for a remedy to be pure it must be effective, efficacious, and be capable of permanently evoking the disorder, not merely the symptoms, to subside from the root or source. Otherwise the remedy is impure. The body is treated as a whole, with no remedy being the same for different individuals with similar conditions.

Treatment Protocols

The interrelationship of the individual to his environment is considered when prescribing treatment. The healing power of food in Ayurvedic medicine is categorized not by carbohydrates or fat content, but by properties of taste such as bitter, salt, sweet, sour, pungent and astringent. Ayurveda also encompasses protocols for detoxification such as fastings and enemas, herbs, drugs, social and mental conditioning, massage, anointing oils and exercise such as yoga, all prescribed on an individual basis.

Ayurvedic preparations are generally contained in a base of brown sugar or honey, which are considered good vehicles for facilitating absorption. Some of the more common ingredients used in Ayurvedic medicine include the following:

Amla (*Emblica officinalis*) and Triphala: Amla is a fruit with high vitamin C content used as the base of many Ayurvedic preparations. Amla, along with Haritaki (*Terminalia chebula*) and Bibhitake (*Terminalia belerica*) are blended together in Triphala, a compound used to balance, cleanse and nourish the body. Triphala is reported to improve vision and liver function, aid digestion, eliminate toxins and rejuvenate the body. Triphala is available at health food stores and is used by many people with hyperthyroidism related to food allergies and digestive issues.

Gotu kola (*Hydrocotyle asiatica*/Brahmi): Gotu kola, which has recently gained popularity in the United States for its vascular strengthening properties, is used to revitalize nerves and brain cells. Also used as a blood purifier and a memory enhancer.

Shatavari (asparagus root): Shatavari is used as a rejuvenative tonic for women, balancing the reproductive system.

Energy Healing

Energy healing dates back to 500 B.C. when the Pythagoreans recorded observing a halo of light energy surrounding the body. In ancient China, Japan and India, sage healers called this same phenomenon ch'i or qi or Prana. In TCM, ch'i is an invisible flowing energy force regulating the body as well as conditions of the environment. Energy, according to TCM, flows or circulates through the body through a system of meridians.

The goal of energy healing is to correct blockages in the flow of ch'i energy along the meridians. In the human body there are 26 or more principal meridians that follow along the front and back of the body. Their midlines correspond to the center of the body. Meridians contain RNA and DNA, which is likely the underlying basis of their action. The following section describes various methods of energy healing.

Acupuncture

Acupuncture points (acupoints) are located at spots where meridians emerge at the surface of the body. Acupuncture restores balance by manipulating acupoints with needles. Although there are 365 different channel points and various systems of charting them, there are approximately 2,000 acupoints. Each acupoint has a mirror image position and a corresponding internal Zang-Fu organ. Zang-Fu organs, while similar to anatomical organs, are more related to clusters of functions working in tandem with other organs to promote whole body healing.

An electro-acupuncture device may also be used to locate regions of reduced skin resistance or blockage. These regions can be further assessed for states of yin and yang. Acupuncture needles are then guided into specific acupoints and, depending on the manipulation and properties of the needle, are capable of performing more than 150 different actions, including healing, releasing energy blockages and restoring strength.

Acupuncture is used to treat the underlying causes of hyperthyroidism and it is used as an adjuvant during surgeries including thyroidectomy in China.

Precautions

Although acupuncture is generally regarded as safe, the technique has certain risks, which although small can be serious. Although most states require acupuncturists to be certified by an exam, experts advise that patients seek a licensed practitioner who is a physician or who has trained at an accredited school.

Acupressure

Acupressure is a form of energy healing that utilizes the same acupoints as in acupuncture, which it refers to as tsubos. Energy flow is manipulated by applying finger pressure to these points. Acupressure isn't as intensive as acupuncture, but is a valuable aid in treating colds, headaches and backaches and boosting energy in patients with hyperthyroidism. Pressure is generally applied for five seconds and then released for five seconds. Sore spots are indicators of ch'i blockage and can be used to diagnose blockage in organs corresponding to the acupoint.

Stress Reduction

Stress depresses immune function by decreasing immune system components that normally stop the autoreactive process before autoantibodies are produced while increasing levels of white blood cells that trigger autoantibody production. Consequently, in stress the immune system remains overactive while its normal regulatory suppressor mechanism is inhibited. Methods for reducing stress such as meditation or breathing exercises also restore immune function.

Role of Stress in Disease

The waxing and waning of symptoms in Graves' hyperthyroidism has been shown to have a psychosomatic component, with exacerbations seen after periods of stress. Stress functions to release two stress hormones, corticotrophin-releasing hormone (CRH) via the hypothalamus, and adrenaline by the adrenal glands. CRH causes the pituitary to release adrenocorticotrophic hormone (ACTH), which causes the adrenal gland to release cortisol. All of these hormones cause other organs to pitch in and aid the body in dealing with the stressor agent. The ultimate effect of chronic stress is an elevated cortisol level and a weakened immune system.

Besides traditional stress reduction methods such as biofeedback, meditation and yoga, effectively dealing with stress involves being prepared for certain anticipated life events (having a plan of action like carrying an umbrella when a thunderstorm is expected). It also involves proper attention to diet, avoiding foods such as refined sugar and processed foods that cause inflammation.

Meditation

Evidence left behind on cave walls indicates that man's yearning for spiritual expression began about 17,000 years ago. Early cultures didn't distinguish spiritual from everyday life and regarded spirituality as respect for the mystery of existence. Meditation, in contrast to religion, fills man's need to illuminate his place in the world without reference to an external entity. Meditation can follow the rules and rituals of various formal disciplines or it can be an uncontrived spontaneous solitary effort to connect with the universe.

Autogenic Training

Autogenic training is a mind-body approach used to heal chronic pain syndromes and stress-related disorders. Stress is known to trigger and exacerbate symptoms in autoimmune diseases, especially thyroid disorders. Autogenic training refers to a series of 6 standard exercises along with breathing exercises, imagery techniques and other helpful tips designed to enhance self-regulatory mechanisms for counteracting the effects of stress. The exercises primarily focus on supplying heaviness and warmth to the extremities. The purpose is to elicit a shift from an anxiety state to the autogenic state, which facilitates and movilizes the recuperative and self-normalizing brain mechanisms. The goals are similar to those of meditation. However, often people are too uptight to hold still long enough to meditate. Autogenic training is a powerful alternative (Sadigh 2012, 30–37).

Yoga

The ancient Hindu word *yoga* means "to yoke" or to "to join." This refers to the joining of the individual soul to Brahman, which is the ultimate reality and the unifying concept of Hinduism. Brahman is the soul or inner essence of all things. There are several distinctive schools or paths in yoga. Each involves physical training and mental disciplines depending on the spiritual level. Yoga masters can help their clients assume postures that are favorable to healing the thyroid gland.

Neural Therapy

Neural or craniosacral therapy is a method that focuses on the movement of energy up and down the spine and assesses how this energy corresponds to the rhythmic pulsations of cerebrospinal fluid. Disruption to the spine's energy flow can be caused by trauma, even circumstances related to birth.

Craniosacral therapy was pioneered by Florida's Dr. John Upledger. While assisting in surgery, Dr. Upledger observed a rhythmic movement of a patient's dura mater. This led him to research what we now know to be the craniosacral system that includes the dura mater, which is attached to facial and skull bones, and the sacrum. Dr. Upledger discovered that he could influence the flow of cerebrospinal fluid by applying pressure to areas of the craniosacral zone and thereby correct energy blockages. Naturopaths frequently employ neural therapy to facilitate healing in hyperthyroidism.

Acetyl-L-Carnitine's Role in Healing Hyperthyroidism

Acetyl-l-carnitine (ACL) is an amino acid that effectively inhibits the activity of excess thyroid hormone and reduces symptoms of hyperthyroidism. Studies dating back to the 1960s in animals and recently in humans suggest that ACL blocks the effects of excess thyroid hormone in some of the body's tissues. ACL does not affect the thyroid gland itself but effectively reduces symptoms of hyperthyroidism. The primary effects of ACL are on the activity of thyroid hormone. ACL is is effective for treating hyperthyroidism related to Graves' disease, toxic multinodular goiter, and the excessive use of thyroid replacement hormone (Benvenga et al. 2004).

Specifically, L-carnitine blocks the entry of excess thyroid hormone into the cell nucleus of liver cells and neurons (cells of the brain and central nervous system), and thereby significantly reduces the physiological effects associated with hyperthyroidism. Overall, study results show that the addition of 1–3 grams of oral carnitine daily is an effective tool for reducing symptoms of nervousness, heat intolerance, insomnia, emotional instability, tremors, and excessive sweating in hyperthyroidism.

ACL's effects are related to its ability to inhibit the entry of both T4 and T3 into the cell nucleus. This is important because entry into the cell nucleus is essential for thyroid hormone to cause the effects commonly associated with hyperthyroidism. In clinical observations, L-carnitine reduces effects in both mild hyperthyroidism and in the severe form of hyperthyroidism known as thyroid storm. Studies showed benefits starting with the second week of treatment using 2–4 grams of L-carnitine daily including reduction of goiter size, I-131 uptake, liver enzyme levels, and an improvement in eye symptoms including ophthalmopathy. In addition L-carnitine has a beneficial effect on muscle function, strength, and bone mineralization.

Because hyperthyroidism depletes the body of L-carnitine and other nutrients, doses of L-carnitine as high as 4 grams daily are not associated with toxicity, teratogenicity (effects on offspring), contraindications or interactions with other drugs. A naturally occurring substance, L-carnitine is a known protector of mitochondrial function in the body's cells. Studies of patients with both hypothyroidism and hyperthyroidism show decreased levels of L-carnitine in muscles. These deficiencies are known to contribute to muscle fatigue in both conditions.

In one study involving 50 patients with hyperthyroidism, L-carnitine caused mild nausea in two patients during the first week of treatment. These symptoms did not require a discontinuation of treatment, and they subsided within a few days. L-carnitine caused no significant alterations in blood counts, serum proteins, bilirubin levels, blood sugar levels or urine chemistry levels (Benvenga et al. 2004).

Anti-Inflammatory Agents

Because inflammation is considered the root cause of most diseases, supplements with anti-inflammatory and antioxidant properties are a welcome addition to any holistic healing protocol. The best supplements for hyperthyroidism include acetyl-1-carnitine for reducing the potency of excess thyroid hormone and CoQ10 for correcting the deficiencies that occur in hyperthyroidism.

Other supplements commonly used depending on specific symptoms include ginger, vitamin B complex, vitamin D, black cumin oil, oregano leaf oil, resveratrol, and *Rhodiola rosea*.

Chronic Infections and Sensory Therapies

A number of infectious agents described in Chapter 2 are known to trigger the development of Graves' disease. Some integrationist physicians believe that untreated or latent infectious agents can cause physiological effects that cause relapses or prevent remission entirely. Practitioners specializing in the treatment of sensory disorders address the methylation defects caused by these infections.

Proline-Rich Peptides

Colostrum and other proline-rich peptides function as signaling peptides by activated macrophages and activated T-cells that control the production of cytokines. As a supplement, proline-rich peptides act as immunomodulators, balancing the immune system and tampering the inflammatory response associated with latent infection.

Correcting Methylation Defects

Methyl groups are carbon chains utilized extensively in the body for transport of fat-soluble nutrients, thereby activating genes. In infection and other chronic states, the methylation pathway is defective. This defect prevents healing and creates an advantageous situation for further assault by environmental and infectious agents. This results in a wide range of conditions including thyroid dysfunction, diabetes, schizophrenia, and attention deficit hyperactivity disorder.

Correcting the defect and strengthening the methylation pathways are goals of sensory therapy. Treatments include CoQ10, acetyl-1-carnitine, and folic/folinic acid. Folate is part of the normal methylation pathway, and deficiencies, which aren't always seen with blood tests, can also lead to deficiencies of neurotransmitters such as dopamine. Impaired methylation also increases histamine levels, contributing to allergic reactions, making methylation correction an important factor in healing autoimmune disorders.

9

Hyperthyroidism in Pregnancy and the Postpartum Period

Pregnancy poses a number of different circumstances. During pregnancy, patients may be on anti-thyroid drug therapy for hyperthyroidism; previously treated for Graves' disease and now hypothyroid; or they may be newly diagnosed. During the postpartum period, hyperthyroidism may develop as a result of postpartum thyroiditis, or it may cause relapse in patients with Graves' disease. Changes to the mother's thyroid function during pregnancy also affect the fetus. The many changes to thyroid function that occur during and after pregnancy are discussed in Chapter 9.

Changes in Laboratory Function Test Ranges

Twenty years ago, when tests for T4 and T3 were primarily used, laboratories listed a different normal range for pregnant patients. Typically, the reference range for T4 and T3 in pregnancy were 1.5 times higher than the usual adult reference ranges. The normal increases in T4 and T3 during pregnancy were due to slight elevations of hormone but primarily due to the significant increase in carrier proteins that occurs during early pregnancy and to the increased half-life of thyroxine-binding-globulin (TBG) that occurs in pregnancy (Graham 2010). In addition, the pregnancy hormone beta HCG is similar to the pituitary hormone TSH. As beta HCG levels rise in early pregnancy, thyroid hormone levels also rise.

Now that thyroid hormone levels are measured with the FT4 and FT3 levels, different ranges are no longer given for pregnant patients. Most methods for FT4 and FT4 aren't influenced by binding proteins and only measure free available hormone, although slight increases can occur due to protein influences. However, while the reference ranges for FT4 and FT3 remain the same, the TSH level falls in early pregnancy, and levels as low as 0.1 mu/L in pregnancy are considered normal (James 2003).

Changes at Midterm

By midterm HCG levels have fallen and thyroid hormone levels also fall. In patients with Graves' disease, the immune system slows down, thyroid antibody levels decline, and, consequently, thyroid hormone levels may fall a great deal. Patients with active Graves' disease often achieve temporary periods of remission at this time. Most Graves' disease patients are able to lower or stop anti-thyroid drugs. Patients on thyroid replacement hormone generally need to increase their dose by 50 percent.

The Reproductive System in Hyperthyroidism

The occurrence of amenorrhea (absence of menstrual periods) resulting from Graves' disease was one of the major symptoms originally reported by Dr. Robert Graves. Since then, other related effects have been noted, including anovulation (absence of ovulation), oligomenorrhea (decreased or scant menses), and menorrhagia (profuse menstrual flow), although this condition is more often seen in hypothyroidism. Prepubertal girls with thyrotoxicosis may experience a slightly delayed menarche.

Reproductive problems of miscarriage, implantation failure and in vitro fertilization failure are associated with autoimmune thyroid disease (AITD) and are more often seen in hypothyroidism. In hyperthyroidism, the body's conversion of androgens to estrogens may be increased due to changes in protein binding. Consequently, circulating estradiol levels are occasionally increased in thyrotoxic men. As a result, men with hyperthyroidism may have symptoms of increased estrogen biologic activity. Gynecomastia (excessive development of breasts in males), spider angiomas and a decrease in libido are frequent complaints.

Fertility and Pregnancy in Patients with Hyperthyroidism

Patients with severe conditions of Graves' disease have greater difficulty conceiving, and the incidence of spontaneous abortion is increased (Larsen et al. 1998, 450). The autoimmune process in Graves' disease is thought to activate natural killer (NK) cells of the CD 56+ variety and the CD 19+5+

variety. The CD 56+ NK cells produce a cytokine called tumor necrosis factor (TNF). TNF causes further inflammation and damage to other organs including the embryo, the womb lining and the placental cells that attach the fetus to the uterus. The CD 19+5+ variety produce antibodies to several hormones, including estradiol, FSH, LH, progesterone and beta HCG, and to neurotransmitters including endorphins, enkaphlins and serotonin (Beer 1999). Women with neurotransmitter autoantibodies are reported to have premature menopause, poor uterine lining responses and poor blood flow responses to the endometrium as the uterus prepares for successful implantation or pregnancy.

Treatment of hyperthyroidism doesn't necessarily bring fertility improvement, although it can. Treated women, especially those who become hypothyroid, are reported to still suffer poor stimulation cycles, infertility, implantation failures, donor egg failures and miscarriages. Proper diagnosis of these immune disturbances is necessary, followed by preconception treatment that may take up to three months. Tissue slides from previous pregnancy loss can also aid in diagnosis. Depending on the immune system effects, treatment may consist of lymphocyte immune therapy, or intravenous immunoglobulin therapy to suppress NK cell activity (Beer 1991).

Hyperthyroidism rarely develops during preganancy. It's estimated that only one to two out of every 1,000 pregnancies will be complicated by hyperthyroidism (Glinoer 2000, 1020). Causes of hyperthyroidism in pregnancy include those found in the general population and others specific for pregnancy. These causes include Graves' disease, toxic adenoma, toxic multinodular goiter, subacute or silent thyroiditis, iodide-induced thyrotoxicosis, transient gestational thyrotoxicosis, thyrotoxicosis facitia, molar disease, and hydatidiform mole.

Graves' Disease Development in Pregnancy

Graves' disease is the most common cause of hyperthyroidism seen in pregnancy. Almost all pregnant Graves' disease patients were previously diagnosed and treated or undergoing treatment. Patients with Graves' disease who plan to become pregnant are advised to start ATD treatment and wait to conceive until after the first 6 weeks when their ATD dose is reduced.

For more than 60 years women have been safely treated with ATDs during pregnancy, and the natural course is for Graves' disease to improve or resolve during the second half of pregnancy. Rarely, Graves' disease can develop or be newly diagnosed during pregnancy. The presence of new onset Graves' disease at this time is often a misdiagnosis in which it is confused with transient gestational thyrotoxicosis, a condition of hyperthyroidism more likely to develop in pregnancy.

In a newly diagnosed case of hyperthyroidism in a pregnant women, certain features suggest the possibility of Graves' disease development. Because the TSH normally falls in early pregnancy, these features can help differentiate Graves' disease from gestational thyrotoxicosis and normal changes. These include:

- Prior individual or family history of autoimmune thyroid disease
- Weight loss (or failure to gain), palpitations, proximal muscle weakness, emotional lability
- Graves' ophthalmopathy or pretibial myxedema
- Thyroid gland enlargement
- Increased severity of normal pregnancy symptoms such as heat intolerance, fatigue, and diaphoresis (increased sweating)
- Pruritis (itching)
- Pulse rate greater than 100
- Widened pulse pressure (Glinoer 2000, 1021).

Treatment of Hyperthyroidism in Pregnancy

Radioiodine, both ablative and diagnostic, is contraindicated in pregnancy because of its potential to affect the fetus. RAI should also be avoided in women planning to become pregnant in the following 6–12 months. RAI is recommended in pregnancy only if rapid control of hyperthyroidism is required and ATDs cannot be used (Bahn et al. 2011).

Surgery during the first and last trimesters is rarely performed since it may induce labor. If surgery is required it should be performed during the late second trimester. Even then, the risk of preterm labor is high at 4.5–5.5 percent (Bahn et al. 2011).

ATDs are most often used in pregnancy, but careful monitoring is needed to adjust for the normal changes that occur during pregnancy. Both methimazole and PTU cross the placental barrier and affect the fetal thyroid. Since PTU crosses the barrier less readily, it is recommended for the first trimester when the fetus relies on the mother's thyroid hormone stores. Another reason for PTU preference is the greater association between methimazole and aplasia cutis in the fetus, although this condition may also rarely occur in mothers using PTU and hyperthyroid mothers not on ATDs. Aplasia cutis causes skin lesions that usually affect the scalp. Methimazole taken by the mother in the first trimester is also associated with a syndrome of MMI embryopathy, including choanal and esophageal atresia (Bahn et al. 2011). In addition, joint pain and drug-related lupus can occur with either methimazole or PTU.

ATD Dosage

The recommended daily dose of PTU in pregnancy is 200 mg or less and for MMI the daily dose is 10 mg or less. The ATD dose can usually be reduced in the second trimester as symptoms spontaneously diminish. The lowest dose needed to keep FT4 within range should be used. With excess ATD in the fetal circulation, goitrous hypothyroidism can occur. Maternal transfer of T4 is seldom sufficient to compensate. Some physicians advise that hormone levels are not as important as the patient's clinical status (Larsen et al. 1998, 451). Furthermore, a modest increase in heart rate is reported to be common in pregnancy and not a reason to increase ATD dosage.

All pregnant patients with hyperthyroidism require careful observation and close monitoring of intrauterine thyroid function, using ultrasound for assessment of fetal growth and fetal heart rate monitoring. Fetal hyperthyroidism can be treated by the use of maternal methimazole, taking advantage of its enhanced ability to cross the placental membrane.

Thyroid Antibodies in Pregnancy

Measurements of TSI antibodies should be monitored in the third trimester in all patients with hyperthyroidism or who have been treated for hyperthyroidism, and in the first and third trimesters in women previously treated with RAI. Antibodies are measured to evaluate the potential for fetal hyperthyroidism (Bahn et al. 2011). At a symposium held during the European Thyroid Association's annual meeting in 1997, it was concluded that when TSH receptor antibodies at levels greater than 300 percent activity are present in early gestation (Rocchi 2005), they should be monitored again at 6 months gestation. If antibody titers have not decreased substantially during the second trimester, the possibility of fetal hyperthyroidism should be considered (Glinoer 2006, 1021). Fetal monitoring, however, is more predictive of thyrotoxicosis than antibody titers. Overall, hyperthyroidism that is due to Graves' disease tends to improve progressively during the course of pregnancy, although exacerbations can occur in the first 3 months.

When hyperthyroidism has been previously treated by ablation, the mother may not have enough remaining thyroid tissue to exhibit symptoms of thyrotoxicosis despite having high titers of stimulating TRAb in her blood. Clues to the presence of fetal hyperthyroidism are fetal heart rate consistently above the normal limit of 160 beats per minute and high antibody titers.

Some doctors also measure TPO antibodies in pregnancy. High levels in the first trimester are associated with an increased risk for miscarriage and postpartum thyroiditis (Stevens 2003; Check 2007, 68). In one study, women with TPO antibodies in the first trimester were treated with levothyroxine, which reduced the miscarriage rate by 75 percent (Glinoer 2006). Thyroid peroxidase antibodies are also considered a marker for subsequent postpartum depression (Kuijpens et al. 2001; Check 2007, 68).

Treatment Precautions and Contraindications

Strong iodine solution should not be used in pregnancy because of its ability to cross over to the placenta. High concentrations of iodine can cause fetal goiter, and an enlarged goiter may interfere with breathing. Block-and-replace therapy should not be used in pregnancy. Although ATDs cross the placental barrier, thyroid hormone does not.

Beta Blockers in Pregnancy

The use of beta blockers is controversial in pregnancy, with some studies showing significant side effects and others showing that beta blockers are not contraindicated in pregnancy (Becks and Burrows 1991, 139). However, there are no adequate, well-controlled studies in pregnant women. Side effects for pregnancy noted in newborns whose mothers were using propranolol at the time of delivery have exhibited bradycardia (abnormal heart rhythm), hypoglycemia and respiratory depression (Becks and Burrows 1991, 139). The category B beta blockers, which showed no effects in pregnancy in animal studies, are considered the safest and include acebutolol, pindalol, and sotalol. The general recommendation is to use the lowest dose of beta blockers that keeps the maternal heart rate to 80–90 beats per minute (Becks and Burrows 1991, 139).

Pregnancy in the Controlled Hyperthyroid or Hypothyroid Patient

About 20 percent of patients with Graves' disease move into spontaneous hypothyroidism, which may be temporary. While this form of hypothyroidism is typically mild, patients are treated with replacement hormone. During pregnancy, hypothyroid patients on thyroid hormone replacement generally require a 50 percent to 100 percent increase in their maintenance doses (Arky 1997).

Thyroid requirements are increased because of increased TBG, increased body mass and increases in deiodination to rT3 rather than T3. Many physicians increase the patient's maintenance dose by 50 percent as soon as pregnancy is confirmed because the increased requirement begins shortly after implantation and lasts until a few weeks following delivery (Larsen et al. 1998, 473).

Euthyroid patients in spontaneous remission from Graves' disease may very rarely have a relapse during pregnancy. This relapse may be due to hormonal changes or it may be triggered by the increased FT4 seen in early pregnancy and the stimulatory effects of the beta HCG hormone. Relapse may be transient with symptoms resolving during the first trimester.

ATD Treatment During Lactation

Small quantities of ATDs are secreted in human breast milk in women using ATDs (Glinoer 2000, 1023). Although there have been no side effects reported in nursing infants, mothers on ATDs have traditionally been advised not to nurse their babies despite no "evidence-based" reason (Glinoer 2000, 1023). Numerous studies have found ATDs to be safe and there have been no reports of increased neonatal TSH levels occurring with the use of either methimazole or PTU during lactation. As long as doses are kept moderate, the risk for the infant is practically negligible (Glinoer 2000, 1023).

Gestational Transient Thyrotoxicosis

Gestational transient thyrotoxicosis (GTT) is a non-autoimmune form of hyperthyroidism of variable severity that occurs in women who have a normal pregnancy. Occurring in 2–3 percent of all pregnancies (Glinoer 2000, 1023) GTT is often seen in association with hyperemesis (extreme morning sickness). GTT differs from thyroid disease in that it occurs in women without a history of thyroid disease who do not have TSH receptor antibodies. It is caused by hypersensitivity to beta HCG's stimulation of the thyroid gland.

GTT is not always clinically apparent or routinely detected. Symptoms include weight loss or the absence of weight increase, tachycardia, and unexplained fatigue, which occurs in about half of the women with GTT. Higher levels of HCG levels, especially when they're of longer duration, are associated with a more severe form of thyrotoxicosis. Therefore, GTT is more common in women pregnant with twins (where HCG levels are often twice as high as usual).

Gestational Trophoblastic Disease

Gestational trophoblastic disease (GTD) is a rare complication of pregnancy that can result in hyperthyroidism. GTD occurs when the normal placental tissue grows abnormally into a large mass of grapelike structures called a hydatidiform mole, which produces abnormally high levels of beta HCG hormone. In this condition, which is managed with ATDs, thyroid function returns to normal as HCG levels fall.

Nodular Hyperthyroidism

One or more thyroid nodules, with accompanying hyperthyroidism, may be recognized for the first time during pregnancy. If a nodule is seen for the first time during the first trimester, a fine-needle aspiration biopsy should be performed. If a malignancy is found, appropriate thyroid surgery is indicated. If a diagnosis of possible follicular neoplasm or suspicious results are reported, surgery can be postponed until after delivery, at which time further studies can be done to tell if a benign autonomously functioning nodule is present. There is no evidence that pregnancy affects the growth of thyroid malignancies (Glinoer 2000, 1024).

Hyperthyroidism in the Postpartum Period

Hyperthyroidism that occurs in the postpartum period can occur as a relapse or exacerbation of Graves' disease. More commonly, hyperthyroidism at this time is caused by postpartum thyroiditis (PPT), a condition with an average prevalence of 7–8 percent (Burman 2012). PPT occurs within one year after delivery or a spontaneous (miscarriage) or induced abortion.

Postpartum Graves' Disease

The autoimmune nature of Graves' disease is affected by the profound autoimmune changes that occur after delivery or abortion. Consequently, there is a greater frequency of onset, recurrence or exacerbation of Graves' thyrotoxicosis during the postpartum period. This occurrence is more frequent among Japanese women with Graves' disease, in whom up to 40 percent of newly diagnosed cases in women of childbearing age, developed their disease during the postpartum period (Glinoer 2000, 1023). This increase is not universal, however. In Belgium only 12 percent of women of childbearing age who developed Graves' disease did so within 2 years of childbirth (Glinoer 2000, 1023).

Differentiating Graves' disease from postpartum thyroiditis may be difficult. The radioiodine uptake is high in Graves' disease and low in postpartum thyroiditis. However, due to precautions against administering this test to women with small children, it is rarely used. Antibody tests are more helpful for diagnosis. A high level of TSI antibodies indicates Graves' disease. However, some women with Graves' disease can develop coexisting conditions of postpartum thyroiditis, further confusing diagnosis. Making the distinction is important since women with Graves' disease can use ATDs and women with PPT are usually not prescribed ATDs since they typically move naturally into hypothyroidism.

Postpartum Thyroiditis

The prevalence of postpartum thyroiditis in the general population ranges from 1 to 17 percent, varying in different geographical regions, and reaching levels as high as 25 percent in women with type 1 diabetes (Glinoer 2000, 1023). PPT can cause conditions of transient hyperthyroidism alone and conditions of transient hyperthyroidism followed by hypothyroidism and then recovery. On average, conditions of PPT resolve within one year. Because PPT is considered a form of Hashimoto's thyroiditis, low levels of TPO and thyroglobulin antibodies are often present. These antibodies are also seen in Graves' disease. However, elevated levels of TSI are typically seen only in Graves' disease.

Changes to the Fetus and Neonate

Hyperthyroidism in pregnancy can affect the fetus and neonate. Although it is generally accepted that it's preferable to be slightly hyperthyroid than slightly hypothyroid in pregnancy, both conditions can have ill effects. The effects of hypothyroidism, however, such as growth and developmental deficits, can be more serious, and miscarriage during the first trimester is highly associated with subclinical hypothyroidism (De Vivo 2010). Changes to the fetus and neonate related to hyperthyroidism are described in Chapter 10.

10

Hyperthyroidism in Children and Adolescents

During fetal development the thyroid gland is the first endocrine gland to develop. At about 11 weeks gestation, the fetus begins producing thyroid hormone. This is a clue to the importance of thyroid hormone in fetal development. The process of development continues throughout infancy, with changes in thyroid hormone levels reflecting the increased mental and physical development of children. Chapter 10 explores the problems that occur when thyroid hormone is produced in excess throughout the early life stages, including childhood and adolescence. While fetal hyperthyroidism is rare and typically transient, the incidence of hyperthyroidism in older children is becoming increasingly common.

The Thyroid Gland in Fetal Development

The first endocrine gland to develop, the thyroid is capable of producing, releasing and circulating low amounts of thyroid hormone to the fetal brain as early as 10 to 11 weeks gestation. The fetal thyroid depends on the mother for its iodine supply, but otherwise, it works independently by about 11 weeks, sending needed hormone to other cells, especially those of the central nervous system.

The development of the thyroid and gastrointestinal tracts are closely related because both of these cell lines develop from the primitive endoderm, the innermost of the embryonic cellular layers that form the digestive tract. This association is demonstrated by their sharing of several functions. For instance, the salivary and gastric glands are also able to concentrate iodine. Although neither the salivary gland nor the gastric glands respond to TSH stimulation, the salivary glands can also iodinate tyrosine.

Embryonic Origin

The thyroid gland is the first endocrine gland to develop in mammals. Human thyroid tissue cells are detected in the embryo one month after conception. A developing embryo has 3 cell layers: the ectoderm, which gives rise to skin and nerves; the mesoderm, which becomes muscle, blood arteries, veins and the heart; and the endoderm, which develops into the stomach lining, the intestines, pancreas, thyroid gland and gastric parietal cells that line the stomach cavity.

The thyroid primordium (early primitive tissue) originates on about day 16 or 17 as epithelial endoderm cells from two distinct regions of the pharynx floor thicken. These thickened cells form a diverticulum (outpocketing of tissue) known as the median thyroid anlage (the thyroid foundation or basement layer). These inchoate or primitive thyroid cells derived from the pharynx floor emerge adjacent to the cells that simultaneously emerge to form the heart.

As fetal development proceeds, the middle of the diverticulum is displaced, projecting inward. The primitive stalk of tissue connecting this embryonic thyroid tissue to the pharynx elongates, forming the thyroglossal duct. While moving inward, the outpocket shape begins to fill with cells, taking on the shape of two lobes. The resulting tissue fuses with the fourth pharyngeal pouch. Because the thyroid develops so close to the emerging heart, its location is influenced by the heart's position. As the heart descends into the chest cavity, the thyroid is pulled to its position near the base of the neck.

Ectopic Thyroid Tissue

As it moves into position, remnants of thyroid tissue can lodge in other locations. Ectopic (away from its normal location) thyroid tissue occurs in 7–10 percent of the population (Basaria and Cooper 1999). Ectopic thyroid tissue can result from abnormal thyroid migration secondary to changes in the heart's development. Therefore, when it is present, ectopic thyroid tissue usually occurs in the sublingual region beneath the tongue or in the region between the neck and heart. Other locations in the head and neck regions where ectopic thyroid tissue may be found include the trachea, submandibular, lateral cervical regions, axilla, palatine tonsils, carotid bifurcation, iris of the eye and pituitary gland. In addition, ectopic thyroid tissue has been found in locations distant from the neck region including the heart, ascending aorta, thymus, esophagus, duodenum, gallbladder, stomach bed, pancreas, mesentery of the small intestine, porta hepatis, adrenal gland, ovary, fallopian tube, uterus and vagina (Ibrahim 2011).

Ectopic thyroid tissue can become goitrous and cause either hypothyroidism or hyperthyroidism. In one study, a Graves' disease patient who had been ablated had a recurrence of hyperthyroidism nine years later in which mediastinal (chest cavity) ectopic thyroid tissue grew (presumably in response to stimulating TRAb) much like a goiter, causing substernal chest pain (Basaria and Cooper 1999).

Fetal Thyroid Maturation

Two months after conception, the thyroglossal duct normally dissolves and fragments. At the junction of the middle and posterior thirds of the tongue, only a small dimpled remnant of the duct called the foramen caecum remains. Cells of the lower portion of the duct differentiate into thyroid tissue that forms the pyramidal lobe of the thyroid gland. At 10 weeks gestation, TBG can be detected in fetal serum.

Thyroid Follicle Development and Thyroxine Synthesis

Three months after conception, early thyroid cells form intricate cordlike arrangements interspersed with vascular connective tissue. These soon take on the shape of follicles that eventually fill with colloid. By 11 weeks, the follicular cells are able to concentrate iodide and synthesize thyroxine. Radioactive iodine given to the mother at this time would be concentrated by the fetal thyroid, and the early fetal thyroid cells would also be ablated. At 10 to 12 weeks, the pituitary begins secreting TSH and the hypothalamus begins secreting TRH. From then on, rapid changes in the thyroid and pituitary take place. By 26 weeks gestation, fetal TSH levels are higher than those of the mother, perhaps because of the fetal pituitary's greater sensitivity to TRH stimulation.

Role of Fetal Thyroid Hormone

As the fetus develops, thyroid hormone plays an instrumental role in the maturation of the skeletal system, the lungs and the brain. Although T4 is primarily converted to rT3, small amounts of fresh T3 are slowly deiodinated in the fetal pituitary, brain and brown adipose or fat tissue. About a week before birth, there's a gradual prenatal surge where T3 levels rise. Two to four hours after birth, these levels abruptly surge (postnatal surge), presumably to meet the increased life demands.

Placental Influences and Hyperthyroidism in Pregnancy

Fetal development is highly influenced by the placenta. Acting as a semi-permeable membrane between the fetal and maternal systems, the placenta regulates what nutrients, hormones, drugs and other chemicals can cross over to the fetus. Besides supplying iodide, the placenta supplies T4 to the fetus during the first half of gestation when the fetal mechanism is not yet fully functioning. In the euthyroid fetus, transfer of placental T4 is marginal, whereas in hypothyroidism, sufficient maternal T4 may cross the placental membrane in sufficient quantities to bring levels up to half of the normal value seen at birth.

The protective placental tissue is rich in the particular deiodinase enzyme that converts T4 into the benign reverse T3 rather than the more potent T3. Considering the small energy requirements of the fetus, T3 isn't needed until delivery approaches. Excess T3 before then could harm the fetal heart and nervous system, a fact the placenta apparently recognizes. Several weeks before delivery, the placental enzymes shift and the outer ring deiodinase predominates, preparing for the postnatal surge.

The Fetal Pituitary-Thyroid Axis and Maternal Influences

The fetal pituitary-thyroid axis, which completes its development during the late stages of fetal development, functions independently of the mother. Transplacental passage of TSH from the mother is negligible, although the transfer of T4 is significant. At amounts that vary during different stages of gestation, maternal T4 spills over to the fetal circulation and accounts for approximately 30 percent of the serum T4 present in cord blood at term. This maternal contribution is important for normal fetal maturation (Fisher and Brown 2000, 960–61).

Thyroid Dysfunction in the Fetus and Neonate

Hyperthyroidism in the fetus is best diagnosed by ultrasonography to determine if goiter is present and by monitoring fetal heartbeat. In mothers who are on ATDs, the mother is generally switched to methimazole if she's on PTU if fetal hyperthyroidism is detected. In children born to mothers with active Graves' disease, the onset of temporary neonatal hyperthyroidism usually begins before birth, although symptoms may not appear obvious until a few days after birth. The onset of neonatal Graves' disease may also be delayed several weeks or longer and is related to the activity of passively transferred maternal TSI antibodies.

Normal Thyroid Function in the Newborn

Mean T4 levels in the newborn are 12 mcg/ml, a level that would be considered high in an adult. The increase may be due to the elevated TBG normally seen in the newborn considering that at term, the newborn's levels of FT4 are slightly less than those in maternal serum. Serum T4, T3 and thyroglobulin also continue to rise during the first few hours after delivery, reaching the hyperthyroid range by 24 hours.

Immediately after birth, neonatal TSH levels rise rapidly, peaking 30 minutes after birth, then dropping to its initial value within 48 hours. This rise is considered a response to the temperature cooling that occurs at delivery and accounts for the increased levels of T4, T3 and thyroglobulin. D2 type deiodinase present in adipose tissue contributes to the conversion of T4 to T3 rather than rT3. By the fifth day of life, levels of rT3 return to normal, although levels of T3 remain increased for the first year of life, then gradually diminish until they reach the normal range. The normal rates of thyroid hormone production are higher per unit of body weight in infants and children than in adults.

Neonatal Hyperthyroidism

Thyrotoxicosis is rarely seen in neonates and accounts for about 1 percent of all cases of childhood hyperthyroidism (LaFranchi and Hanna 2000, 989). The most common cause is Graves' disease, and in neonates this condition is transient. Neonatal Graves' disease is seen in mothers with Graves' disease, including those who have previously had radioiodine ablation, and occasionally in mothers with Hashimoto's thyroiditis. Neonatal Graves' thyrotoxicosis, which occurs equally in boys and girls, occurs in fewer than 2 percent of infants born to mothers who had Graves' thyrotoxicosis during or before pregnancy (LaFranchi and Hanna 2000, 989). However, mild cases may escape detection.

Besides Graves' disease, neonatal hyperthyroidism may be caused by other rare conditions. TSH receptor mutations and conditions of resistance to thyroid hormone, which is also caused by a genetic mutation, are other causes. Germline mutations in the transmembrane region of the TSH receptor cause a constitutive activation of the receptor, which results in thyrotoxicosis. These mutations may be inherited as an autosomal dominant trait or occur sporadically as new mutations. Another cause of neonatal thyrotoxicosis is McCune-Albright syndrome, which is caused by a genetic mutation affecting signaling pathways.

Neonatal Graves' disease is caused by the placental passage of stimulating TSH receptor antibodies (TSI) from mothers who continue producing these antibodies late into gestation, typically with total TRAb or TBII levels reaching 500 percent activity (LaFranchi and Hanna, 2000, 989). TSI antibodies stimulate the fetal/neonatal thyroid gland to produce excess thyroid hormone.

However, once they are produced TSI antibodies, similar to other IgG immunoglobulins, stay in the blood circulation for only 2–3 months, after which they're broken down into amino acids and excreted. Consequently, neonatal thyrotoxicosis from Graves' antibodies is self-limited to 6–12 weeks, although this period may be extended if levels of TSI are unusually high. Neonatal Graves' disease does not lead to Graves' disease or TSI production. The immune system of children less than 2 years is generally too immature to produce thyroid antibodies.

Symptoms of Neonatal Hyperthyroidism

Hyperthyroid infants are often premature and appear to have stunted intrauterine growth. Goiter is usually present, and the infant appears extremely restless, irritable, hyperactive, unusually alert and anxious. Growth and development, especially of the nervous system, are impaired by neonatal thyrotoxicosis. Microcephaly (condition characterized by a small head, which is usually associated with mental defects), ventricular enlargement, frontal bossing or triangular facies, poor weight gain, heart enlargement, jaundice, enlarged liver, enlarged spleen, diarrhea, vomiting, cardiac decompensation, tachycardia and an elevated temperature are all symptoms that may be present, and the eyes may appear exophthalmic (LaFranchi and Hanna 2000, 989). The onset, severity, and duration of symptoms in neonatal Graves' disease are variable. Neonates born to mothers on ATDs may not show symptoms for a few days after birth. Rarely, blocking TSH receptor antibodies may also be present and block symptoms of thyrotoxicosis for several weeks.

Treatment of Neonatal Hyperthyroidism

Anti-thyroid drugs, either methimazole or carbimazole, remain the treatment of choice in neonatal Graves' disease although, recently, iodinated cholecystographic agents, sodium ipodate, or iopanoic acid have come into use and appear beneficial. In one study, all neonates treated with iopanoic acid showed clinical improvement within 24 to 72 hours with no adverse effects (Earles et al. 2004).

In severe cases, propranolol is used to reduce cardiac symptoms, and glucocorticoid steroids are used to decrease the conversion of T4 into T3. Thyrotoxic infants with genetic mutations or McCune-Albright syndrome have permanent conditions of hyperthyroidism. They're initially treated with ATDs and after age 5 treated with more aggressive therapies.

In most neonates with Graves' disease, improvement with ATDs or iodinated contrast agents is rapid, and treatment can be tapered and withdrawn after several weeks or months. If hyperthyroidism persists, it is usually due to another cause besides Graves' disease. However, in patients with an impressive family history of Graves' disease, neonatal hyperthyroidism may persist into childhood, although TSH-stimulating antibodies are no longer detectable.

Hypothyroidism in the Fetus and Neonate

Antithyroid drugs used to treat the mother may cross the placental barrier, causing hypothyroidism in the newborn or fetus. PTU does not cross to the placenta as readily as methimazole, making it the treatment of choice for the first trimester. However, with the recent black box warnings to PTU, many patients are treated with methimazole or carbimazole throughout their pregnancies.

In addition to ATDs, blocking TSH receptor antibodies may rarely cross into the fetal circulation and bind to the TSH receptor, interfering with the actions of TSH. Since the thyroid-hypothalamic-pituitary axis isn't defined until late in pregnancy, the effects and any resulting hypothyroidism occur near the end of the gestational period.

Iodine deficiency may also cause hypothyroidism in patients with disorders that impair iodine absorption. Neonatal hypothyroidism in these infants occurs as a consequence of maternal iodine deficiency or from a maternal diet high in goitrogens or soy. Transient hypothyroidism may also occur in babies who are exposed to substances high in iodine content, such as X-ray dyes and certain skin cleansers, around the time of their birth. In these instances, hypothyroidism may persist for several days to several months.

ATD-Induced Maternal Hypothyroidism

Maternal hypothyroidism is associated with fertility problems and an increased risk of miscarriage, especially in the first trimester, and pre-term labor. Poor outcome is associated with the severity of the hypothyroidism. Maternal hypothyroidism may also have an adverse effect on fetal development. Maternal thyroxine is transferred to the fetal circulation more readily during the first half of pregnancy. Fetal requirements are critical since T4 contributes to the development of the central nervous system. In maternal hypothyroidism, inadequate maternal T4 exacerbates the effects of fetal hypothyroidism, contributing to irreversible nervous system disorders. A TSH level higher than 2.0 miu/L is considered a sign of hypothyroidism in pregnancy (Check 2007).

Hyperthyroidism in Children and Adolescents

When thyrotoxicosis occurs in children and adolescents, the culprit is usually Graves' disease. The proportion of hyperthyroid children having Graves' disease is higher than the proportion seen in hyperthyroid adults. Other causes of hyperthyroidism in children include autonomously functioning nodules and, very rarely, conditions of silent, subacute or bacterial thyroiditis, TSH receptor mutations, excess iodine, HCG secreting tumors, exogenous thyroid hormone use, resistance to thyroid hormone, and toxic multinodular goiter. Pituitary causes of thyrotoxicosis in childhood include pituitary adenoma and pituitary resistance to T4. Hyperthyroidism may very rarely occur in infancy, but overall it is seldom seen in children less than 5 years old (LaFranchi and Hanna 2000, 990).

Many other disorders, including diabetes, nutrient deficiencies, and attention deficit hyperactivity disorder (ADHD) can have symptoms mimicking those of hyperthyroidism in children. In addition, many symptoms wax and wane and are typical of childhood and aren't noticed unless they're dramatic. Family history is generally the best clue when children develop one or more symptoms suggestive of hyperthyroidism. Common symptoms that prompt an office visit include emotional lability, hyperactivity, increased appetite (although weight loss is not as common as in adults) goiter, eye changes, difficulty sleeping, weight gain (due to an excessive appetite), and frequent outbursts. Prepubertal children often experience symptoms for a longer time than pubertal children before they're diagnosed.

Many parents of children with Graves' disease report that changes in appearance, energy or behavior led them to consult a physician. In several instances, another relative who hadn't seen the child in a while remarked on the changes, which in day-to-day life easily go unnoticed.

Symptoms and Signs in Hyperthyroid Children and Adolescents

The following signs and symptoms are listed in the order of their frequency and range from 99 percent of patients with goiter to 13 percent of patients with diarrhea.

- Goiter
- Tachycardia
- Nervousness
- Increased pulse pressure
- Hypertension
- Exophthalmos
- Tremor
- Increased appetite
- Weight loss
- Thyroid bruit
- Increased perspiration
- Hyperactivity
- Heart murmur
- Palpitations
- Heat intolerance
- Fatigue
- Headache
- Diarrhea (LaFranchi and Hanna 2000, 991)

Prevalence of Childhood Hyperthyroidism

Because Graves' disease accounts for more than 95 percent of childhood cases of hyperthyroidism in the United States, the frequency of Graves' disease closely approximates the frequency of all cases of hyperthyroidism. Prevalence of Graves' disease is approximately 0.02 percent in childhood, accounting for fewer than 5 percent of the total U.S. cases of Graves' disease (Ferry 2011).

About 5 percent of all patients with Graves' disease are less than 15 years old (Behrman et al. 2000, 1709–12). The peak incidence is adolescence. In children born to mothers with Graves' disease, the onset of hyperthyroidism occurred between 6 weeks and 2 years of age. Aside from transient neonatal hyperthyroidism caused by antibody transfer, childhood Graves' disease occurs 4 to 5 times more often in females than males.

In one Italian study, researchers described three girls in whom Graves' disease developed before age 3 (presumably between an age of 6 to 12 months), although they weren't diagnosed until a mean age of 3 years. These children presented with goiter, exophthalmos, tachycardia, and hyperactivity. Two of the children consequently had impaired verbal expression and one child had severe mental retardation that is still evident. The children had been previously brought in to the pediatric clinic for symptoms of hyperthyroidism including poor language development, but they weren't tested for Graves' disease. The study's authors emphasize the need for psychological assessment in evaluating hyperthyroidism and greater awareness of the consequences on growth and development in the first two years of life (Segni et al. 1999).

In two of the children in this study, there was no maternal history of diagnosed Graves' disease, although one mother had isolated exophthalmos, and in one child the mother had been diagnosed with Graves' disease during pregnancy. Symptoms in all three children included goiter, exophthalmos, tachycardia and hyperactivity, and they all turned out to have consistently high levels of stimulating TRAb.

In addition, one child showed severe psychomotor delay and had undergone surgery for craniosynostosis. Craniosynostosis, a condition in which two or more cranial bones mesh to form a single bone, is a known complication of thyrotoxicosis in children. It is attributed to the higher sensitivity to thyroid hormones of membranous bone (bone attached to membrane) compared to enchondral bone, which is bone that is connected to bone (Segni et al. 1999).

Graves' Ophthalmopathy in Children

Exophthalmos is noticeable in most all children with Graves' disease but it is usually mild. Symptoms of Graves' opthalmopathy seen in children and adolescents include lagging of the upper eyelid on downward gaze, impairment of convergence or alignment, upper eyelid retraction, "staring eyes" and infrequent blinking. Infiltrative congestive ophthalmopathy is very rare in children and adolescents, and symptoms usually disappear when euthyroidism is restored. The administration of steroids is restricted to rare severe cases (Behrman 2000, 1712).

Diagnosis and Treatment

The diagnosis of hyperthyroidism in children is similar to that of adults. The TSH, FT4 and FT3 tests are used to diagnose hyperthyroidism. Antibody tests are used to confirm Graves' disease, with more than 90 percent of children having TSI, TPO and thyroglobulin antibodies (LaFranchi and Hanna 2000,

993). Measurements of radioiodine uptake and radionucolide imaging are seldom needed in children (LaFranchi and Hanna 2000, 992).

Treatment of Pediatric Graves' Disease

Treatment options listed in Chapters 6 and 7 are used in children as well as adults. However, because of the risks involved with radioiodine, treatment in children is generally restricted to antithyroid drug therapy or surgery. Alternative healing options are occasionally used in very mild cases or as adjunctive therapy in children on ATDs. Because some children will go into remission, methimazole therapy is still considered first-line treatment for most children (Bahn et al. 2011).

However, whatever treatment is used, the results are reported to be less satisfactory than in adults. Both problems with compliance and the fact that the thyroid cells divide and grow faster in children make treatment more of a challenge.

Children should have baseline CBCs and liver function tests or a metabolic profile before starting antithyroid drug therapy. The starting dosage of methimazole is 0.25 to 1.0 mg/kg/24 hr. given once or twice daily. Smaller initial doses are used in early childhood. After 4–8 weeks, when the FT4 level falls into range, the dose is typically reduced by 50 percent. Over time, the dose is reduced, with the lowest dose needed that keeps FT4 near the high end of the range, regardless of the TSH level, which remains low for many months. Some patients achieve remission within 1–2 years, especially when the offending trigger (often exposure to allergens) is removed, although drug therapy may be necessary for five years or longer. Most children with Graves' thyrotoxicosis are treated with ATD therapy for long periods (LaFranchi and Hanna 2000, 992). Reasons for this choice are the high incidence of remission in children, and in addition, many physicians, patients and their families have concerns that radioiodine therapy may yet prove to have some long-term side effects (LaFranchi and Hanna 2000, 992).

In children treated with an antithyroid drug, with follow-up periods of 8 to 22 years, about 10 percent eventually developed hypothyroidism caused by chronic autoimmune thyroiditis, either by a move into Hashimoto's thyroiditis or by the production of blocking TSH receptor antibodies, which can cause temporary or permanent conditions of autoimmune atrophic thyroiditis (LaFranchi and Hanna 2000, 993). Hypothyroidism in children following ATD therapy is generally mild compared to the hypothyroidism caused by surgery or radioiodine, and it is frequently a temporary condition.

Precautions

Pediatric patients and their caretakers should be informed of side effects of antithyroid drugs (see Chapter 7) and the necessity of stopping the medication immediately and informing their physician if they develop pruritic rash, jaundice, pale stools, dark urine, arthralgias, abdominal pain, nausea, fatigue, fever or pharyngitis (Bahn et al. 2011, 613).

Remission Using ATDs

Remission refers to a freedom from disease and its symptoms. In Graves' disease, patients older than 13 years, boys, patients with a higher body mass index, and patients with small goiters and modestly elevated T3 levels are reported to have earlier remissions. If relapse occurs after remission, it usually occurs 3–6 months from the discontinuation of therapy. At this time, ATDs are generally resumed. While ATDs can evoke remission, treatment with surgery or radioiodine corrects hyperthyroidism but does not bring about remission. Remission occurs when the immune system heals and stops producing TSI antibodies at a rate capable of causing hyperthyroidism.

Radioiodine and Surgery

Because of the enhanced carcinogenic potential of radiation in the thyroid glands of growing children and the lack of long-term studies, many endocrinologists do not recommend the use of radioiodine ablation for children with Graves' disease (Larsen et al. 1998, 451). Also, children and adolescents are considered to be at the greatest risk for genetic damage, damage which may take 30 years or more to show up. Of the various molecules that radiation may damage within the cell, DNA is said to be the most critical since damage to a single gene may irreparably alter or kill the cell (Upton 1998, 1293). A recent study from the University of Rochester Medical Center shows that the risk of thyroid cancer persists for 58 years or longer after childhood radiation (Adams 2010).

Although surgery is a viable option, thyroidectomy in children is associated with a higher risk of hypothyroidism than is seen in adults. This is probably related to the natural course of the disease compounded by the effect of declining thyroid hormone levels on growth. Also, surgical complications such as recurrent laryngeal nerve damage or hypoparathyroidism have lifelong consequences.

Beta adrenergic blocking agents are used during the early course of treatment in children with heart rates in excess of 100 beats per minute. As the ATD therapy begins to work and euthyroidism occurs (based on an FT4 level within the reference range), the dose of beta blockers is typically lowered and eventually withdrawn.

Treatment for Hyperthyroidism in Nodular Disease

True solitary nodules occur in 0.22–1.25 percent of the pediatric population (Hebra 2012). In adults, the prevalence is closer to 4 percent. A number of different thyroid masses can suggest nodules but turn out not to contain nodules. Upon close examination, thyroid masses often turn out to cause asymmetric enlargement of one lobe and often are devoid of nodules. Examples include unilateral agenesis, Hashimoto's thyroiditis, or other abnormalities such as lymph node or thyroglossal duct cysts. Ectopic thyroid tissue may also cloud the issue.

However, true nodules in children need to be evaluated and examined carefully because the presence of malignancy in pediatric nodules is higher than in the adult population. Malignancy in pediatric nodules is estimated to be 14–25 percent (Hebra 2012). In addition, thyroid cancer is much more aggressive in children and has a greater association with early metastasis to regional lymph nodes and surrounding organs, most commonly lung and bone.

Thyroid Masses and Nodules in Children

Benign tumors are the most common cause of thyroid nodules in children. Solitary nodules are more likely to be malignant than multiple nodules. Nodules are 2–3 times more common in girls than in boys. Nodules are usually discovered when the thyroid is palpated by a physician during a physical examination and a mass is felt. A palpated mass may be solid, cystic, or mixed. Ultrasound can determine the type of mass. Benign cysts can be evacuated successfully by aspiration, and there is usually no recurrence. However, the identification of a cyst does not exclude neoplastic changes, especially if the mass contains mixed tissue.

If a palpated mass is diagnosed as a truly solitary solid thyroid nodule, scintigraphy is used to help tell if the activity is hot, warm or cold. However, it can be difficult to determine, and fine needle aspiration (FNA) biopsy is the only way to confirm nodular activity.

Hot Nodules

In the pediatric population, hot nodules are rarely seen and comprise 5 percent of all nodules (Hebra 2012). Hot nodules have self- or autonomous regulation and, while suppressing the rest of the gland, are able to cause hyperthyroidism and thyrotoxicosis. While hot nodules are seen less often in children, they're more likely to cause hyperthyroidism, in which case they're called toxic nodules.

Warm Nodules

Warm nodules are usually functioning adenomas, although they may be malignant. Warm nodules show some function on scintigraphy but the patient remains euthyroid (normal thyroid function). These nodules are often watched for signs of growth, fixation to tissues or enlarged lymph nodes, signs that suggest possible malignancy. Most observed nodules are watched for changes.

Solitary Cold Nodule

Solitary cold nodules are the most common type of nodule in children, comprising 40–70 percent of all pediatric nodules. Solitary cold nodules also have the highest rate (17–36 percent) of malignancy (Hebra 2012). Still, most cold nodules are benign and are identified as follicular adenomas or Hashimoto's thyroiditis, ectopic thyroid tissue, or Hurthle cell hyperplasia. When nodules are found during the early hyperthyroid phase of Hashimoto's thyroiditis, they may cause transient conditions of hyperthyroidism. Cold nodules are common in Hashimoto's thyroiditis, and this disorder can be confirmed by the presence of TPO and thyroglobulin antibodies. It's unclear if an association with Hashimoto's thyroiditis increases the rate of malignancy. Regardless, nodules found in Hashimoto's thyroiditis and also in Hurthle cell adenomas should be analyzed by FNA biopsy or surgically removed because of their tendency to progress to malignancy.

Papillary and follicular cancers are the most common types of cancer. While medullary, undifferentiated, and anaplastic cancers are rarely seen in children, medullary thyroid cancer usually is found in children with multiple endocrine disorders (see Chapter 2).

Treatment of Toxic Adenoma

Anti-thyroid drugs are often used to shrink nodules and reduce thyroid hormone disease in children with hyperthyroidism caused by nodules. Alternative techniques include percutaneous ethanol injection (PEI), thermal ablation, and radiofrequency ablation. The cure rate with PEI has been reported to be as high as 93 percent (Bahn et al. 2011). Complications are rare and include transient laryngeal nerve damage, abscess, and hematoma.

Immunological Studies in Hyperthyroid Children and Adolescents

Because of the frequent appearance of autoimmune thyroid disease in patients with systemic autoimmune diseases such as systemic lupus erythematosus, Sjogren's syndrome, and rheumatoid arthritis, Bulgarian researchers conducted a study to assess the frequency of thyroid antibodies, thyroid inflammation and thyroid lesions in children and adolescents with rheumatological disorders. The results showed that 44 percent of subjects with juvenile arthritis had thyroglobulin or TPO antibodies. Of these children with thyroid antibodies, 85.2 percent were euthyroid (normal thyroid function), 11.1 percent had compensated hypothyroidism, and 3.7 percent had Hashitoxicosis, a disorder characterized by Hashimoto's thyroiditis in the presence of stimulating TSH receptor antibodies. Hashitoxicosis causes transient symptoms of hyperthyroidism in patients with hypothyroidism.

Hyperthyroidism in Adolescents

Similar to what is seen in children, hyperthyroidism in adolescents is most often caused by Graves' disease. However, hyperthyroidism in adolescence has a significantly higher prevalence at 0.6 percent (Gruters 1999). Autonomously functioning nodules also occur at a higher rate in adolescents than children.

Similar to hyperthyroidism in children, conditions of infiltrative ophthalmopathy are rare, and eye symptoms are generally a result of excessive thyroid hormone. Remission rates in adolescents are significantly higher than in children, which is likely due to better compliance. Adolescents are also more likely to follow dietary protocols and exercise programs that help heal the immune system in Graves' disease.

The unique challenge to health care providers in diagnosing and treating adolescents is that hyperthyroidism can adversely affect growth and development during puberty. Because symptoms associated with hyperthyroidism are common in this age group, diagnosis is often delayed (Hanna and LaFranchi 2002).

11

Graves' Ophthalmopathy and Other Extrathyroidal Manifestations

Graves' ophthalmopathy (GO) is the most common cause of orbital disease in adults. It develops in 25–50 percent of patients with Graves' disease (Griepentrog and Garrity 2009). Although the associated hyperthyroidism is easily managed, treatment of the eye symptoms remains challenging. Advances in the last decade have brought several new treatment options and a better understanding of factors that influence GO development, and the role antioxidant nutrients and stress reduction play in healing this condition.

A better understanding of the dermal manifestations of Graves' disease and their relationship to GO have also led to better treatments and preventive measures. These topics are explored in Chapter 11.

Eye Changes in Hyperthyroidism

Hyperthyroidism can affect the eyes, causing a characteristic stare, eye dryness, eyelid lag, and eye tremor called Graves' ophthalmopathy or thyroid eye disease (TED). These symptoms resolve when thyroid hormone levels are corrected, and they're related to the effects of excess thyroid hormone on eye tissues. The majority of symptoms related to excess thyroid hormone are upper eyelid elevation and spastic signs.

Thyroid hormone affects all of the cells in the body, typically speeding up metabolic functions. The increased activity of the sympathetic nervous system also contributes to the eye symptoms. Up to 90 percent of patients with active Graves' disease exhibit a prominent stare related to sympathetic nervous system stimulation, which is attributed to increased levels of epinephrine and norepinephrine resulting from excess thyroid hormone. Besides the fixed stare, other symptoms caused by thyroid hormone excess include dryness, tearing, puffiness, and twitching. Patients with thyrotoxicosis, upon close examination, often show a widening of the palpebral fissure, and lag of the globe on upward or downward gaze, causing a pop-eyed appearance. These abnormalities may cause the eye to appear exophthalmic, but measurement may show that there is no actual proptosis (Moore 2003, 48).

In Graves' hyperthyroidism, and other autoimmune thyroid conditions including Hashimoto's thyroiditis and Hashitoxicosis, patients can also develop an autoimmune, infiltrative congestive form of Graves' ophthalmopathy. The congestive form of GO can also occur in the absence of thyroid dysfunction in a condition called euthyroid Graves' disease. Patients with congestive eye disease can also develop other extrathyroidal (occurring away from the thyroid gland) symptoms in the skin, causing pretibial myxedema, and, in the soft tissues of the fingers and toes, causing thyroid acropachy.

Graves' Ophthalmopathy

Some ophthalmologists do not consider the signs and symptoms related to excessive thyroid hormone as true conditions of Graves' ophthalmopathy since they resolve quickly and do not have an autoimmune origin. In the following sections of this chapter, the term Graves' ophthalmopathy refers to the congestive, infiltrative form of GO.

Congestive, Infiltrative Graves' Ophthalmopathy

Congestive Graves' ophthalmopathy is an autoimmune disorder that runs its own course independent of the thyroid disorder. This condition is caused by an immune system defect that leads to the production of pro-inflammatory cytokines and TSH receptor antibodies that target TSH receptor protein on orbital cells.

Researchers at Wright State University in Dayton, Ohio, have completed studies that confirm that TSH receptor protein is targeted in Graves' ophthalmopathy. This protein is found in both skin and orbital tissue of both normal and Graves' patients. In patients with autoimmune thyroid disorders, but not normal patients, messenger RNA (mRNA) is present, and the fibroblasts are activated, suggesting that activated fibroblasts are distributed throughout the body in Graves' disease (Warwar 1999).

The Autoimmune Process in GO

In the eye, activated fibroblasts (early precursor tissue cells) differentiate into adipocytes rather than normal orbital cells. Adipocytes produce glycosaminoglycan (GAG), which accumulate in the orbital cavity, causing the proptosis (eye bulging, proptosis) characteristic of congestive GO. Autoreactive T cells contribute to inflammation.

Cytokines such as interferon-gamma, which are released by T cells and macrophages, stimulate orbital fibroblasts a well as adipocytes to produce GAG. Cytokines also cause the

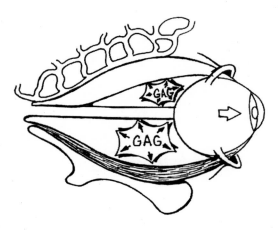

Congestive Graves' ophthalmopathy (courtesy Marvin G. Miller).

orbital fibroblasts to express HLA-DR. HLA-DR is normally only expressed on lymphocytes, monocytes and endothelial cells. Its presence on fibroblasts is aberrant, allowing these cells to present autoantigens to receptive T cells. This perpetuates the autoimmune inflammatory response.

Normal Progression of Graves' Ophthalmopathy

Most researchers agree that ophthalmopathy in Graves' disease is self-limiting. The course of GO characteristically worsens over an initial period of 3–6 months, followed by a lengthy plateau that may last several years. Many patients experience spontaneous improvement after a cycle of periodic flare-ups (exacerbations). Graves' ophthalmopathy usually develops within 18 months after the diagnosis of hyperthyroidism. When it develops before hyperthyroidism occurs, GO is called euthyroid Graves' disease.

The Natural Progression of Graves' Ophthalmopathy

Graves' ophthamopathy is an inflammatory ocular disorder with a wide range of symptoms. The most common symptoms include staring, proptosis, dryness, grittiness, diplopia (double vision), and eyelid retraction. Graves' ophthamopathy may affect the extraocular muscles and connective tissue that supports the eye; the blood vessels and nerves that serve the eye; and the eyelids that protect the eye.

In Graves' ophthamopathy, inflammation or congestion affects the connective tissues, fat deposits, and the muscles of the eye. In addition, one or more of the six ocular muscles that move the eye become enlarged. Normally, these muscles cannot be seen on the surface. They originate behind the eye at the peak of the eye socket and attach to the eye just behind the cornea. A thin film called the conjunctiva covers the eye muscles.

The fatty tissue present in the eye also enlarges in Graves' ophthalmopathy as it becomes filled with fluid, white blood cells, and GAG deposits. The increased volume of both the eye muscles and orbital fat causes increased retrobulbar pressure within the bony cage or eye socket surrounding the eye. This compression cause the eye tissues to become inflamed, reddened and swollen. Crowding displaces the eyeball, pushing it forward. When eye muscles become rigid and fixed in place due to this crowding, diplopia occurs. In addition, the muscles may press on the optic nerve, threatening vision.

Phases of Graves' Ophthalmopathy

Responding to immune system influences, Graves' ophthalmopathy runs its own self-limiting course, which can be divided into 3 phases: an active, progressive phase; a plateau phase, in which symptoms taper off; and a resolution phase, in which symptoms typically resolve. Most patients experience a spontaneous remission of symptoms during the resolution phase (Moore 2003, 30).

During the active, progressive phase of GO, vision-threatening complications may arise, including optic neuropathy and corneal ulceration. The active phase typically runs for 3 to 6 months, although in some patients it may last up to 5 years. The active phase is associated with a worsening or development of diplopia, photophobia (light sensitivity), excessive watering, and aching orbits sometimes associated with eye movements. Signs of activity include TSI elevations, an obvious fluid-filled distending eyelid, red eyelid, red eye or bright red vessels, and swollen conjunctiva.

Measures to reduce orbital inflammation have the greatest efficacy during this progressive or "hot" stage. However, it is important not to have orbital decompression surgery at this time unless vision is threatened and unresponsive to corticosteroid treatment. Surgery during the active phase interferes with the normal healing process that occurs in the resolution phase. Surgery performed too early leads to the need for additional surgeries. Many patients treated too early surgically before the autoimmune nature of Graves' ophthal-mopathy was fully understood have had more than 20 corrective surgeries.

In the plateau phase, disease activity is reduced. Inflammation subsides and symptoms begin to resolve. During this phase, patients often worry about changes to their appearance and become frustrated and impatient. However, surgery and orbital radiotherapy aren't beneficial at this time because the tar-gets of these therapies are no longer active, rendering treatment ineffective.

During the resolution phase (inactive, dry phase) most changes resolve. However, the extraocular muscles may heal by progressive fibrosis or scarring, resulting in fibrotic contractures and diplopia. After symptoms appear inactive for six months, recurrence of eye disease is infrequent although it may coincide with poor control of thyroid hormone levels. Thyroid hormone levels that are too low for the body's need cause symptoms of hypothyroidism and encourage thyroid antibody production. Low levels of FT4 and FT3 contribute to the worsening and development of Graves' ophthalmopathy.

Euthyroid Graves' Disease

Euthyroid Graves' disease is an autoimmune condition that causes the characteristic eye symptoms of Graves' ophthalmopathy, which is more com-monly known as thyroid eye disease (TED), in the absence of thyroid dys-function. Most patients with euthyroid Graves' disease go on to develop thyroid disease within 12–18 months after eye symptoms develop (Char 1991, 99). Most of these patients develop Graves' disease, an autoimmune thyroid disorder, although a smaller number of patients may develop autoimmune hypothyroidism. About 15–20 percent of patients with euthyroid Graves' dis-ease never develop thyroid dysfunction (Char 1991, 99). However, even though patients with euthyroid Graves' disease are considered to have normal thyroid function based on blood tests for thyroid function, they can have transient symptoms of both hypothyroidism and hyperthyroidism.

Patients with euthyroid Graves' disease typically have high levels of both stimulating and blocking TSH receptor antibodies (TRAb). While stimulating TRAb (TSI) stimulate thyroid cells to produce excess thyroid hormone in Graves' disease, the blocking TRAb in euthyroid Graves' disease prevent TSI from causing hyperthyroidism. Each of these antibodies cancels out the effects of the other on thyroid function. However, because they are both capable of eliciting an immune response in eye muscle (orbital) tissue, they contribute to signs and symptoms of TED.

The most significant changes in TED involve congestion and infiltration of orbital muscle, causing the eyeball to appear swollen. The eye muscle in

TED also has limited motion caused by this congestion, causing limited upward or downward gaze. Muscle restriction also contributes to double vision (diplopia). The muscle fibers in TED do not change, but deposits of white blood cells and immune system chemicals lodge between the fibers, causing orbital congestion. Typical symptoms in TED include eyelid retraction, puffiness (orbital edema), proptosis or exophthalmos (bulging forward of the eyeball), lid lag, photophobia (light sensitivity), conjunctival inflammation, double vision, redness, optic nerve compression, and keratitis.

Individuals with Hashitoxicosis are at high risk for Graves' ophthalmopathy (thyroid eye disease or TED). TSH receptor antibodies are known to contribute to trigger Graves' ophthalmopathy and worsen symptoms. Patients in the early phases of Hashitoxicosis may have normal thyroid function tests because of blocking TSH receptor antibodies preventing TSI from reacting with thyroid cells. Consequently, individuals with Hashitoxicosis and eye disease may be misdiagnosed as having euthyroid Graves' disease.

Diagnosis of Graves' Ophthalmopathy

Diagnosis is straightforward in hyperthyroid patients. In euthyroid patients, a vigilant effort is generally made to detect an underlying thyroid disorder. On the other hand, some patients with thyrotoxicosis may have eye problems unrelated to thyroid disease, for instance, coexisting conditions of myasthenia gravis. And some patients with Graves' ophthalmopathy remain euthyroid in conditions of euthyroid Graves' disease, which may be difficult to diagnose without imaging tests.

Ocular findings are most specific for GO when they occur bilaterally and in certain combinations. The concurrence of bilateral lid retraction with proptosis and restrictive eye movement is virtually diagnostic. Markedly asymmetric or unilateral occurrence of most of these symptoms suggests a different origin for the ocular disease.

The Objective Eye Examination

The eye exam begins with an assessment of visual acuity in each eye. The pupillary responses to light are evaluated. When both a reduction in visual acuity and an afferent pupillary defect are present, optic neuropathy is likely and formal field testing is mandatory. The eyes are then inspected for periorbital edema, lid edema and lid lag. Diplopia field testing and the Lancaster or Hess screens are used to determine the degree of extraocular muscle impairment.

Bilateral proptosis in itself is not diagnostic of Graves' ophthalmopathy. It may result as a consequence of shallow orbits as in Crouzon's disease, or be due to large globes (seen in severe myopia), or to retroocular fat accumulation as occurs in exogenous steroid administration. Other causes include Cushing's syndrome, obesity, lithium therapy, cirrhosis, orbital pseudotumor, Wegener's granulomatosus, lymphoma and metastatic tumors (Burch et al. 2000, 532–34).

Even though unilateral proptosis is less specific, Graves' ophthalmopathy is its single most common cause, representing 15 percent to 28 percent of cases (Burch et al. 2000, 532). Axial proptosis, in which the eye is displaced in an anterior direction, is a frequent finding in Graves' ophthalmopathy. Other ocular deviations, such as those in which the eye position appears down and out, down and in, or elevated with proptosis, are typically seen in other pathologic processes (Char 1991, 100).

The eye signs of Graves' disease have been classified by the American Thyroid Association as a mnemonic system in which the first letters of each category constitute the term NOSPECS.

Class 0 — No physical signs or symptoms

Class 1 — Only signs, no symptoms (signs limited to upper lid retraction, stare, lid lag, and proptosis to 22 mm)

Class 2 — Soft tissue involvement with periorbital edema, congestion or redness of the conjunctiva and swelling of the conjunctiva (chemosis)

Class 3 — Proptosis >22 mm as measured by Hertel exophthalmometry

Class 4 — Extraocular muscle involvement, most commonly the inferior rectus with involvement impairing upward gaze

Class 5 — Corneal involvement (keratitis)

Class 6 — Sight loss from optic nerve involvement [Char 1991, 100].

NOSPECS represents a useful system for evaluation. Objective measurements for each eye separately (as recommended) include documentation of maximus lid fissure width, assessment of exposure keratitis and extraocular muscle function, measurement of intraocular pressure, and measurements of visual acuity, fields and color vision.

However, some ophthalmologists do not rely on NOSPECS or any of its modifications for categorization or treatment decisions. Their reasoning is that patients often progress from one class to another without proceeding through the interval steps, awarding the system no prognostic value. Also, the separate components comprising Graves' ophthalmopathy may vary in their severity or not be equal in terms of visual or cosmetic debility (Char 1991,

101). Consequently, there is no gold standard for grading the severity or activity of GO. This has led to difficulty in comparing treatments (Griepentrog and Garrity 2009). The following grading systems are also used to classify GO.

Classification of GO by Werner

This is a numbered system created by Sydney Werner:

1. No symptoms or signs
2. Signs only, such as upper lid retraction, staring vision, lid lag; no symptoms
3. Soft tissue involvement (symptoms and signs)
4. Exophthalmos: (a) extraocular muscle involvement; includes diplopia; (b) corneal involvement; (c) vision loss (optic neuropathy)

Criteria of Mourits —
The Clinical Activity Score (CAS)

In this system, one point is given for any disease manifestation, with 0 indicating no activity and 10 indicating a very high disease activity. After two consecutive clinical examinations the CAS can be determined. In this classification, patients with scores greater than 3 have active disease and show a better response to treatment than those with lower scores.

- Spontaneous retrobulbar pain
- Painful oppressive feeling on or behind the globe
- Pain with eye movements, including attempted up, side or down gaze
- Erythema (redness) of the eyes, eyelids or conjunctiva
- Swelling
- Chemosis (edema of the bulbar conjunctiva)
- Edema of the eyelids
- Increase in proptosis of 2 mm or more over a 1–3 month duration
- Impaired eye function
- Decrease in visual acuity of 1 or more lines on the Snellen chart over 1–3 months
- Decrease of eye movements equal or greater than 5 degrees over 1–3 months

Other Autoimmune Associations

Although lid retraction and proptosis are most commonly associated with Graves' disease, they may also be seen in Hashimoto's thyroiditis and the autoimmune condition myasthenia gravis. Euthyroid Graves' disease is also associated with specific changes. Most patients with this condition are likely to develop diplopia, experience problems closing lids, and have limited eyeball movements, corneal involvement and unilateral proptosis. Other causes of proptosis include the following non-neoplastic conditions:

- Myopia in hypokalemic periodic paralysis
- Posterior commissure brain lesions; Cushing's syndrome
- Myasthenia gravis; Wegener's granulomatosis
- Lymphoma, idiopathic inflammatory pseudotumors
- (Parinaud's syndrome) Chronic obstructive lung disease
- Congenital anomalies such as uremia
- Cirrhosis — superior vena cava syndrome
- Medication (lithium, steroids, etc.); sympathomimetic amine drugs (Adderall, some diet pills, and antihistamines)
- Contralateral ptosis — nerve III lesions
- Myopia
- Carotid cavernous fistula; infection
- Hydrocephalus status after lid surgery (Char 1991, 97–99)

Imaging Studies in Graves' Ophthalmopathy

Not all patients with GO require imaging studies for diagnosis or treatment, especially if there is thyroid involvement, no apparent corneal staining and good vision. The primary indication for radiographic evaluation is to confirm the diagnosis when there is uncertainty. When imaging studies are required, magnetic resonance imaging (MRI), computed tomography (CT) and ultrasonography are the methods commonly employed.

Proptosis may be measured by a variety of instruments such as the Hertel exophthalmometer. However, the most sensitive measurements are made by high resolution orbital imaging. The typical imaging pattern in Graves' ophthalmopathy demonstrates enlarged recti muscles, usually with the tendons spared and varying amounts of orbital fat. In up to 30 percent of cases, only a single muscle is involved and occasionally the only abnormality is an increase in orbital fat (Burch et al. 2000, 533–34). Both CT and MRI allow measurements of extraocular muscle thickness and provide good visualization in the critical area at the orbital apex. MRI using a 1.5 tesla unit and orbital surface coils provides optimal spatial resolution of the orbit. Although proptosis is typically bilateral (affecting both eyes) in GO, unilateral (affecting one eye) proptosis can occur. However, with imaging tests patients who appear to have unilateral proptosis show signs of proptosis in both eyes.

A disadvantage to MRI is that image reformation in different planes is not always available. Also, it is more expensive and takes longer. An advantage is that is provides better anatomic detail, and, with a fat saturation-gadolinium-DTPA protocol, is unparalleled for delineation of subtle compressive optic neuropathy. MRI after gadolinium–DPTA administration can distinguish between muscles that are swollen due to fatty degeneration, fibrosis and edema. T2 weighted MRI images may also demonstrate active inflammation.

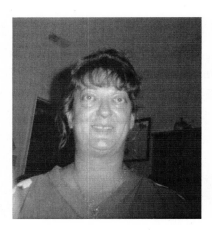

Post-RAI Graves' ophthalmopathy (courtesy Lisa Reynolds).

CT imaging may also be used to estimate the volume of extraocular muscle and retroocular fat tissue. Advantages to CT are that it is faster and less expensive. CT imaging, with axial and coronal views, is the preferred study due to its ability to provide bony detail. Ultrasonography, the first method in use for high-resolution orbital imaging, is least applicable for determining visualization in the critical area of the orbital axis.

Factors Influencing the Development of Graves' Ophthalmopathy

Treatment for Graves' Disease

Graves' disease treatment may affect the natural course of Graves' ophthalmopathy. Because radioiodine therapy evokes prolonged, dramatic increases in serum TSI levels, Graves' ophthalmopathy is often triggered, and in existing conditions there may be an exacerbation of symptoms. Patients given high ATD doses can develop hypothyroidism, which causes an exacerbation of symptoms along with the development of periorbital edema (swelling around the eyes and eyelids).

Cigarette Smoking

It's long been known that both Graves' disease and Graves' ophthalmopathy are associated with smoking. Smoking is associated with decreased levels of interleukin-1-alpha receptor antagonist. From this, researchers postulate that smoking may exacerbate inflammation in Graves' ophthalmopathy by lowering interleukin-1-alpha receptor antagonists levels and increasing the relative activity of interleukin-1-alpha. Interleukin-1-alpha stimulates GAG production (Warwar 1999, 359).

Environmental Triggers of Thyroid Disease

Environmental triggers that contribute to the development of Graves' disease are known to contribute to Graves' ophthalmopathy. These include excess dietary iodine, including iodine used in contrast dyes used in imaging studies and dietary supplements; stress; low selenium levels; exposure to allergens; and cigarette smoke.

Dr. Charles Soparkar, an ophthalmologist specializing in GO, reports that stress worsens symptoms in patients with GO and that he sees this effect frequently in his practice. He also reports that symptoms worsen when patients are dehydrated and that adequate fluid intake is essential (Moore 2003, 132). Stress reduction techniques such as yoga, tai chi, biofeedback, and meditation modulate the immune system, inhibit the activity of autoreactive cells (reducing thyroid antibody production), and reduce inflammation.

Treatment of Graves' Ophthalmopathy

Treatment of Graves' ophthalmopathy depends on the patient's overall condition, specific eye symptoms and disease severity. Most patients have minor disturbances that can be treated with local protective measures such as tinted glasses, eye drops containing 1 percent methylcellulose, prisms, protective eye patches, eye gels, artificial tear ointments and taping the eyelids shut at night. Patients with only minor eye signs such as stare and lid lag or light sensitivity (photophobia) or excessive tearing (epiphora) are best treated with artificial tears or lubrication ointments (such as Lacri-Lube) to prevent or heal corneal surface injury.

While most patients with GO do not require aggressive treatment because their conditions are mild and self-limited, when conditions are moderate to severe, treatment may be needed. Patients who are candidates for therapy include those with the following conditions:

• Sight-threatening ophthalmopathy
• Corneal perforation risk
• Advanced soft-tissue inflammation
• Ophthalmoplegia (paralysis of one or more extraocular muscles)

- History of globe subluxation (dislocation)
- Moderate to severe proptosis
- Optic neuropathy or optic nerve compression risk
- Distressing appearance
- Diplopia that requires abnormal head position to correct

Non-Surgical Treatment Options

Treatment works to reduce the swollen soft tissues, allowing for more space in the orbital cavity, and to improve symptoms. Current treatment options include the short-term use of diuretics to decrease fluid content, corticosteroids to suppress the immune system and reduce inflammation, orbital radiation therapy to reduce soft tissue inflammation and proptosis and improve eye muscle function, prisms to reduce diplopia, and 1 percent methylcellulose drops to prevent dryness. Antioxidant nutrients, especially bioflavonoids and vitamin B_2, are also reported to improve Graves' ophthalmopathy. Plasmapheresis, by reducing levels of thyroid antibodies in the blood circulation, has resulted in improvement, and the immunosuppressive drug cyclosporine has shown promising results.

Prisms

Prism lenses applied to the lens of glasses are used to correct double vision. Prisms can be ground into lenses or pressed on with frunell press-on prisms. Both work well and the eyes do not need to move in all directions for them to work.

Ocreotide

Ocreotide, a chemical that exerts pharmacologic actions similar to the natural hormone somatostatin, has proved effective in some individuals with Graves' ophthalmopathy. Patients who have somatostatin receptors in their eye muscle and who have localization of nuclear isotopes on Octreoscan-111 scanning have shown improvement when treated with octreotide 300 mcg daily over 12 weeks. However, the use of ocreotide is considered investigational, and side effects make its use prohibitive for most patients.

Corticosteroids

Steroids are typically administered in the early stages of Graves' ophthalmopathy before extensive fibrosis has occurred. Taken orally in doses up to 80 mg per day, prednisone proves effective in most patients. Side effects include high blood pressure, insomnia, weight gain, depression, relapse of eye symptoms after stopping treatment and incomplete reversal of the disease in some cases.

Besides their anti-inflammatory and immunosuppressive effects, corticosteroids may directly inhibit GAG synthesis and also its release from fibroblasts. Corticosteroids relieve pain involved with soft tissue inflammation, reduce orbital swelling and edema, and ameliorate the pain of compressive optic neuropathy.

In one protocol, corticosteroids are given at the time of radioiodine ablation. Although this prevents an immediate exacerbation of Graves' ophthalmopathy, there are no long-term studies to evaluate the extent of protection, and patients using this protocol are known to develop Graves' ophthalmopathy several years after RAI.

Immunosuppressants and Anti-inflammatory Agents

Cyclosporine A inhibits the proliferation of helper T cells, thyroid antibodies and cytokines, which contribute to the development of GO. Cyclosporine A is often used with corticosteroids, which allows for a reduction in the steroid dosage. Side effects of cyclosporine A include diplopia, hypertension and infection.

Colchine is an anti-inflammatory agent that has been found to decrease the expression of pro-inflammatory cytokines and reduce antibody secretion. It's known to provide favorable effects in some patients with GO.

Pentoxyfilline is an immunosuppressant used to reduce soft-tissue inflammation, but not proptosis or ophthalmoplegia.

Methotrexate is a chemotherapeutic agent used in the treatment of GO and other orbital inflammatory diseases.

Intravenous immunoglobulins (IVIG) has shown favorable results in some patients. IVIG works to dissolve immune complexes and block the production of new antibodies. However, it's an expensive therapy and availability depends on a sufficient donor population.

Plasmapheresis, a procedure using therapeutic phlebotomy (unit of blood is drawn, plasma is removed, and the cells transfused back into the patient) is another controversial treatment used in GO. The idea behind it is that circulating immunoglobulins in the plasma are removed and their levels diminished. The drawbacks are that it is expensive and any improvement is transient since antibody production is an ongoing process.

Orbital Supervoltage Radiotherapy
(External Beam Radiation)

External beam orbital irradiation has been used to treat GO for more than 60 years. It works by killing the retrobulbar lymphocytes that produce thyroid antibodies. It is generally administered in a dose of 20 Gy given in 10 fractions over two weeks. Irradiation may help reduce soft-tissue inflammation and ameliorate compressive optic neuropathy. The benefits continue to occur for up to 6 months following the last treatment. However, about one-third of patients experience no benefits, and improvement in those who do respond is limited. Side effects include transient worsening of soft-tissue inflammation, loss of hair at the temples, rare conditions of retinopathy and cataracts.

Conflicting reports of the efficacy occur because radiotherapy is often used in combination with steroids. However, good responses have occurred in patients using radiotherapy with or without steroids. In general, patients who show a good response to steroids prove to be good candidates for orbital radiotherapy. Radiotherapy seems to work best in patients with a short history of eye disease and is not recommended for patients with coexisting diabetic retinopathy, due to the increased risk of cataract development following radiotherapy.

In one study, the field of binocular single vision was enlarged in 11 of 17 patients after irradiation, compared with 2 of 15 patients in the control group (Mouritis 2000). Still, 75 percent of the patients receiving orbital irradiation later required strabismus surgery. The conclusion of this study indicated that in patients with moderately severe Graves' ophthalmopathy, radiotherapy is only effective at treating motility impairment.

Eye Surgeries

With advances in understanding the autoimmune nature of GO, patients are no longer rushed into having surgery. Surgery is indicated in patients with advanced soft tissue inflammation, ophthalmoplegia, moderate to severe proptosis or optic neuropathy.

Surgery is generally postponed until the active eye disease (the hot phase) has subsided unless there is progressive optic nerve involvement. With the exception of orbital decompression, most of the surgeries discussed can be performed on an outpatient basis or as a same-day surgery.

Surgical Protocol

The wide range of problems seen in GO is best managed by a team of physicians specializing in different aspects of GO. Such a team might include a neuro-ophthalmologist (specialist in ophthalmology and neurology), an eye muscle specialist (strabismologist), and an oculoplastic surgeon (specialist in GO and plastic surgery).

Orbital decompression is the standard surgical approach for GO and is usually performed first, followed by extraocular muscle surgery or correction of double vision if indicated, which is, in turn, followed by eyelid surgery if indicated.

If this sequence is deviated from, the benefits of an operation may be lost either by the recurrence of the disease or by the effects of a later procedure. For instance, orbital decompression may influence the ocular motility and change the lid aperture. Adjustment or recession of the inferior rectus muscle may alter upper and lower lid retraction. Among the following list of surgeries there may be several customized variations.

Eye Muscle Surgeries

Occasionally, eye muscle enlargement causes a decrease in mobility resulting in diplopia, which may improve spontaneously. If intervention is required, various procedures are available to realign the eyes. Usually, no skin incisions are required and outpatient surgery under general anesthesia is performed. Eye muscle surgery is generally performed after orbital decompression since this procedure may change eye muscle functions. Soreness following surgery is usually mild and lasts for 1–3 days.

Eyelid Surgeries

The eyelids in GO may become puffy and fluid filled (periorbital edema), and the skin below the eye may sag from stretching. Occasionally, the eyelids may retract away from the iris, exposing excess white sclera. Or the eyelids may droop, interfering with the visual range. Corrective surgery is usually performed under local anesthesia. Incisions are usually small and easily camouflaged. Pain is usually mild, lasting one day, although bruising may persist for up to 14 days. Ice-cold compresses are used during the first 2 days post-op, followed by warm compresses for the duration until bruising is healed.

Human Tissue Graft

Banked human tissue graft (e.g., AlloDerm) is used to elevate the lower eyelids in patients with lower eyelid retraction associated with Graves ophthalmopathy. However, insurance companies consider this therapy experimental and investigational. The "En-glove" lower eyelid retraction surgical technique offers a minimally invasive approach for the release of the lower eyelid retractors and allows for volume augmentation using either AlloDerm or dermis-fat spacer graft. In one small study, researchers concluded that "Englove" lower eyelid retraction surgical technique offers a minimally invasive approach for the release of the lower eyelid retractors and allows for volume augmentation using either AlloDerm or dermis-fat spacer graft. (Chang et al. 2011).

Orbital Decompression Surgery

The orbit refers to the bony chamber that houses the eye, the optic nerve and the eye muscles. In GO, enlarged orbital muscles and increased fat may cause orbital nerve compression. Orbital decompression reduces the amount of tissue within the orbit or enlarges the orbit by removing some of the bony supporting walls and expanding the orbit into nearby spaces, most commonly the sinuses. Because patients with GO often have sinus problems, some physicians recommend having simultaneous sinus surgery. Furthermore, orbital decompression increases the risk of sinus disease, and sinus disease can lead to visual disturbances (Soparkar 1999).

Orbital decompression can be considered at any point in which expansion of the bony orbital volume is desired. A second variety of orbital decompression, used on patients with significant orbital fat, removes only orbital fat without removing any bone. This variety is used only after the eye disease has remained stable for at least 6 months.

Several other surgeries for orbital decompression have evolved over the years, including 1-, 2-, 3-, and 4-wall decompression. All varieties require a skin incision of 5–10 mm at the corner of the eye. There may be temporary discomfort (1–3 days), although bruising may persist for 14 days. Orbital decompression surgery is frequently complicated by a worsening of preexisting diplopia regardless of the method employed. Additional surgery is often required after an appropriate length of time to allow for swelling to subside and stabilization of the myopathy.

In addition, lower lid retraction may accompany proptosis. Lower lid retraction frequently occurs after adjustment of the inferior rectus muscle and may be worsened by orbital decompression. One surgery used to correct lower lid retraction involves placing a graft from the upper lid into the lower lid. One surgical procedure used for upper lid retraction is eyelid lengthening, with or without removal of excess skin or fat deposits (dermatochalasis). Alternately, plastic weights may be inserted in the eyelid and later removed if needed.

Antioxidant Nutrients in Graves' Ophthalmopathy

Patients have long reported improvement after incorporating antioxidants into their therapeutic protocols. Common antioxidants used in GO include vitamin B_2, flaxseed oil (using 1000 mg twice daily to increase eye moisture), vitamins A and C, selenium, and melatonin.

In one study, the drug allopurinol, which is commonly used for gout, was used along with nicotinamide, a form of vitamin B_3, using 300 mg daily of both drugs in patients with GO. Both allopurinol and nicotinamide have antioxidant properties. Improvement was seen in 82 percent of patients all of whom were cigarette smokers. The greatest improvement was seen in soft tissue inflammation. No side effects of the antioxidants were noted (Bouzas et al. 2000).

Other Complementary Therapies

Low-Dose Naltrexone (LDN)

Used in low doses, the opiate antagonist naltrexone is found to improve immune function by boosting endorphin circulation. The effects are similar to those seen in acupuncture (see Chapter 8). The use of LDN in treating patients with multiple sclerosis (MS) was first proposed in the mid–1980s by Dr. Bernard Bihari, a New York City neurologist. In his clinical practice, the Harvard-educated Bihari found that a low dose of naltrexone (1.5–4.5 mg daily) taken at bedtime offered benefits to patients with MS and other autoimmune conditions including Graves' disease, Graves' ophthalmopathy, and rheumatoid arthritis. Since then, additional studies and anecdotal reports have confirmed Bihari's findings and demonstrated the effectiveness of naltrexone for Crohn's disease, Parkinson's disease and other conditions.

The effects of naltrexone are also thought to be attributed to the removal of the regulatory effects on the immune system exerted by endogenous opioid peptides, which could activate Th2 and suppress Th1 cytokines. Low-dose naltrexone is frequently used in patients with GO and in patients with Graves' disease using anti-thyroid drug therapy.

Bee Pollen

Naturally harvested bee pollen and its propolis extract taken orally are reported to have beneficial effects on Graves' ophthalmopathy. Dr. Vogel confirms the benefits of bee pollen for eye symptoms, but he recommends that patients wait to use it until their thyrotoxicosis symptoms are under control since he has observed that bee pollen can raise blood pressure (Vogel 1991).

The Dermopathy of Graves' Disease

The skin conditions associated with Graves' disease may be related to thyrotoxicosis or autoimmunity, or they may occur as a distinct peculiarity of Graves' disease. However, while excess thyroid hormone affects nail and hair growth, an autoimmune connection is strongly suggested in the major dermopathy, pretibial myxedema (PTM), which is almost always accompanied by GO. Likewise, the rare condition of acropachy is nearly always seen in patients with GO.

Skin Changes Related to Thyrotoxicosis

Changes in metabolic rate due to thyrotoxicosis may affect the skin and its appendages (hair and nails). Many GD patients report increased acne, which is caused by nutrient deficiencies as well as increased sebum production. Also, the epidermal and dermal tissues of the skin are target organs since they have their own thyroid hormone receptors. Epidermal cell division and breakdown (with results similar to exfoliation) are increased in thyrotoxicosis, which partially accounts for the youthful appearance (smooth, moist skin) often seen in hyperthyroid patients.

The skin in thyrotoxicosis is usually warm and moist with a velvety texture. Episodic flushing may occur over the face and the throat, and telangiectac vessels (spider veins and capillaries) may also develop in these areas. The face, palms and elbows may appear ruddy. Milaria bumps (small blister-like bumps that usually appear on the forehead) may occur as a result of increased sweating and poral occlusion. Pigment alterations (both hyperpigmentation and hypopigmentation) sometimes occur in the skin of patients with thyrotoxicosis. The hyperpigmentation, which is diffuse and may occur in various parts of the body, may involve genitalia, body creases and scars.

Hair Changes

Thyrotoxicosis causes increased hair growth by accelerating the growth cycle in hair follicles. However, moderate hair loss occasionally occurs in some thyrotoxic patients with no relation to disease severity. Axillary hair may also decrease. The hair in thyrotoxicosis is usually fine and soft and is reported to hold a permanent wave poorly, probably because of changes in the protein content.

Almost 25 percent of patients with alopecia areata, a condition of hair loss and thinning, are reported to have thyroid hormone abnormalities or elevation of TPO antibody levels or both, suggesting that autoimmune disease may be associated with this condition (Burch et al. 1996, 536).

Fingernail Changes

The fingernails in thyrotoxicosis become shiny, soft and brittle because of alterations in the keratin matrix and supporting dermal layers. The rate of nail growth is increased, and longitudinal striations associated with a flattening of the surface contour result in a scoop or shovel appearance. Many patients have onycholysis (distal separation from its underlying bed, also called Plummer's nails). The nail changes in hyperthyroidism resolve spontaneously as thyroid hormone levels improve.

Pretibial Myxedema (PTM)

Pretibial myxedema (PTM), which is also known as infiltrative dermopathy and localized myxedema, is a skin disorder that typically affects the anterior (front) surface of the skin on the lower legs in the pretibial area (near the shins). PTM is usually confined to the pretibial area including the front of the lower legs, the top of the feet and the toes, although it may involve the arms, face, shoulders and trunk.

PTM, which occurs in about 2 percent to 3 percent of the patients with Graves' disease, is almost always associated with GO, usually of severe degree (Greenspan 1998, 223). Although more than 90 percent of individuals with PTM have a history of thyrotoxicosis, it can also occur in patients with no evidence of thyrotoxicosis or who have Hashimoto's or atrophic autoimmune thyroiditis (Fatourechi 2000, 548).

Older patients are reported to be at more risk of developing pretibial myxedema, and pretibial myxedema frequently occurs in females in their 50s. Females are 3.5 times more likely to be affected than males. The onset of localized myxedema is most frequently seen 12 to 24 months after the diagnosis of thyrotoxicosis (Fatourechi 2000, 548).

Approximately 4 percent of patients with clinically evident GO develop PTM, and 12 percent to 15 percent of patients with severe GO are affected (Farourechi 2000, 548). In one study, 88 percent of patients with PTM had proptosis (Fatourechi 2000, 548). Almost all patients with PTM have high concentrations of TSH receptor antibodies and are reported to have more severe conditions of Graves' disease.

Symptoms in Pretibial Myxedema

PTM usually begins with raised waxy reddish-brown plaques and papules that develop on the front of the shin. The lesions are thought to be only of cosmetic importance, although large lesions can cause nerve entrapment. The affected area differs from normal skin by virtue of the skin being raised and thickened with a peau d'orange appearance that may be pruritic (itchy) and hyperpigmented.

The lesions of PTM are usually discrete with a sometimes waxy, nodular configuration, but in some instances they appear to have merged in with the normal tissue surface. The lesions and affected tissue have accumulations of GAG, the same substance found in the retroorbital tissue of patients with GO. GAG is produced by activated dermal fibroblasts.

In PTM, GAG is diffusely dispersed in the reticular part of the dermis and rarely in the innermost papillary dermis. PTM is structurally similar to hypothyroid myxedema, but in PTM, hyperkeratosis (resulting in thicker, leathery skin), greater abundance of GAG (rendering a swollen appearance), and mononuclear cell infiltration are more often seen.

The localized myxedema of Graves' disease may appear in several clinical forms:

- diffuse, nonpitting edema (most common occurrence)
- raised lesions on a background of nonpitting edema
- sharply diffuse nodular lesions
- the relatively rare elephantiasic form, consisting of nodular lesions mixed with lymphedema that do not ulcerate.

Treatment of PTM

Usually treatment isn't needed, but in severe cases, application of a high-potency fluorinated corticosteroid cream offers improvement. Nightly application of this cream covered by cellophane or plastic film has been reported to reduce symptoms. Systemic corticosteroid therapy may also help in severe conditions. Plasmapheresis has also helped patients with extremely severe lesions transiently improve. In severe cases, intravenous immunoglobulins are sometimes used, although their effects are also transient and the procedure is costly.

Thyroid Acropachy

Acropachy is a dermatological condition seen in Graves' disease characterized by soft connective tissue swelling that usually affects the hands and feet. It is the least common exta-thyroidal manifestation of Graves' disease. Acropachy usually appears in combination with GO or PTM. Although patients with acropachy usually have a history of thyrotox-icosis, the disorder may occur in euthyroid patients and in patients with autoimmune hypothyroid-ism. Acropachy often occurs years after radioiodine treatment for hyperthyroidism.

Symptoms of acropachy are rarely the first symptoms of Graves' disease to occur. The usual order is thyroid dysfunction, fol-lowed by GO, dermopathy and acropachy. Only 7 percent of patients with PTM exhibit thyroid

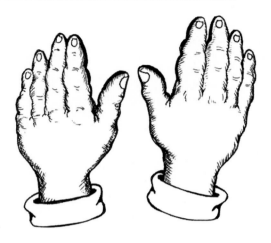

Thyroid acropachy, a dermatological condi-tion seen in Graves' disease, characterized by soft connective tissue swelling (courtesy Marvin G. Miller).

acropachy (Fatourechi 2000, 552). Acropachy represents the sole instance in Graves' disease in which males and females are affected equally. Although it usually occurs 2–3 years after symptoms of hyperthyroidism, acropachy can occur as late as 40 years after the onset of thyroid dysfunction (Fatourechi 2000, 552).

PATHOLOGY AND DIAGNOSIS

Acropachy typically causes asymmetric soft tissue swelling of the hands and feet, usually in association with clubbing of the fingers and toes, which is considered a different disorder (elephantiasis in PTM). Although tissue swelling is pronounced in acropachy, the joints remain unaffected. The skin is commonly pigmented and leathery with equal involvement of upper and lower extremities. Although it is generally considered painless, some patients with acropachy have lymphatic obstruction, extreme swelling, loss of function and considerable pain.

Imaging studies reveal fusiform soft tissue swelling of the digits along with subperiosteal bone formation. The metacarpals, the proximal and middle phalanges of the fingers, and the metatarsal and proximal phalanges of the toes are usually targeted, whereas the long bones of the extremities are rarely involved. The skin is similar to that seen in PTM with fibroblast activation and GAG deposits.

The pathology of thyroid acropachy remains unclear but the disease process suggests that there is autoimmune activation of periosteal bone fibroblast cells. (Fatourechi 2000, 552–3) Treatment consists of local corticosteroid therapy covered by occlusive compression dressings.

Exophthalamos, Pretibial Myxedema and Osteoarthropathy (EMO) Syndrome

In 1967, a syndrome of exophthalmos, pretibial myxedema and osteoarthropathy or acropachy (EMO syndrome) occurring together in patients with Graves' disease was first reported. EMO occurs in about 1 percent of patients with Graves' disease and it is rarely seen in Hashimoto's thyroiditis (Applehans et al. 2004). Most patients with EMO have high titers of thyroid-stimulating antibodies. EMO typically occurs in patients who have radioiodine ablation for thyroid malignancies and Graves' disease. One recent study also reports an association with unilateral fibromatosis of the hand in association with myxedema of the hand (Applehans et al. 2004). EMO has been previously associated with a heart condition called papillary fibroelastoma.

Future Treatment Options

There are no perfect treatments for the extrathyroidal manifestations of Graves' disease although there are some promising potential therapies. In the future it may be possible to block receptor binding of TSH receptor antibodies and/or insulin growth factor (IGF-1) autoantibodies with specific monoclonal antibodies. Studies show that receptors for IGF-1 are present on orbital fibroblast cells, where they also contribute to the production of GAG (Griepentrog and Garrity 2009). Research also suggests that a subpopulation of activated orbital fibroblast present in both orbital fat and connective tissue may be the major source of GAG production.

It's been noted that some patients with GO display adipose expansion as the primary manifestation of their disease, whereas others exhibit predominantly expansion of the muscle component. The predominance of one subpopulation of orbital fibroblasts within the orbit may help to explain this observation.

The underlying changes in pretibial myxedema and thyroid acropachy that lead to tissue swelling appear to follow a similar pathway with increased GAG production by fibroblasts. These effects can be mimicked in tissue studies by stimulation of dermal fibroblasts. Another potential therapy would be to block orbital preadipocyte cells from differentiating into mature adipocytes (Griepentrog and Garrity 2009).

Glossary

AARDA American Autoimmune and Related Disease Association.

acetyl-l-carnitine ACL) An amino acid that effectively inhibits the activity of excess thyroid hormone and reduces symptoms of hyperthyroidism.

acetylcholine receptor antibodies Autoantibodies to the acetylcholine receptor that block triggering impulses at cholinergenic synapses, interfering with muscle contraction; usually seen in myasthenia gravis.

ACL *see* acetyl-l-carnitine.

acropachy Dermal manifestation of Graves' disease causing an inflammatory process in soft connective tissue, especially of the fingers and toes.

ACTH Adrenocorticotropic hormone or corticotrophin, which is made by the pituitary gland to regulate the hormone production of the adrenal glands.

acupoints Locations on the body that are the focus of acupuncture and acupressure. Several hundred acupuncture points are considered to be located along meridians (connected points across the anatomy which affect a specific organ or other part of the body).

acupressure A form of energy healing that utilizes the same acupoints as in acupuncture. Energy flow is manipulated by applying finger pressure to these points.

acupuncture A practice of restoring balance by manipulating acupoints with needles.

Addison's disease An autoimmune condition causing adrenal gland insufficiency.

adenohypophysis Anterior region of the pituitary gland or hypophysis.

adenoma A small noncancerous growth.

adenosine diphosphate (ADP) An ester of adenosine that is reversibly converted to ATP for the storing of energy by the addition of a high-energy phosphate group.

adenosine triphosphate (ATP) Nucleotide of adenosine involved in energy metabolism and required for RNA synthesis; ATP occurs in all of the body's cells and stores energy in the form of high energy phosphate bonds.

adenyl or adenylate cyclase Enzyme that catalyzes the formation of cyclic AMP from ATP

ADP *see* adenosine diphosphate.

adrenal glands Endocrine glands located on top of the kidneys that secrete several important hormones including cortisol into the blood.

adrenaline A hormone produced by the adrenal glands in response to dangerous or unexpected situations. Adrenaline increases heart rate, expands blood vessels and air passages, and makes other subtle changes that help one react instantly.

adrenergic A substance resembling epinephrine in physiological effect; sympathomimetic.

adrenocorticotropic hormone *see* ACTH.

agranulocytosis Acute blood disorder characterized by a severe reduction in circulating granulocytic white blood cells accompanied by lesions of the throat and other mucous membranes of the GI tract and skin.

AITD Autoimmune thyroid disease.

albumin Major plasma protein that serves as a transport medium, carrying anions, fatty acids, drugs and hormones to cells throughout the body.

allele One of a pair of genes that normally occupies a particular locus.

allopathy Method of treating disease by the use of agents that produce effects antagonistic to or incompatible with those of the disease treated.

alopecia Autoimmune condition causing baldness or loss of hair, mainly on the head, either in defined patches or completely; the cause is unknown.

alpha-lipoic acid *see* lipoic acid.

amenorrhea Absence of menstrual periods.

amiodarone hydrochloride Coronary vasodilator used in the control of ventricular and supraventricular arrhythmias; Cordarone.

amphetamine Racemic drug that stimulates the central nervous system.

ANA *see* antinuclear antibodies.

anaphylaxis Hypersensitive reaction to an allergen with symptoms ranging from respiratory distress to death.

angioedema The rapid edema (swelling) of the deep layers of skin.

anovulation The absence of ovulation.

antagonists A drug that counteracts the effects of another chemical by mimicking the other drug and binding to its receptor, blocking its action.

antibody Immunoglobulin produced by B cells after antigenic stimulation and capable of reacting with the antigen that caused its production.

anticonvulsant Substance capable of preventing or arresting seizures.

antigen Substance capable of inducing a specific immunologic response and of reacting with the specific antibody produced by that response.

antigen-presenting cells (APCs) Cells capable of presenting antigen to T and B cells.

antigenic determinant Portion of an antigen that determines the specificity of the immune response.

antinuclear antibodies (ANAs) Antibodies directed against nuclear antigens, such as DNA or histones, and associated with a number of autoimmune syndromes.

antiparietal cell antibody Antibodies directed against the parietal cells lining the stomach cavity.

antiphospholipid disease Autoimmune disorder associated with coagulation abnormalities and miscarriage.

antipyretics Substances such as aspirin used for checking or preventing fever.

antithyroglobulin antibodies (ATG) A test to measure antibodies to a protein called thyroglobulin, which is found in thyroid cells. See *antibody*.

antithyroid Relating to an agent that inhibits thyroid hormone production.

apathetic hyperthyroidism Form of hyperthyroidism commonly seen in the elderly characterized by depression and an absence of typical hyperthyroid symptoms.

APECED *see* autoimmune polyendocrinopathy.

apical Referring to the apex or highest point.

APL *see* antiphospholipid disease.

aplasia cutis Localized failure of development of skin, usually seen on the scalp and less frequently on the trunk and limbs.

apoptosis Normal condition of programmed cell death.

APS *see* autoimmune polyglandular syndrome.

Armour Thyroid Medication made from desiccated pig thyroid that contains all four thyroid hormones, T1, T2, T3, and T4.

arrhythmia Any disturbance in the rhythm of the heartbeat.

ashwagandha Traditional Ayurvedic herb that can help heal and strengthen glands, including the thyroid and adrenal glands.

ATD Antithyroid drug.

atenolol A beta blocker that's effective at slowing a rapid heartbeat caused by hyperthyroidism.

ATG Antithyroglobulin antibodies.

atrial Relating to the atrium (upper heart chambers).

atrial fibrillation An irregular heartbeat in which the upper chambers of the heart (the atria) beat inconsistently and rapidly.

atrophy Reduction in cells leading to general destruction of a tissue or organ.

autoantibodies Abnormal antibodies that attach to parts of the body, causing autoimmune disease.

autoantibody Antibody directed to self antigens.

autoimmune disease Pathological changes resulting from a disordered immune reaction that targets self components.

autoimmune neonatal hyperthyroidism Rare condition caused by the transplacental passage of thyroid-stimulating immunoglobulins.

autoimmune polyendocrinopathy (APECED) A rare autosomal recessive illness that classically occurs in children under 10.

autoimmune polyglandular syndrome (APS) Disorder characterized by a cluster of autoimmune disorders. There are three classes of this syndrome, two of which include autoimmune thyroid disease.

autoimmune thrombocytopenic purpura Autoimmune idiopathic disorder characterized by platelet autoantibodies resulting in thrombocytopenia, a condition of decreased platelets and disturbances of the normal clotting mechanism.

autoimmune thyroid disease (AITD) A number of different autoimmune disorders directed at thyroid cell components, causing abnormal thyroid function.

autoimmunity Condition of immunologic reactivity to self antigens.

autonomously functioning thyroid nodule (AFTN) Characterized by the ability to function without TSH.

autoreactive Intermediate step in autoantibody production; autoreactive cells are either destroyed by the body or they go on to form autoantibodies.

autoregulation Mechanism in which the body regulates levels of certain substances such as iodine in an effort to maintain health.

Ayurveda Ancient Indian medical discipline based on imbalances in doshas.

B cell (B lymphocyte) Immune system white blood cell involved in the humoral response.

basal metabolic rate (BMR) Measurement of the body's rate of oxygen consumption used as a test of thyroid function.

basal temperature test An old-fashioned test used to identify hypothyroidism via body temperature. It's been made obsolete by modern lab tests.

basophil A cell, especially a white blood cell, having granules that stain readily with basic dyes.

benzodiazepines Medications that are effective at managing anxiety caused by hyperthyroidism, including Valium, Xanax, Dalmane, and Tranxene.

beta blockers Beta adrenergic blocking agents are medications such as propranolol used to block the adrenergic response that is associated with cardiac symptoms such as increased heart rate.

beta–human chorionic gonadotropin (beta–HCG) A hormone secreted in women during pregnancy and in individuals with various gonadotropin-secreting malignancies.

betaine HCl Medication used to combat low stomach acid.

bilateral Affecting both sides of the body or two paired organs.

biliary Pertaining to bile, the bile ducts or the gallbladder.

binding proteins Serum proteins that bind substances such as hormones, transporting and carrying these substances through the body.

biopsy *see* fine needle aspiration biopsy and coarse needle biopsy.

biosynthesis Synthesis or production of chemical compounds such as thyroid hormone within the body.

blast cell Large immature (early stage in development) lymphoid cell with a large nucleus that differentiates into one of the basic cell lines.

blastocyst A structure formed in the early development of vertebrates.

blepharoplasty Plastic surgery of the eyelid.

block-and-replace therapy A technique for managing hyperthyroidism in which a doctor blocks the disease with antithyroid medication while simultaneously replacing any lack of hormones with thyroid medication.

BMR *see* basal metabolic rate.

Brocq-Duhring disease *see* dermatitis herpetiformis.

bromocriptine A medication used to slow the growth of, and often shrink, an adenoma on the pituitary gland.

bullous pemphigoid An acute or chronic autoimmune skin disease, involving the formation of blisters, more appropriately known as bullae, at the space between the skin layers epidermis and dermis.

calcitonin Hormone made in the C cells of the thyroid gland that controls calcium levels in the blood by slowing the loss of calcium from bones.

cAMP *see* cyclic adenosine monophosphate.

cardiolipin Phospholipid occurring primarily in mitochondrial inner membranes.

catecholamine Chemically related neurotransmitters, such as epinephrine and norepineprine, that stimulate the sympathetic nervous system.

cell-mediated immunity (CMI) Immunity mediated by T cells without a requirement for B cells or antibodies.

cerebral Relating to the cerebrum, the main portion of the brain.

chemosis Edema of the bulbar conjunctiva, causing corneal swelling.

chi The body's vital life or energy source in Eastern medicine; also qi.

cholecystokinin A hormone that stimulates the digestion of fat and suppresses hunger.

choriocarcinoma A quick-growing form of cancer that occurs in a woman's uterus (womb).

choroid plexus Part of the brain that secretes cerebrospinal fluid.

chronobiology The science of the effect of time, especially rhythms, on life systems.

circumventricular Pertaining to the area around or in the area of a ventricle, as are the circumventricular organs.

cirrhosis A chronic disease of the liver in which fibrous tissue invades and replaces normal tissue.

Class I MHC antigens Histocompatibility antigens encoded by A, B and C MHC loci in humans and by other loci in animals.

Class II MHC antigens Histocompatibility antigens encoded by HLA-DR, HLADP and HLA-DQ antigens in humans and by other loci in animals.

Class III MHC antigens Histocompatibility markers C2, C4 and complement factor B encoded by genes within the MHC.

clinical Pertaining to a clinic or to the bedside; pertaining to or founded on actual observation and treatment of patients, as distinguished from theoretical or basic sciences.

clonal Referring to cell proliferation.

clonal deletion Removal of clones, primarily as a protective mechanism that is largely responsible for the deletion of self-reactive lymphocytes.

CMV *see* cytomegalovirus.

coarse needle biopsy Procedure in which tissue is aspirated through a large-bore needle and evaluated.

coenzyme Q10 *see* CoQ10.

cold nodule *see* thyroid nodule.

colloid Gelatinous substance made up of a system of particles with linear dimensions. Thyroglobulin is the major constituent of thyroid colloid.

complement Complex series of immune system proteins activated by antigen-antibody complexes and other substances.

comprehensive metabolic panel (CMP) A very common test that identifies the levels of a variety of critical chemicals in the bloodstream.

computed tomography scanning (CT or CAT scan) A technique of cross-sectional images in which X-rays are passed through the body at different angles and analyzed by a computer.

congenital Existing as a result of birth; hereditary disorders.

conjunctiva The clear membrane covering the white of the eye and the inside of the eyelid that produces a fluid that lubricates the cornea and eyelid.

contralateral Relating to the opposite side, as when pain is felt or paralysis occurs on the side opposite to that of the lesion.

COPD Chronic obstructive pulmonary disease.

CoQ10 Coenzyme Q10, which is produced by the human body and is necessary for the basic functioning of cells. CoQ10 levels are reported to decrease with age and to be low in patients with hyperthyroidism.

corticosteroids Natural steroid hormones or synthetic drugs that are used to replace natural hormones; functions to suppress the immune system and help prevent inflammation; includes glucocorticoids and mineralcorticoids.

corticotrophin-releasing hormone (CRH) Secreted by the hypothalamus in response to stress.

coupling The mechanism by which the thyroid hormone precursors MIT and DIT link to form T3 and T4.

cretinism Condition of stunted growth and mental retardation caused by severe hypothyroidism.

CRH *see* corticotrophin-releasing hormone.

cricoid Pertaining to a ring-shaped cartilage at the lower part of the larynx.

CT *see* computed tomography scanning.

CTL Cytotoxic T lymphocyte.

Cushing's syndrome Adrenal gland disorder causing excess cortisol production.

cyclic adenosine monophosphate (cAMP) A chemical acting as a second messenger in the hormonal response.

cytokine Hormone-like, low molecular weight messenger proteins, which regulate the intensity and duration of immune responses.

cytomegalovirus Any of several viruses that cause cellular enlargement and formation of eosinophilic inclusion bodies especially in the nucleus and include some acting as opportunistic infectious agents in immunosuppressed conditions.

cytotoxic Detrimental or destructive to cells.

cytotoxic T cells T cells with the ability to kill other cells.

D gene region Diversity segment of the genome that encodes part of the hyper-variable region of the immunoglobulin heavy chain.

deiodination The loss or removal of iodine from a compound as seen in the conversion of T4 to T3; monodeiodination.

deletion Chromosomal aberration in which a portion of a chromosome is lost. It may also refer to loss of a DNA segment in mutations.

dendritic Threadlike extensions of the cytoplasm of neurons.

deoxyribonucleic acid (DNA) Any of various nucleic acids that are usually the molecular basis of heredity, localized especially in cell nuclei, and are constructed of a double helix held together by hydrogen bonds between purine and pyrimidine bases which project inward from two chains containing alternate links of deoxyribose and phosphate.

dermatitis herpetiformis Autoimmune disorder characterized by celiac disease and a chronic skin disorder characterized by itchy, occasionally blistering eruptions and hyperpigmention; also known as Brocq-Duhring's disease.

dermatitis multiformis *see* dermatitis herpetiformis.

dermopathy Disorder affecting or involving the skin.

dexamethasone Synthetic glucocorticoid far more potent than cortisol used for treating symptoms of adrenal insufficiency.

diabetes mellitus (IDDM) Autoimmune disorder of insulin dependent or juvenile diabetes mellitus caused by various antibodies that attack pancreatic cells.

diaphoresis Perspiration, especially when artificially induced or excessive.

diethylstilbesterol (DES) Synthetic, nonsteroidal estrogen compound with estrogenic activity greater than estrone.

diiodotyrosine (DIT) An intermediate in the biosynthesis of thyroid hormone.

diphenylhydantoin phenytoin (Dilantin) An anticonvulsant used in the treatment of seizure disorders, which may interfere with thyroid hormone metabolism.

diplopia Visual disturbance in which an object appears double; double vision.

DIT *see* diiodotyrosine.

DNA *see* deoxyribonucleic acid.

dopamine A chemical neurotransmitter that transmits messages in the brain, which is known to inhibit the secretion of TSH.

dysbiosis An imbalanced intestinal ecology that results in a dysfunctional intestinal lining, sometimes referred to as leaky gut syndrome.

dyshormonogenesis Defect in one or more of the several chemical steps that take place in the manufacture of thyroid hormones.

dysphagia Difficulty in swallowing.

dysphonia Altered voice production.

dysphoria A mood of general dissatisfaction.

dyspnea Difficulty breathing; shortness of breath.

dystonia Uncontrolled muscle movement due to disordered muscle tonicity.

EAC *see* erythema annulare centrifugum.

EBV Epstein-Barr virus.

ectopic Located away from its normally occurring position.

edema An abnormal accumulation of fluid in the tissue spaces, cavities or joint capsules of the body, causing swelling of the area.

EFA *see* essential fatty acids.

effector Substances such as cytokines that are released during the immune response that act as messengers, inciting other changes.

electrocardiograph A galvanometric device that detects variations in the electric potential that triggers the heartbeat, used to evaluate the heart's rhythms.

encephalopathy A general term referring to an inflammatory brain disease that alters the brain's structure or function.

endocrine glands Glands that secrete hormones internally into the blood or lymph.

endocytosis Movement of external substances into a cell, usually by pinocytosis.

endoderm The innermost cell layer of the embryo in its gastrula stage.

enteropathy Any intestinal disorder, for example gluten sensitivity enteropathy (GSE), which is also known as celiac disease.

enzymes Enzymes are complex proteins that cause a specific chemical change in all parts of the body. For example, they can help break down the foods we eat so the body can use available nutrients.

epinephrine A hormone secreted by the adrenal medulla upon stimulation by the central nervous system in response to stress.

epitope *see* antigenic determinant.

ER Emergency room.

erythema Abnormal redness of the skin and mucous membranes accompanied by fever and pain.

erythema annulare centrifugum (EAC) One of the figurate or gyrate erythemas. It is characterized by a scaling or nonscaling, nonpruritic, annular or arcuate, erythematous eruption.

essential fatty acids (EFA) Fatty acids that humans must ingest because the body requires them for good health but cannot create them. They are required for biological purposes.

estradiol An estrogenic hormone produced by the maturing Graaffan follicle that causes proliferation and thickening of the endometrium.

estrogen Relating to any of several major female sex hormones (estriol, estradiol, or estrone) produced primarily by ovarian follicles.

euthyroid Graves' disease Condition in which the characteristic eye disease of GD, Graves' ophthalmopathy, is evident although thyroid function is normal.

euthyroid hyperthyroxinemia Condition in which the serum total or the free thyroxine concentrations are abnormally elevated without evidence of thyroid disease.

euthyroidism A condition in which the thyroid gland is functioning normally as reflected in normal thyroid function tests.

exophthalmos Protrusion of the eyeball from the orbit; proptosis.

extraocular Adjacent to but outside the eyeball.

extrathyroidal Outside of or away from the thyroid gland itself.

Fas protein Surface protein that acts as a regulator of apoptosis when it's produced at the expense of Fas ligand.

fibroadipose Having both fibrous and adipose or fatty characteristics.

fibroblast Immature fibrous connective tissue cell that differentiates into chrondoblasts, collagenoblasts, orbital tissue cells and osteoblasts.

fibromyalgia A condition characterized by muscle and joint pain.

fibrosis Formation of fibrous tissue (such as muscle, tissue containing fibers).

fibrotic Characterized by fibrosis.

fine needle aspiration (FNA) A technique that allows a biopsy of various bumps and lumps; also called fine needle biopsy. It allows for the retrieval of enough tissue for microscopic analysis and thus makes an accurate diagnosis of a number of problems, such as inflammation or cancer.

FNA *see* fine needle aspiration.

folic acid Water-soluble vitamin that is converted to a coenzyme essential to purine and thymine biosynthesis and thyroid function.

follicle Sac or pouch-like depression or cavity; basic structural unit of the thyroid gland.

follicular cells Cells of the thyroid follicles.

free thyroxine (T4) Unbound thyroxine that has been cleaved from its binding protein and is now capable of causing cellular effects.

free triiodothyronine (T3) Unbound triiodothyronine that has been cleaved from its binding protein and is now capable of causing cellular effects.

FT3 *see* free triiodothyronine (T3).

FT4 *see* free thyroxine (T4).

GAG *see* glycosaminoglycan.

galactorrhea An abnormally persistent flow of milk.

GD Graves' disease.

genome The total genetic constitution of a cell or organism.

gestational hyperthyroidism A clinical condition characterized by thyrotoxicosis and debilitating nausea and vomiting during pregnancy.

gestational transient thyrotoxicosis (GTT) A non-autoimmune form of hyperthyroidism of variable severity that occurs in women who have a normal pregnancy.

gestational trophoblastic disease (GTD) A rare complication of pregnancy that can result in hyperthyroidism.

gland An organ that that synthesizes a substance for release of substances such as hormones or breast milk, often into the bloodstream (endocrine gland) or into cavities inside the body or its outer surface (exocrine gland). See endocrine glands.

glucagon A hormone secreted by the pancreas that acts in opposition to insulin in the regulation of blood glucose levels.

glucocorticoid Any of a class of steroid hormones that are produced by the adrenal cortex under conditions of stress and that inhibit immune reactions.

glycoprotein Any of a group of complex proteins, as mucin, containing a carbohydrate combined with a simple protein.

glycosaminoglycan (GAG) Any of a class of polysaccharides that form mucins when complexed with proteins. GAG is responsible for the congestive dermal and orbital infiltration in GD.

GO *see* Graves' ophthalmopathy.

goiter Enlargement of the thyroid gland.

goitrogen Substance that inhibits thyroid hormone production.

gonadal Referring to the gonads or reproductive organs.

granulomatous Characterized by aggregates of white blood cells.

Graves' ophthalmopathy (GO) Characteristic eye disorder associated with Graves' disease that has two components, a spastic disorder and a congestive infiltration.

GTD *see* gestational trophoblastic disease.

GTT *see* gestational transient thyrotoxicosis.

halothane A colorless liquid used as an inhalant for general anesthesia.

haploids Having a single set of chromosomes.

haplotype Set of alleles on a single chromosome that are inherited as a closely linked set, generally considered in terms of MHC genes.

hapten Antigenic determinant of low molecular weight that can act as an immunogen when coupled to an immunogenic carrier molecule.

haptenic determinants Part of the antigen that determines its antigenic specificity.

Hashimoto's encephalopathy A rare condition associated with Hashimoto's thyroiditis and Graves' disease. The disease occurs primarily in the fifth decade of life and may present in two types—a sudden vasculitic type or a progressive subacute type associated to cognitive dysfunction, confusion and memory loss.

Hashimoto's thyroiditis (HT) An autoimmune disorder of the thyroid gland, which may induce thyroid enlargement (goiter) and hypothyroidism.

Hashitoxicosis A temporary episode of hyperthyroidism in a patient with HT.

hCG Human chorionic gonadotropin.

helper T cells (Th) Subset of T cells, usually bearing CD4, which functions by cooperating with B cells or other T cells.

hematology The study of blood.

hematopoietic Pertaining to the formation of blood cells; of bone marrow origin.

heparin Synthetic substance with anticoagulant properties used medically to prevent or dissolve blood clots.

hirsutism Abnormal hairiness, usually associated with females having a male pattern of hair growth.

histocompatability The condition of having similar immune system antigens such that cells or tissues transplanted from a donor to a recipient are not rejected.

HIV Human immunodeficiency virus (AIDS virus).

HLA (human leukocyte antigens) Human MHC region and its products located on the short arm of chromosome 6, encompassing the immune system genes.

homeostasis The tendency of an organism to maintain health via the coordinated response of its parts to any threatening situation or stimulus.

hormone Substances secreted by endocrine glands that affect the functions of specifically receptive organs or tissues.

HPP *see* hypokalemic periodic paralysis.

HT *see* Hashimoto's thyroiditis.

hTG Thyroglobulin.

humoral Term applied to soluble substances in body fluids. In immunology, it generally refers to immunoglobulins or complement components (or both).

hyaluron Major glycosaminoglycan seen in GD.

hydatidiform mole A rare mass or growth that forms inside the uterus at the beginning of a pregnancy. It is a type of gestational trophoblastic disease (GTD).

hypercalcemia Condition of excess serum calcium.

hyperdefecation Condition of increased bowel movements.

hyperglycemia An abnormally high level of glucose in the blood.

hyperkinesis An abnormal amount of uncontrolled muscular action; spasm.

hypermetabolism Increased metabolic state.

hyperplasia Abnormal multiplication of cells.

hypertension High blood pressure. Blood pressure is the force of blood pushing against the walls of arteries as it flows through them.

hyperthyroid eye disease Ocular problems from hyperthyroidism, and especially Graves' disease, including "lid lag," sensitivity to light, feeling painful dryness or grittiness in the eyes, double vision, and eyelids retracting while eyes enlarge and protrude.

hyperthyroidism A sustained period of thyrotoxicosis.

hypertrophy Abnormal increase in cell size.

hypoglycemia An abnormally low level of glucose in the blood.

hypokalemia A lower-than-normal amount of potassium in the blood.

hypokalemic periodic paralysis Condition of low serum potassium characterized by muscle weakness that may progress to paralysis.

hypomanic Overexcited state resembling mania but to a lesser intensity.

hyponatremia Abnormally low blood sodium level.

hypophysis The pituitary gland.

hypothalamic-pituitary-thyroid axis Thyroid regulatory system in which there is a negative feedback, which aims to maintain normal thyroid hormone levels.

hypothalamus The ventral part of the diencephalon in the brain.

hypothyroidism A sustained period of reduced thyroid hormone.

I iodine.

I-123 Radioiodine isotope 123.

I-131 Radioiodine isotope 131.

IDDM Insulin dependent diabetes mellitus (type 1 or juvenile diabetes).

IFN *see* interferons.

IFN-alpha Interferon, type (alpha).

immune complexes Molecular complexes composed of antigen and antibody, with or without complement.

immune response The reaction of the immune system against foreign substances. When the reaction occurs against the body's own cells or tissues, it is called an autoimmune reaction.

immune system A network of organs, cells and chemicals that protects the body from foreign substances and destroys infected and malignant cells.

immunity The state of being immune from a particular disease.

immunoassays A laboratory method for detecting a substance by using an antibody reactive with it.

immunogen Substance capable of inducing an immune response.

immunoglobulin Protein composed of H and L chains that functions as an antibody.

immunomodulator Substance capable of modulating or balancing the immune system.

immunosuppressive Capable of depressing the immune system.

indole-3-carbinol A natural compound found in cruciferous vegetables — such as broccoli, cauliflower, cabbage, Brussels sprouts, and kale — that can interfere with the thyroid's hormone production and so may be useful in combating hyperthyroidism.

infection Invasion by and subsequent overgrowth of pathogenic microorganisms, including bacteria, viruses, and parasites, in a bodily part or tissue, which may produce subsequent tissue injury and spread to other organs.

interferons (IFN) Cytokine with multiple immune regulatory functions.

interfollicular Space between follicles.

interleukin (IL) Cytokine with diverse immunologic and inflammatory activities.

iodine A mineral essential for the production of thyroid hormone.

iodotyrosine Compound formed when an iodine atom combines with tyrosyl residues or the amino acid tyrosine.

intrathyroidal Situated or occurring within the thyroid.

islet of Langerhans Any of the clusters of endocrine cells in the pancreas that are specialized to secrete insulin, somatostatin or glucagon.

isoenzyme Subset of an enzyme with certain characteristic functions but with slight difference in chemical structure.

K cell Killer lymphocyte capable of antibody dependent cytotoxicity.

kampo Japanese herbal healing tradition with roots in China.

karyotype The chromosomes of a cell, usually displayed as a systematized arrangement of chromosome pairs in descending order of size.

keratitis Inflammation of the cornea.

ketoacidosis State of imbalance in the body's normal acid-base mechanism characterized by ketones in the blood or urine and an acid Ph.

KI potassium iodide.

labile Open to change; adaptable, unstable.

lacrimination The secretion of tears, especially in abnormal abundance.

LAF Lymphocyte activating factor.

leptin Hormone that enhances metabolism while decreasing appetite and caloric intake.

leukocytes White blood cells.

levothyroxine Monosodium salt of the levo isomer of the thyroid hormone thyroxine commonly used in hormone replacement therapy.

LGL Large granulocytic lymphocyte.

ligand Molecule capable of binding to another molecule.

linkage disequilibrium Tendency of certain genes on a chromosome to be inherited as a group and occurring more often than would be seen by chance.

lipoic acid A natural antioxidant found in various foods and available as a dietary supplement.

lipolytic Effect of breaking down fat.

long-acting thyroid stimulator (LATS) Thyroid-stimulating antibody associated with Graves' disease.

Lugol's solution Liquid solution of strong saturated potassium iodine.

lumen Cavity within a tube or tubular organ.

lupus erythematosus Any of several autoimmune diseases, especially systemic lupus.

lymphocyte Nongranular white blood cell important in antibody production.

lymphokine *see* cytokine.

lymphoma A tumor arising from any of the cellular elements of lymph nodes.

lysosome A cell organelle containing enzymes that break down proteins and other large molecules into smaller constituents.

lysozyme An enzyme that is destructive of bacteria and functions as an antiseptic, found in tears, leukocytes, mucus, egg albumin and certain plants.

macrophage Large white blood cell that ingests foreign particles and infectious microorganisms by a process called phagocytosis.

magnetic resonance imaging (MRI) A process of producing images of the body regardless of intervening bone by means of a strong magnetic field and low-energy radio waves.

major histocompatibility complex (MHC) Cluster of genes on the short arm of chromosome 6 associated with many aspects of immune responsiveness and autoimmunity; in humans, MHC genes are known as HLA antigens.

malignant Tending to metastasize; cancerous.

MAS *see* multiple autoimmune syndrome.

melanocytes A cell that produces the dark pigment melanin.

menorrhagia Excessive menstrual discharge.

meridians In traditional Chinese medicine, qi energy flows through the body along a system or network of meridians.

metabolism The body's energy level, which is set by the hypothalamus and enforced by the thyroid's hormones.

metastatic A secondary cancer, or one that has spread from one area of the body to another.

methimazole One of the primary antithyroid agents used in the United States; recently made available in a generic form; brand name Tapazole.

metoprolol Type of cardioselective beta adrenergic blocking agent; Lopressor.

MG *see* myasthenia gravis.

MHC *see* major histocompatibility complex.

MIT *see* monoiodotyrosine.

mitochondrion An organelle in the cell cytoplasm that has its own DNA and that produces enzymes essential for energy metabolism.

mitral valve The valve between the heart's left atrium and left ventricle that prevents blood from flowing back into the atrium when the ventricle contracts.

molecular mimicry Cross-reactivity between an antigen and a tissue component; a mechanism for autoimmunity.

monoclonal antibodies Set of identical immunoglobulins produced by one B cell alone.

monoiodotyrosine (MIT) Thyroid hormone intermediary precursor with one iodine atom.

MRI *see* magnetic resonance imaging.

mRNA Messenger RNA.

MS Multiple sclerosis, an autoimmune nervous system disorder.

mucopolysaccharide Former name of glycosaminoglycan.

mucosal immune system Lymphoid tissues associated with the gastrointestinal and respiratory mucosa.

multiple autoimmune syndrome (MAS) Presence of more than two autoimmune diseases in one patient.

myasthenia gravis A disease of impaired transmission of motor nerve impulses, characterized by episodic weakness and fatiguability of the muscles.

myocardial infarction Heart attack.

myopathy Any abnormality or disease of muscle tissue.

myopia A condition of the eye in which parallel rays are focused in front of the retina, causing nearsightedness.

myxedema A condition of hypothyroidism characterized by thickening of the skin, blunting of the senses and intellect, and labored speech.

natural killer (NK) cells Cells that provide rapid responses to virally infected cells and respond to tumor formation, acting at around 3 days after infection.

Nature-Thyroid Medication made from desiccated pig thyroid that contains all four thyroid hormones: T1, T2, T3 and T4.

naturopathy A method of treating disease that employs no surgery or synthetic drugs to assist the natural healing process.

neonatal Relating to the period immediately succeeding birth and continuing through the first 28 days of extrauterine life.

neoplasm An abnormal tissue that grows by cellular proliferation more rapidly than normal and continues to grow after the stimuli that initiated the new growth cease. Neoplasms show partial or complete lack of structural organization and functional coordination with the normal tissue, and usually form a distinct mass of tissue that may be either benign (benign tumor) or malignant (cancer).

nephritis Inflammation of the nephrons in the kidneys.

neurohypophysis Posterior region of the pituitary gland.

neutrophilic Characterized by white blood cells with granular cytoplasm.

nitrofurantoin Synthetic antibacterial agent.

NK *see* natural killer (NK) cells.

nodule A small node, which can be detected by touch (palpating).

nucleoprotein Any of the class of conjugated proteins occurring in cells and consisting of a protein, usually a histone combined with a nucleic acid.

nucleoside Consisting typically of deoxyribose or ribose combined with adenine, guanine, cytosine, uracil or thymine.

ocreotide Somatostatin analog used in the treatment of GO.

oligomenorrhea Scant menses; infrequent menstrual cycles.

onycholysis Separation of the nail from its nail bed; symptom of Graves' disease.

ophthalmopathy Any disease of the eye.

ophthalmoplegia Paralysis of eye muscles, particularly on upward gaze.

optic neuropathy Disorder or compression of the optic nerve.

oral tolerization Autoimmune disease therapy using glandular extracts.

orbital decompression Type of surgery used to reduce congestive infiltration of GO.

orbital fibroblasts Immature orbital tissue cells.

orbital pseudotumor Nonmalignant growth resembling a tumor found in the eye region.

organification Process by which iodide ions are converted to iodine.

organotherapy A newly emerging branch of homeopathy especially suited for the treatment of organ-specific diseases.

oxyphil Abnormal white blood cell seen in long-term Graves' disease.

painless sporadic thyroiditis Clinically and pathologically similar to postpartum thyroiditis but occurs in the absence of pregnancy. It appears to be autoimmune in origin; the thyroid contains a lymphocytic infiltrate partially resembling Hashimoto's disease but without the fibrosis, Askanazy cells, and extensive lymphoid follicle formation.

palpable Perceptible to touch.

pancytopenia Suppressed platelet count.

parafollicular Surrounding the thyroid follicle, as in the basement cavity.

parathyroid Gland situated near the thyroid gland.

parathyroid hormone (PTH) Secreted by the chief cells of the parathyroid glands as a polypeptide containing 84 amino acids. It acts to increase the concentration of calcium in the blood.

parenchyma Functional tissue of an organ, distinct from its stroma.

Parry's disease Disorder of hyperthyroidism arising in association with toxic multinodular goiter.

PCA *see* antiparietal cell antibody.

peau d'orange Characteristic skin texture with the roughness of an orange.

peptide A compound containing two or more amino acids in which the carboxyl group of one acid is linked to the amino group of the other.

perchlorate A salt or ester of perchloric acid, as potassium perchlorate.

peripheral Away from the normal location or point of origin.

peripheral lymphoid organs or tissues Lymphoid aggregates or tissues excluding the thymus and bone marrow, the latter considered to be the source of lymphoid stem cells.

pernicious anemia (PA) A severe anemia associated with inadequate intake or absorption of vitamin B_{12}, caused by an autoimmune mechanism.

phagocytes Cells able to ingest particles, including microbes.

phagocytosis The ingestion by a cell of a microorganism, cell particle or other matter surrounded and engulfed by the cell.

pharmacodynamics The pharmacological or active mode of drugs.

pharmacopeia or **pharmacopoeia** A government or educational publication containing a list of drugs, their formulas, production methods and effects.

pheochromocytoma Condition caused by a tumor of the adrenal gland(s) that secretes hormones that affect one's blood pressure.

phospholipid Any of a group of fatty compounds composed of phosphoric esters and present in living cells.

photophobia Abnormal sensitivity to or intolerance of light, as in iritis.

phytochemistry The branch of biochemistry dealing with plants and plant processes.

phytomedical Chemical or medicinal properties of plants.

pineal gland An endocrine organ in the posterior forebrain that secretes melatonin; involved in biorhythms and gonadal development.

pinocytosis Process of cellular ingestion of soluble material.

PIP2 Phospholipase C.

pituitary Endocrine gland that regulates thyroid function.

plasma cells Mature B cells capable of intensive antibody production and secretion.

plasmapheresis Procedure in which blood cells are returned to the bloodstream of the donor and the plasma is removed to reduce antibody levels.

platelet Small, irregularly shaped clear cell fragments; thrombocytes.

Plummer's disease Toxic multinodular goiter.

Plummer's nails *see* onycholysis.

polyaromatic hydrocarbons (PAH) Chemicals such as chloroform that are suspected of being hormonal disruptors.

polymyositis A connective tissue disorder with symptoms resembling fibromyalgia.

polypeptide A chain of amino acids linked together by ten or more peptide bonds and having a molecular weight of up to about 10,000 kD.

postablative hypothyroidism Hypothyroidism resulting from ablative treatment of hyperthyroidism by surgery or by RAI.

postpartum thyroiditis (PPT) A transient condition causing a small, painless goiter and a very low radioiodine uptake test result.

prana Vital life force in Eastern medicine.

pretibial Referring to the skin of the lower leg near the shin over the tibia.

pretibial myxedema A skin condition affecting usually the lower legs and feet.

primary lymphoid tissue Site of lymphocyte proliferation, generally the bone marrow.

procainamide A medicine commonly used in the treatment of cardiac arrhythmias.

propranolol A beta-blocking drug; Inderal.

proptosis Protrusion of the eyes; exophthalmos.

Propylthiouracil (PTU) First anti-thyroid compound used in the United States.

prostaglandins Hormone-like substances released during the inflammatory response.

proteolysis Cleaving of hormone from its carrier protein.

psychosomatic Of or pertaining to a physical disorder that is caused or notably influenced by emotional factors.

PTH *see* parathyroid hormone.

PTU *see* propylthiouracil.

pyramidal lobe Remnant of the embryonic thyroglossal duct occasionally seen in the middle region of the thyroid gland.

qi *see* chi.

RA Rheumatoid arthritis, an autoimmune rheumatic disorder.

radioimmunoassay One of a group of tests for detecting antigen or antibody where one of the reagents is labeled with a radioactive isotope.

radioiodine Any of nine radioisotopes of iodine used as radioactive tracers in research and clinical diagnosis and treatment.

radioiodine ablation Therapeutic destruction of thyroid cells by I-131 used to reduce the amount of functional thyroid cells that produce thyroid hormone.

radioiodine uptake test and scan (RAI-U) Diagnostic measurement of radioiodine and its pattern of distribution quantified after ingestion of a known oral dose of radioiodine.

RAI Radioiodine.

RAI-U Radioiodine uptake test and scan.

resistance to thyroid hormone (RTH) The syndrome of resistance to thyroid hormone is defined by a normal or elevated TSH level with elevated circulating levels of free thyroid hormone resulting from an underlying condition of reduced target tissue responsiveness.

resorcinol A water-soluble vitamin A derivative used as a skin medication.

retinoid Any of a group of substances related to and functioning like vitamin A.

retrobulbar Behind the orbital cavity.

retrosternal Behind the sternum.

retrovirus RNA virus that uses reverse transcriptase for replication.

reverse transcriptase Enzyme in microorganisms that catalyzes the transcription of DNA from RNA.

rhabdomyolysis An acute, fulminating, potentially fatal disease of skeletal muscle that entails destruction of muscle, as evidenced by myoglobinemia and myoglobinuria.

rheumatoid factor (RF) Immunoglubulin, usually IgM, directed against IgG, often seen in patients with rheumatoid arthritis or other rheumatic disease.

riboflavin A vitamin B complex factor essential for proper thyroid function.

Riedel's thyroiditis Rare, chronic proliferating inflammatory condition usually involving one thyroid lobe, although it may extend to both lobes and also the trachea.

RNA Ribonucleic acid.

rT3 Reverse T3.

salicylate A salt or ester of salicylic acid; aspirin.

sarcoidoisis A disease in which abnormal collections of chronic inflammatory cells form as nodules in multiple organs.

Schmidt's syndrome Original name of type 2 APS (or APS2). Characterized by adrenal insufficiency along with one or more additional autoimmune endocrine disorders.

scintiscan Method of measuring the scanning pattern after RAI-U.

sclerosis An induration, or hardening associated with inflammation.

secondary lymphoid tissue Sites in the body where lymphocytes proliferate in response an immune stimulus.

selenium A mineral essential for the conversion of T4 to T3.

sella turica A depression on the upper surface of the sphenoid bone, lodging the pituitary gland.

sertaline Zoloft; an antidepressant.

silent thyroiditis Swelling (inflammation) of the thyroid gland, in which the person alternates between hyperthyroidism and hypothyroidism.

sinus tachycardia Abnormal heart pattern.

Sjogren's Syndrome Autoimmune disorder characterized by oral and ocular dryness.

SLE Systemic lupus erythematosus.

somatostatin A polypeptide hormone produced in the brain and pancreas.

spironolactone Medication used to lower blood pressure.

sporadic Denoting a temporal pattern of disease occurrence in an animal or human population in which the disease occurs only rarely and without regularity.

SREAT *see* steroid-responsive encephalopathy associated with autoimmune thyroiditis.

SSKI Saturated solution of potassium iodide.

steatorrhea Passage of fat in large amounts in the feces, due to failure to digest and absorb it; occurs in pancreatic disease and the malabsorption syndromes.

steroid-responsive encephalopathy associated with autoimmune thyroiditis (SREAT) Condition of Hashimoto's encephalopathy that can cause memory impairment, cognitive changes, dementia, and associated neurological symptoms.

steroidogenic Having properties of a steroid hormone.

sterol Any of a group of solid, mostly unsaturated, polycyclic alcohols, as cholesterol and ergosterol, derived from plants or animals.

stroma Network of supporting tissue or matrix of an organ.

struma ovarri Condition characterized by ectopic thyroid tissue acting as an ovarian tumor.

subacute Somewhat or moderately acute.

subacute thyroiditis (SAT) A self-limited thyroid condition associated with a triphasic clinical course of hyperthyroidism, hypothyroidism, and return to normal thyroid function.

subclinical Pertaining to an early stage of a disease; having no noticeable clinical symptoms and only one abnormal lab marker.

sulfonamide Sulfa drug commonly used as an antibiotic, which has ATD properties.

superantigens Potent T cell stimulatory molecules that bind to MHC class II molecules.

suppressor T cells Subset of T cells able to inhibit T cell or B cell reactivity. May be antigen-specific or antigen-nonspecific.

suppurative thyroiditis A rare and potentially life-threatening infection of the thyroid gland.

surface receptors Protein on the cell on the surface membrane that actively reacts with specific hormones or drugs.

sympathomimetic Mimicking stimulation of the sympathetic nervous system.

T3 *see* triiodothyronine.

T4 *see* thyroxine (tetraiodothyronin).

T cell receptor Antigen-specific complex on a T cell that denotes specificity.

T cells (T lymphocyte) Lymphocytes subgroup that regulates the immune response.

tachycardia Excessively rapid heartbeat.

TBG *see* thyroxine-binding globulin.

TBII Thyrotroin-binding inhibitory.

TBPA Thyroxine binding prealbumin.

TCM Traditional Chinese medicine.

TCR T cell receptor.

technetium A synthetic element obtained in the fission of uranium.

TED Thyroid eye disease.

teratoma A true neoplasm made up of different types of tissue, none of which is native to the area in which it occurs; usually found in the ovary or testis.

TgAb *see* antithyroglobulin antibodies.

TGI *see* thyroid growth-stimulating immunoglobulin.

thiamine A crystalline, water-soluble vitamin B compound; vitamin B_1.

thiocyanate Medicine used to treat heart problems that has antithyroid properties.

thrombocyte Blood component that aids coagulation; see *platelet*.

thymoma Tumor of the thymus.

thymus gland A ductless gland lying at the base of the neck, formed mostly of lymphatic tissue and aiding in the production of T cells.

thyrocytes Pituitary cells that produce thyrotropin.

thyroglobulin antibodies Antibodies mainly directed against the thyroglobulin stored in the thyroid gland.

thyroglossal duct Embryonic duct connecting the mouth to the thyroid.

thyroid crisis or **storm** An acute exacerbation of the symptoms of thyrotoxicosis.

thyroid gland One of the largest endocrine glands; found in the neck; controls how quickly the body uses energy, makes proteins, and controls how sensitive the body is to other hormones.

thyroid growth-stimulating immunoglobulin Autoantibodies with the ability to increase DNA synthesis in thyrocytes.

thyroid module Abnormal solid or fluid-filled growth that appears as a lump in thyroid tissue.

thyroid peroxidase Enzyme involved in the production and metabolism of thyroid hormone.

thyroid peroxidase (thyroperoxidase) antibodies (TPO) An enzyme necessary for thyroid hormone production and metabolism. TPO antibodies are markers of inflammation.

thyroid stimulating hormone (TSH *see* thyrotropin.

thyroid stimulating immunoglobulins (TSI) Antibodies that cause hyperthyroidism in Graves' disease.

thyroidectomy Surgical excision of all or a part of the thyroid gland.

thyroiditis Inflammation of the thyroid gland.

thyromegaly Enlarged thyroid.

thyrotoxic myopathy Cardiac muscle involvement associated with thyrotoxicosis.

thyrotoxicosis Effects of excess thyroid hormone on the body's tissues.

thyrotrope A type of basophil in the adenohypophysis that secretes thyrotropin.

thyrotroph A cell in the anterior lobe of the pituitary that produces thyrotropin.

thyrotropin Pituitary hormone which regulates thyroid hormone production and release; also known as thyroid-stimulating hormone (TSH).

thyrotropin receptor antibodies Antibodies responsible for symptoms of autoimmune thyroid disease; stimulating antibodies cause the symptoms of Graves' disease.

thyrotropin-releasing hormone (TRH) A hormone of the hypothalamus that controls the release of thyrotropin by the pituitary gland.

thyroxine (tetraiodothyronin) A hormone of the thyroid gland that regulates the metabolic rate of the body; preparations of it are used for treating hypothyroidism; T4.

thyroxine-binding globulin (TBG) The most important thyroid hormone carrier protein, it carries about 70 percent of thyroxine.

torticollis A condition in which the neck is twisted and the head inclined to one side, caused by spasmodic contraction of the muscles of the neck.

toxic multinodular goiter (TMG) Involves an enlarged thyroid gland that contains rounded growths called nodules. These nodules produce too much thyroid hormone.

TPO *see* thyroid peroxidase.

TPO Ab thyroid peroxidase (thyroperoxidase) antibodies.

TRAb *see* thyrotropin receptor antibodies.

transcription Synthesis of RNA from a DNA template.

translation Synthesis of a polypeptide protein from an RNA template.

transplacental Across or passing through the placenta over to the fetal circulation.

transthyretin Protein which transports thyroid hormone through the blood.

TRBAb Thyrotropin receptor-blocking antibodies.

tremulousness Characterized by trembling, as from fear, nervousness, or weakness.

TRH *see* thyrotropin-releasing hormone.

triiodothyronine A thyroid hormone, similar to thyroxine but more potent: preparations of it are used in treating hypothyroidism; T3.

tRNA Transfer RNA.

trophic Hormonal effect produced in a different gland.

TSAb Thyrotropin receptor-stimulating antibodies.

TSBAb Thyrotropin receptor blocking antibodies.

TSH Thyroid-stimulating hormone (thyrotropin).

TSI Thyroid-stimulating immunoglobulins (stimulating TRAb).

TTR *see* transthyretin.

tumor Solid or fluid-filled masses of tissue; also known as neoplasms.

tumor necrosis factors (TNFs) Cytokines able to cause tumor cell lysis and other effects, including inflammation.

Turner's syndrome An abnormal congenital condition resulting from a defect on or absence of the second sex chromosome.

tyrosine Amino acid that combines with iodine to form thyroid hormone.

tyrosol residues Tyrosine fragments present in thyroglobulin.

ultrasonography (ultrasound) A diagnostic imaging technique utilizing reflected ultrasonic waves to delineate, measure, or examine internal body structures or organs.

unilateral proptosis Proptosis involving only one eye.

uremia Renal disorder caused by the presence in the blood of excessive urea.

urticaria (hives) Pruritic skin eruption with edematous wheals.

variable (V) region Amino-terminus end of an H or L chain where the amino acid sequence differs from one antibody to another.

varicella Chickenpox virus.

vitiligo A skin disorder characterized by patches of unpigmented skin.

xenobiotics Nonliving substances with biologic properties.

yin and yang The opposing polarities such as hot and cold which govern man as well as the universe in Eastern medicine.

zoster Shingles virus.

References

Abad, Marina. 2009. "Thyroid Nodules: Function Tests and Fine-Needle Aspirations Help Increase Early Diagnoses." *Advance for Medical Laboratory Professionals*, November 17, http://laboratorian.advanceweb.com/Article/Thyroid-Nodules.aspx. Accessed November 10, 2012.

Abraham, P., Avenell, A., Park, C., Watson, W., and Bevan, J. 2005. "A Systematic Review of Drug Therapy for Graves' Hyperthyroidism." *European Journal of Endocrinology*, 153 (October): 489–98. http://www.eje-online.org/content/153/4/489. Accessed July 6, 2012.

Adams, M.J. 2010. "Decades After Childhood Radiation, Thyroid Cancer a Concern." *Alert Newsletter of the University of Rochester Medical Center*, December 16.

Appelans, C., Breukmann, F., Bastian, A., Altmeyer, P., and Kreuter, A. 2004. "Fibromatosis of the Hand Associated with EMO Syndrome: A Case Report." *BMC Dermatology*. http://www.biomedcentral.com/1471-5945/4/17. Accessed June 4, 2012.

Arky, Ronald, ed. 1997. *Physician's Desk Reference*. 51st ed. Montvale, NJ: Medical Economics Company, 1410–12, 2647–48.

Arturi, F., Scarpelli, D., Coco, A., Sacco, R., Bruno, R., Filetti, S., and Russo, D. 2003. "Thyrotropin Receptor Mutations and Thyroid Hyperfunctioning Adenomas Ten Years After Their First Discovery: Unresolved Questions," *Thyroid*; 13(4): 341–43.

Auger, Manon. 2003. "Fine Needle Aspiration Cytology of the Thyroid," American Society for Clinical Pathology (ASCP) Commission on Continuing Education, Annual Meeting Course, New Orleans, September.

Aziz, Douglas. 1997. *Use and Interpretation of Tests in Endocrinology*. Santa Monica, CA: Specialty Laboratories.

Bahn, Rebecca, Burch, Henry, Cooper, David,

Garber, Jeffrey, Greenlee, M., Klein, Irwin, Laurberg, Peter, McDougall, I. Ross, Montori, Victor, Rivkees, Scott, Ross, Douglas, Sosa, Julie, and Stan, Marius N. 2011. "Hyperthyroidism and Other Causes of Thyrotoxicosis: Management Guidelines of the American Thyroid Association and American Association of Clinical Endocrinologists: The American Thyroid Association and American Association of Clinical Endocrinologists Task Force on Hyperthyroidism and Other Causes of Thyrotoxicosis," *Thyroid* 21: 6 Mary Ann Liebert, Inc. doi: 10.1089/thy.2010.0417. http://thyroidguidelines.net/sites/thyroidguidelines.net/files/file/THY_2010_0417.pdf. Accessed July 1, 2012.

Baran, Daniel T. 2000. "The Skeletal System in Thyrotoxicosis," in *Werner & Ingbar's The Thyroid: A Fundamental and Clinical Text*, 8th edition, edited by Lewis E. Braverman and Robert D. Utiger. Philadelphia: Lippincott Williams & Wilkins, 659–66.

Bartalena, Luigia, and Hennemann, Georg. 2010. "Graves' Disease: Complications," in *Thyroid Disease Manager*, http://www.thyroidmanager.org/chapter/graves-disease-complications. Accessed April 10, 2012.

Basaria, S., and Cooper, D. 1999. "Graves' Disease and Recurrent Ectopic Thyroid Disease," *Thyroid* 12: 1261–64.

Bassi, V., Santinelli, C., Iengo, A., and Romano, C. 2010, December. "Identification of a Correlation Between *Helicobacter pylori* Infection and Graves' Disease." *Helicobacter*, 15 (6): 558–62.

Bayer, Monika. 1991. "Effective Laboratory Evaluation of Thyroid Status," in *The Medical Clinics of North America, Thyroid Disease*, 75 (1) Edited by Francis Greenspan. Philadelphia: W.B. Saunders.

BBC News, World Edition. 2002, November 3.

"Gene Breakthrough in Graves' Disease," http://news.bbc.co.uk/2/hi/health/2386305. stm. Accessed May 1, 2012.

Becks, G., and Burrows, G. 1991, January. "Thyroid Disease and Pregnancy," in *Medical Clinics of North America, The Thyroid* 75 (1): 121–39.

Beer, Alan. 1998. *Thyroid Disorders and Reproductive Problems of Miscarriage, Implantation and In Vitro Fertilization Failure*, Chicago: Reproductive Medicine Program.

Behrman, R., Kliegman, R., and Jenson, H. *Nelson Textbook of Pediatrics*, 16th ed. Philadelphia: W.B. Saunders.

Beir, V. 1990. "Health Effects of Exposure to Low Levels of Ionizing Radiation," National Research Council Publication. Washington, DC: National Academy Press.

Benvenga, S., Amato, A., Calvani, M., and Trimarchi, F. 2004, November. "Effects of Carnitine on Thyroid Hormone Action," *Annals of the New York Academy of Sciences*, 1033: 158–67.

Bhatti, Atiq. 2010. "What Is Organo Therapy?" Academy for Homeopathic Knowledge. http://www.dratiq,cin/acadent/organo.html. Accessed September 1, 2012.

Blumental, Mark, ed. 1998. *The Complete German Commission E Monographs Therapeutic Guides to Herbal Medicines*, The American Botanical Council in Cooperation with Integrative Medicine Communications. Boston: American Botanical Council.

Boelaert, K., Newby, P.R., Simmonds, M.J., Holder, R.L., Carr-Smith, J.D., Heward, J.M., Manji, N., Allahabadia, A., Armitage, M., Chatterjee, K.V., Lazarus, J.H., Pearce, S.H., Vaidya, B., Gough, S.C., Franklyn, J.A. 2010, February. "Prevalence and Relative Risk of Other Autoimmune Diseases in Subjects with Autoimmune Thyroid Disease." *American Journal of Medicine* 123 (2): 183–89.

Bouzas, E.A., Karadimas, P., Mastorakos, G., and Koutras, D.A. 2000, May. "Antioxidant Agents in the Treatment of Graves' Ophthalmopathy." *American Journal of Ophthalmology* 129 (5): 618–22.

Boyages, Steven. 2000. "The Neuromuscular System and Brain in Thyrotoxicosis," in *Werner & Ingbar's The Thyroid: A Fundamental and Clinical Text*, 8th edition, edited by Lewis E. Braverman, and Robert D. Utiger. Philadelphia: Lippincott Williams & Wilkins, 631–33.

Braga-Basaria, Milena, and Shehzad Basaria. 2003. "Marine-Lenhart Syndrome: Images in Thyroidology," *Thyroid* 13 (10): 991–93.

Braverman, Lewis E., and Robert D. Utiger, 2000. "Introduction to Thyrotoxicosis," in *Werner & Ingbar's The Thyroid: A Fundamental and Clinical Text*, 8th edition, edited by Lewis E. Braverman and Robert D. Utiger. Philadelphia: Lippincott Williams & Wilkins, 515–17.

Brix, T., Kyvik, K., and Hegedus, L. 1998. "What Is the Evidence of Genetic Factors in the Etiology of Graves' Disease?: A Brief Review." *Thyroid* 8: 627–34.

Brokken, L., Scheenhart, J., Wiersinga, W., and Prummel, M. 2001. "Suppression of Serum TSH by Graves' Ig: Evidence for a Functional Pituitary TSH Receptor." *The Journal of Clinical Endocrinology & Metabolism* 86 (10): 4814–17.

Brokken, L., Wiersinga, W., and Prummel, M. 2003. "Thyrotropin Receptor Autoantibodies Are Associated with Continued Thyrotropin Suppression in Treated Euthyroid Graves' Disease Patients." *The Journal of Clinical Endocrinology & Metabolism* 88 (9): 4135–38.

Brown, Valerie. 2003, September. "Disrupting a Delicate Balance: Environmental Effects on the Thyroid." *Environmental Health Perspectives* 111 (12): 642–49.

Bunevicius, Robertas, and Prange, Arthur, Jr. 2006. "Psychiatric Manifestations of Graves' Hyperthyroidism: Pathophysiology and Treatment Options," *CNS Drugs* 20 (1): 897–909.

Burch, H., Burman, K., and Cooper, D. 2012, December. "A 2011 Survey of Clinical Practice Patterns in the Management of Graves' Disease." *Journal of Clinical Endocrinology and Metabolism* 97 (12): 4549–58.

Burch, H., Colum, A., and Gorman, A. 1996. "Graves' Ophthalmopathy," in *Werner & Ingbar's The Thyroid: A Fundamental and Clinical Text*, 8th edition, edited by Lewis E. Braverman and Robert D. Utiger. Philadelphia: Lippincott Williams & Wilkins, 533–46.

Burch, H., Colum, A., Gorman, A., Bahn, R., and Garrity, J. 2000. "Ophthalmopathy," in *Werner & Ingbar's The Thyroid: A Fundamental and Clinical Text*, 8th edition, edited by Lewis E. Braverman and Robert D. Utiger. Philadelphia: Lippincott Williams & Wilkins, 531–48.

Burger, Joanna. 1995. "Ionizing Radiation," in *Environmental Medicine*, edited by Stuart Brooks. St. Louis, MO: Mosby–Year Book, 527–40.

Burman Kenneth. 2012, November 5. "Postpartum Thyroiditis." *Wolters Kluwer UpToDate Health*, http://www.uptodate.com/contents/postpartum-thyroiditis. Accessed December 28, 2012.

Cain, H., Pannall, P., Kotase, D., and Norman, R. 1991. "Choriogonadotropin-Mediated Thyrotoxicosis in a Man," *Clinical Chemistry* 37 (6): 1127–31.

Carani, C., Isidori, A.M., Granata, A., Carosa,

E., Maggi, M., Lenzi, A., and Jannini, E. 2005, December. "Multicenter Study on the Prevalence of Sexual Symptoms in Male Hypo- and Hyperthyroid Patients," *Journal of Clinical Endocrinology and Metabolism* 90 (12): 6472–79.

Carnell, N.E., and Valente, W.A. 1998, August. "Thyroid Nodules in Graves' Disease: Classification, Characterization, and Response to Treatment." *Thyroid* 8 (11): 647–52.

Centanni, M., Marignani, M., Gargano, L., Corleto, V., Casini, A., Delle Fave, G., Andreoli, M., and Annibale, B. 1999. "Atrophic Body Gastritis in Patients With Autoimmune Thyroid Disease: An Underdiagnosed Association," *Archives of Internal Medicine* 159: 1726–30.

Chang, H.S., Lee, D., Taban, M., Douglas, R.S., and Goldberg, R.A. 2011, March-April. "Englove" Lysis of Lower Eyelid Retractors with AlloDerm and Dermis-Fat Grafts in Lower Eyelid Retraction Surgery. *Ophthalmic Plastic and Reconstructive Surgery* 27 (2): 137–41.

Char, Devron. 1991, January. "The Ophthalmopathy of Graves' Disease," in *Medical Clinics of North America, The Thyroid* 75 (1): 97–101.

Check, William. 2007, February. "Untangling Thyroid Problems, Test by Test," *CAP Today* 21 (2): 1, 64–70.

Chen, Chun-Rong, Pichurin, Pavel, Nagayama, Yuji, Latrofa, Francesco, Rapoport, Basil, and McLachlan, Sandra. 2003, June 15. "The Thyrotropin Receptor Autoantigen in Graves' Disease Is the Culprit as Well as the Victim," *Journal of Clinical Investigation*, 111 (12): 1897–1904.

Chiovatoe, L., et al. 1988. "Outcome of Thyroid Function in Graves' Patients Treated with Radioiodine: Role of Thyroid-Stimulating and Thyrotropin-Blocking Antibodies and of Radioiodine-Induced Thyroid Damage." *Journal of Clinical Endocrinology and Metabolism* 83 (1): 40–46.

Chopra, Inder J., and Sabatino, Laura. 2000. "Nature and Sources of Circulating Thyroid Hormones" in *Werner & Ingbar's The Thyroid: A Fundamental and Clinical Text*, 8th edition, edited by Lewis E. Braverman and Robert D. Utiger. Philadelphia: Lippincott Williams & Wilkins, 121–35.

Clark, C.D., Bassett, B., and Burge, M.R. 2003. "Short-Term Ingestion of Kelp Has a Weak Antithyroid Effect in Normal Subjects." *Endocrine Practice* 9: 363–69.

Colborn, Theo, Dumanoski, Dianne, and Myers, John. 1996. *Our Stolen Future.* New York: Penguin.

Conway, Carolyn. 1999, April 27. "Radiation Carcinogenic Even without Hitting Cell Nucleus," *UniSci Science and Research News.*

Cooper, David S. 2000. "Treatment of Thyrotoxicosis," in *Werner & Ingbar's The Thyroid: A Fundamental and Clinical Text*, 8th edition, edited by Lewis E. Braverman and Robert D. Utiger. Philadelphia: Lippincott Williams & Wilkins, 691–715.

Cooper, David S. 2005, March 3. "Antithyroid Drugs." *The New England Journal of Medicine* 352: 905–17.

Dabbs, D. 2004, June 31. "Can Cytomorphology Differentiate Between Benign Nodules and Tumors Arising in Graves' Disease?" *Diagnostic Cytopathology* (1): 64–67.

Daniels, G. 1999, January-February. "Hyperthyroidism: Multiple Possibilities in the Female Patient," *International Journal of Fertility and Women's Medicine* 44 (1): 6–11.

Das, P.K., Wherrett, D., and Dror, Y. 2007, August. "Remission of Aplastic Anemia Induced by Treatment for Graves' Disease in a Pediatric Patient." *Pediatric Blood Cancer* 49 (2): 210–12.

Davies, Terry. 2000. "Graves' Disease," in *Werner & Ingbar's The Thyroid: A Fundamental and Clinical Text*, 8th edition, edited by Lewis E. Braverman and Robert D. Utiger. Philadelphia: Lippincott Williams & Wilkins, 518–30.

Davies, Terry, Ando, T., Lin, R., Tomer, Y., and Latif, R. 2005, August 1. "Thyrotropin Receptor–Associated Diseases: from Adenomata to Graves' Disease." *The Journal of Clinical Investigation* 115 (8): 1972–83. http://www.ncbi.nlm.nih.gov/pmc/articles/PMC1180562. Accessed May 27, 2012.

DeGroot, Leslie J. 2010. "Graves Disease and the Manifestations of Thyrotoxicosis," in *Thyroid Disease Manager*, http://www.thyroidmanager.org/chapter/graves-disease-and-the-manifestations-of-thyrotoxicosis. Accessed May 2, 2012.

DeGroot, Leslie J. 2012. "Diagnosis and Treatment of Graves' Disease," in *Thyroid Disease Manager*. http://www.thyroidmanager.org/chapter/diagnosis-and-treatment-of-graves-disease. Accessed May 2, 2012.

Demir, T., Akinci, G., Comlekci, A., Karaoglu, O., Ozcan, M., Yener, S., Yuksel, F., Secil, M., and Yesil, S. 2009. "Levothyroxine (LT4) Suppression Treatment for Benign Thyroid Nodules Alters Coagulation," Clinical Endocrinology Division of *Medscape*, http://www.medscape.com/viewarticle/712917. Accessed June 1, 2012.

Despres, Normand, and Grant, Andrew. 1998. "Antibody Interference in Thyroid Assays: A Potential for Clinical Misinformation," *Clinical Chemistry* 44 (3): 440–54.

De Vivo, A., Mancuso, A., Giacobbe, A., Moleti, M., Maggio, S.L., De Dominici, R., Priolo,

A.M., and Vermiglio, F. 2010, June. "Thyroid Function in Women Found to Have Early Pregnancy Loss." *Thyroid* 20 (6): 633–37.

Doi, Y., Goto, A., Murakami, T., Yamashita, H., Yamashita, H., and Noguchi, S. 2004, September. "Primary Thyroid Lymphoma Associated with Graves' Disease," *Thyroid* 14 (9): 772–76.

Dong, Betty. 2000, February. "How Medications Affect Thyroid Function." *Western Journal of Medicine* 172 (2): 102–06. http://www.ncbi.nlm.nih.gov/pmc/articles/PMC1070767. Accessed December 10, 2012.

Djrolo, F., Gervaise, N., Combe, H., Linassier, C., Lhuintre, Y., and Lecomte, P. 2001, November. "Maltoma of the Thyroid and Graves' disease," *Annals of Endocrinology* 62 (5): 442–45.

Dluhy, Robert. 2000. "The Adrenal Cortex in Thyrotoxicosis," in *Werner & Ingbar's The Thyroid: A Fundamental and Clinical Text*, 8th edition, edited by Lewis E. Braverman and Robert D. Utiger. Philadelphia: Lippincott Williams & Wilkins, 637–41.

Donovan, Jennifer. 1997, March 12. "Hyperactivity Linked to Thyroid Hormones." *Science Daily*, http://www.sciencedaily.com/releases/1997/03/970312165726.htm. Accessed March 3, 2012.

Duffy, William. 1965. *You Are All Sanpaku*, English version of original text by Sakurazaw Nyoiti (George Oshawa). Secaucus, NJ: Citadel Press.

Earles, S.M., Gerrits, P.M., and Transue, D.J. 2004, February. "Iopanoic Acid in the Management of Neonatal Graves' Disease." *Journal of Perinatology* 24 (2): 105–08.

Emiliano, A., Governale, L., Parks, M., and Cooper, David. 2010, May. "Shifts in Propylthiouracil and Methimazole Prescribing Practices: Antithyroid Drug Use in the United States from 1991 to 2008." *Journal of Clinical Endocrinology and Metabolism* 95 (5): 2227–33.

Fakhouri, F., Noel, L.H., and Zuber, J. 2003, June. "The Expanding Spectrum of Renal Diseases Associated with Antiphospholipid Syndrome," *American Journal of Kidney Disease*, 1205–11.

Faria, A.M., and Weiner, H.L. 2006, June–December. "Oral Tolerance: Therapeutic Implications for Autoimmune Diseases." *Clinical and Developmental Immunology* 13 (2–4): 143–57.

Fatourechi, Vahab. 2000. "Localized Myxedema and Thyroid Acropachy," in *Werner & Ingbar's The Thyroid: A Fundamental and Clinical Text*, 8th edition, edited by Lewis E. Braverman and Robert D. Utiger. Philadelphia: Lippincott Williams & Wilkins, 548–55.

Felz, Michael, and Stein, Peter. 1999, October

15. "The Many Faces of Graves' Disease, Part 2: Practical Diagnostic Testing and Management Options," *Postgraduate Medicine* 106 (5): 45–52.

Ferry, R. 2011, November 3. "Pediatric Hyperthyroidism," *eMedicine, Medscape Reference*, http://emedicine.medscape.com/article/921707-overview. Accessed March 3, 2012.

Fisher, Delbert. 1998. *The Quest Diagnostics Manual: Endocrinology Test Selection and Interpretation*, 2nd ed., Teterboro, NJ: Quest Diagnostics.

Fisher, Delbert, and Brown, Rosalind. 2000. "Thyroid Physiology in the Perinatal Period and during Childhood," in *Werner & Ingbar's The Thyroid: A Fundamental and Clinical Text*, 8th edition, edited by Lewis E. Braverman and Robert D. Utiger, editors. Philadelphia: Lippincott Williams & Wilkins, 959–71.

Franklyn, J., et al., 1998, March. "Mortality After the Treatment of Hyperthyroidism with Radioactive Iodine." *The New England Journal of Medicine* 338 (11): 712–16.

Franklyn, J., et al., 1999, June 19. "Cancer Incidence and Mortality After Radioiodine Treatment for Hyperthyroidism: A Population-Based Cohort Study." *Lancet* 353 (9170): 2111–15.

Franklyn, J., Sheppard, M., and Maisonneuve, P. 2005. "Mortality Is Slightly Increased After Radioiodine Therapy in Patients with Hyperthyroidism." *Clinical Thyroidology* 17 (3): 45.

Franklyn, Jayne. 2000. "Metabolic Changes in Thyrotoxicosis," in *Werner & Ingbar's The Thyroid: A Fundamental and Clinical Text*, 8th edition, edited by Lewis E. Braverman and Robert D. Utiger, editors. Philadelphia: Lippincott Williams & Wilkins, 667–72.

García, B., Gimeno Orna, J.A., Aguillo Gutiérrez, E., Altemir Trallero, J., Cabrejas Gómez, C., Ilundaín González, A., Lázaro Puente, F., Ocón Bretón, J., Faure Nogueras, E. 2010, February. "Prevalence and Predictive Factors of Parietal Cell Antibody Positivity in Autoimmune Thyroid Disease." *Endocrinology and Nutrition* 57 (2): 49–53.

Gartner, R., Gasnier, B.C., Dietrich, J.W., Krebs, B., and Angswurm, M.W. 2002, April. "Selenium Supplementation in Patients with Autoimmune Thyroiditis Decreases Thyroid Peroxidase Antibodies Concentrations." *Journal of Clinical Endocrinology & Metabolism* 87 (4): 1687–91.

Gemsenjager, E., and Girard, J. 1981, October 17. "Preclinical Hyperthyroidism in Thyroid Invasion by Tumors of Other Organs," *Schweizerische Medizinische Wochenschrift* 111 (42): 1563–64.

Giana, C., Fierabracci, P., Bonacci, R., Gigliotti,

A., Campani, D., De Negri, F., Cecchetti, D., Martino, E., and Pinchera, A. 1996, March. "Relationship Between Breast Cancer and Thyroid Disease: Relevance of Autoimmune Thyroid Disorders in Breast Malignancy." *Journal of Clinical Endocrinology and Metabolism* 81(3): 990–94.

Giovinale, M., Fonnesu, C., Soriano, A., Cerquaglia, C., Curigliano, V., Verrecchia, E., De Socio, G., Gasbarrini, G., Manna, R. 2009. "Atypical Sarcoidosis: Case Reports and Review of the Literature," *European Review of Medical Pharmacology and Science* 13 Suppl 1: 37–44.

Glinoer, Daniel. 2000. "Thyroid Disease during Pregnancy," in *Werner & Ingbar's The Thyroid: A Fundamental and Clinical Text*, 8th edition, edited by Lewis E. Braverman and Robert D. Utiger. Philadelphia: Lippincott Williams & Wilkins, 1013–27.

Glinoer, Daniel. 2006, July. "Miscarriage in Women with Positive Anti-TPO Antibodies: Is Thyroxine the Answer?" Editorial in *Journal of Clinical Endocrinology and Metabolism* 91 (7): 2500–02. http://jcem.endojournals.org/content/91/7/2500.full. Accessed November 8, 2012.

Gofman, John. 1991. *Radiation & Human Health*. San Francisco: Sierra Club Books.

Gong, J.K. 1999, December. "A Lifelong, Wide-Range Radiation Biodosimeter: Erythrocytes with Transferring Receptors." State University of New York at Buffalo, Occupational and Environmental Safety Services, *Health Physics* 77 (6): 713.

Goodman, Louis, and Gilman, Alfred. 1955. *The Pharmacological Basis of Therapeutics*. 2nd edition. New York: Macmillan.

Goodman, Louis, and Gilman, Alfred. 2006. *The Pharmacological Basis of Therapeutics,* 11th edition. Edited by Laurence Brunton. New York: McGraw-Hill.

Graham, Kelly. 2010, July 28. "Pregnancy and the Thyroid." *Advance for Medical Laboratory Professionals*, 1–2.

Graves, L., Klein, R., and Walling, A. 2003. "Addisonian Crisis Precipitated by Thyroxine Therapy: A Complication of Type 2 Autoimmune Polyglandular Syndrome," *Southern Medical Journal* 96 (8): 824–27.

Greenspan, Francis. 1991. *Basic and Clinical Endocrinology*. 3rd edition. Norwalk, CT: Appleton & Lange.

Greenspan, Francis. 1997. *Basic and Clinical Endocrinology.* 5th edition. Norwalk, CT: Appleton & Lange.

Gripentrog, G., and Garrity, J.A. 2009. "Update on the Medical Treatment of Graves' Ophthalmopathy." *International Journal of General Medicine*, 263–69.

Gruters, A. 1999. "Ocular Manifestations in Children and Adolescents with Thyrotoxicosis," *Experiments in Clinical Endocrinology and Diabetes* 107 Suppl 5: S172–74.

Hamburger, J. 1980. "Evolution of Toxicity in Solitary Nontoxic Autonomously Functioning Thyroid Nodules," *Journal of Clinical Endocrinology and Metabolism* 50: 1089–93.

Hanna, C.E., and LaFranchi, S.H. 2002. "Adolescent thyroid disorders." *Adolescent Medicine* 13 (1): 13–35.

Hebra, Andre. 2012, November 8. "Solitary Thyroid Nodule," *Medscape Reference, Drugs, Diseases & Procedures.* http://emedicine.medscape.com/article/924550. Accessed January 4, 2013.

Henry, J. 1991. *Clinical Diagnosis & Management by Laboratory Methods*. Philadelphia: W. B. Saunders Company.

Hidaka, Yoh, Kimura, Masahiro, Izumi, Yukiki, Takano, Roru, Tastsumi, Keita, and Amino, Nobuyuki. 2003. "Increased Serum Concentration of Eosinophil-Derived Neurotoxin in Patients with Graves' Disease," *Thyroid* 12 (2): 129–32.

Hirano, T. 1981, November 27. "Association of Graves' Disease with Turner's Syndrome," *Journal of the American Medical Association* 246 (21): 2429.

Hoffman, William S. 1961. *The Biochemistry of Clinical Medicine*. 2nd edition. Chicago: The Yearbook Publishers.

Huber, A., Jacobson, E., Jazdewski, K., Concepcion, E., and Tomer, Yaron. 2008, March. "Interleukin (IL)-23 Receptor Is a Major Susceptibility Gene for Graves' Ophthalmopathy: The IL-23/T-Helper 17 Axis Extends to Thyroid Autoimmunity," *Journal of Clinical Endocrinology and Metabolism* 93 (3): 1077–81.

Ibrahim, N.A., and Fadeyibi, I. 2011. "Ectopic Thyroid: Etiology, Pathology and Management," *Hormones* 10 (4): 261–69.

Idris, I., and O'Malley, B.. 2000, May. "Thyrotoxicosis in Down's and Turner's Syndromes: The Likelihood of Hashimoto's Thyroiditis as the Underlying Aetiology," *International Journal of Clinical Practice* 54 (4): 272–73.

Ingbar, David. 2000. "The Pulmonary System in Thyrotoxicosis," in *Werner & Ingbar's The Thyroid: A Fundamental and Clinical Text*, 8th edition, edited by Lewis E. Braverman and Robert D. Utiger. Philadelphia: Lippincott Williams & Wilkins, 605–16.

James, Erin. 2003, February 24. "Testing for Autoimmune Thyroid Disease in Pregnant Patients." *Advance for Medical Laboratory Professionals* 15 (5): 3–7.

Jialal, I., Winter, W., and Chan, D. 1999. *Handbook of Diagnostic Endocrinology*. Washington, DC: AACC Press.

Kabadi, U., and Premachandra, B. 2007, October. "Serum Thyrotropin in Graves' Disease: A More Reliable Index of Circulating Thyroid-Stimulating Immunoglobulin Level than Thyroid Function?" *Endocrine Practice* 13 (6): 615–19.

Kahn, Katherine. 2011, December 20. "Risk for Graves' Disease Nearly Tripled in Vietnam Vets Exposed to Agent Orange," *Medscape Medical News*, April 27, http://www.medscape.com/viewarticle/720864. Accessed December 20, 2011.

Kang, G.Y. 2011, October 26. "Thyroxine and Triiodothyronine Content in Commercially Available Thyroid Health Supplements." Abstract presented at the American Thyroid Association Annual Meeting, Boston, MA.

Kano, H., Inoue, M., Nishino, T., Yoshimoto, Y., and Arima, R. 2000, December. "Malignant Struma Ovarii with Graves' Disease," *Gynecologic Oncology* 79 (3): 508–10.

Kasagi, K., Hidaka, A., Nakamura, H., Takeuchi, R., Missaki, T., and Lida, Y. 1993. "Thyrotropin receptor antibodies in hypothyroid Graves' disease," *Journal of Clinical Endocrinology and Metabolism* 76: 504.

Kashiwai, T., Hidaka, Y., Takano, T., Tatsumi, K., Izumi, Y., Shimaoka, Y., Tada, H., Takeoka, K., and Amino, N. 2003. "Practical Treatment with Minimum Maintenance Dose of Antithyroid Drugs for Prediction of Remission in Graves' Disease." *Endocrine Journal* 50 (1): 45–49.

Kelley, D., and Meyers, Arlen. 2011, December 6. "Evaluation of Solitary Thyroid Nodules," eMedicine/Medscape, emedicine.medscape.com/article/850823-overview. Accessed June 1, 2012.

Kelly, Jeannie Chen. 2012, February 23. "Struma Ovarii," *Medscape*, http://emedicine.medscape.com/article/256937-overview. Accessed April 10, 2012.

Khan, Ali Nawaz. 2012, February 13. "Thyroid Nodule Imaging," *Medscape*, http://emedicine.medscape.com/article/385301-overview. Accessed August 1, 2012.

Klein, Irwin, and Levey, Gerald S. 2000. "The Cardiovascular System in Thyrotoxicosis," in *Werner & Ingbar's The Thyroid: A Fundamental and Clinical Text*, 8th edition, edited by Lewis E. Braverman and Robert D. Utiger. Philadelphia: Lippincott Williams & Wilkins, 596–604.

Kopp, Peter. 2010. "Thyrotoxicosis of Other Etiologies," in *Thyroid Disease Manager*. http://www.thyroidmanager.org/chapter/thyrotoxicosis-of-other-etiologies. Accessed December 9, 2012.

Kubota, S., Tamai, H., Ohye, H., Fukata, S., Kuma, K., and Miyauchi, A. 2004, April.

"Transient Hyperthyroidism After Withdrawal of Antithyroid Drugs in Patients with Graves' Disease." *Endocrinology Journal* 51 (2): 213–17.

Kuijpens, J.L., Vader, H.L., Drexhage, H.A., Wiersinga, W.M., van Son, M.J., and Pop, V.J. 2001, November. "Thyroid Peroxidase Antibodies During Gestation Are a Marker for Subsequent Depression Postpartum." *European Journal of Endocrinology* 145 (5): 579–84.

Kumar, Vijay. 2007, February. "Pernicious Anemia," *Medical Laboratory Observer* 28–30.

LaFranchi, S., and Hanna, C.E. 2000. "Graves' Disease in the Neonatal Period and Childhood," in *Werner & Ingbar's The Thyroid: A Fundamental and Clinical Text*, 8th edition, edited by Lewis E. Braverman and Robert D. Utiger. Philadelphia: Lippincott Williams & Wilkins, 989–997.

Larsen, P., Davies, T., and Hay, Ian. 1998. "The Thyroid Gland," in *Williams' Textbook of Endocrinology*. 9th edition. Edited by Jean Wilson. Philadelphia: W.B. Saunders.

Lee, Stephanie. 2003. "New Dimensions in TSH Control," *Thyroid Today* http://www.thyroidtoday.com/TTLibrary/current/AACE%20Newsletter.pdf. Accessed June 15, 2012.

Leger, J., Gelwane, G., Kaguelidou, F., Benmerad, M., and Alberti, C. 2012, January. "Positive Impact of Long-Term Antithyroid Drug Treatment on the Outcome of Children with Graves' Disease: National Long-Term Cohort Study." *Journal of Clinical Endocrinology and Metabolism* 97 (1): 110–19.

Ljunggren, J., Torring, O., Wallin, G., Taube, A., Tallstedt, L., Hamberger, B., and Lundell, G. 1998, August. "Quality of Life Aspects and Costs in Treatment of Graves' Hyperthyroidism with Antithyroid Drugs, Surgery, or Radioiodine: Results from a Prospective Randomized Study." *Thyroid* 8 (8): 653–59.

Longcope, Christopher. 2000. "The Male and Female Reproductive Systems in Thyrotoxicosis," in *Werner & Ingbar's The Thyroid: A Fundamental and Clinical Text*, 8th edition, edited by Lewis E. Braverman and Robert D. Utiger. Philadelphia: Lippincott Williams & Wilkins, 652–58.

Majeroni, Barbara, and Patel, Parag. 2007. "Autoimmune Polyglandular Syndrome, Type II," *American Family Physician* 75: 667–67.

Malik, R., and Hodgson, H. 2002. "The Relationship Between the Thyroid Gland and the Liver," *Oxford Journals QJM: An International Journal of Medicine* 95 (9): 559–69, http://qjmed.oxfordjournals.org/content/95/9/559.long. Accessed November 10, 2012.

Mancini, G.M., Corbo, A., and Gaballo, S. 2006, July 17. "Relationships Between Plasma CoQ10 Levels and Thyroid Hormones in

Chronic Obstructive Pulmonary Diseases." Presentation from the Fourth Conference of the International CoQ10 Association, Los Angeles, CA.

Mao, Chaoming, Wang, Shu, Xiao, Yichuan, Xu, Jingwei, Jiang, Quian, Jin, Min, Jiang, Hua Guo, Xiahuo, Ning, Guang, and Zhang, Yanyun. 2011. "Impairment of Regulatory Capacity of CD4+CD25+ Regulatory T Cells Mediated by Dendritic Cell Polarization and Hyperthyroidism in Graves' Disease," *The Journal of Immunology,* prepublished online March 11, doi. 10.4049/j.immunol/0904135, http://www.ihs.ac.cn/upload/2011031701.pdf. Accessed May 16, 2012.

McLachlan, S., and Rapoport, B. 1996. "Genetic Factors in Thyroid Disease," in *Werner and Ingbar's The Thyroid.* 7th edition, edited by Lewis E. Braverman and Robert D Utiger. Philadelphia: Lippincott-Raven, 474–87.

McLachlan, Sandra, and Rapoport, Basil. 2003. "Graves' Disease: The Th1/Th2 Paradigm versus the 'Hygiene' Hypothesis and Defective Immune Regulation," Guest Editorial in *Thyroid* 13 (2): 127–28.

Metso, S., Suvinen, A., Huhtala, H., Salmi, J., Oksala, H., and Jaatinen, P. 2007. "Increased Cardiovascular and Cancer Mortality After Radioiodine Treatment for Hyperthyroidism." *Journal of Clinical Endocrinology and Metabolism* 92: 2190–96.

Michigishi, T., Mizukami, Y., Shuke, N., Stake, R., Noguchi, M., Aburano, T., Tonami, N., and Hisada, K. 1992. "An Autonomously Functioning Thyroid Carcinoma Associated with Euthyroid Graves' Disease." *The Journal of Nuclear Medicine* 33(11): 2024–26.

Mishra, A., and Mishra, S.K. 2001, October. "Thyroid Nodules in Graves' Disease: Implications in an Endemically Iodine Deficient Area," *Journal of Postgraduate Medicine* 47 (4): 244–47.

Mohan, M., and Ramesh, T. 2003. "Multiple Autoimmune Syndrome," *Indian Journal of Dermatology, Venereology and Leprology* 69 (4): 298–299.

Moore, E. 2003. *Thyroid Eye Disease: Understanding Graves' Ophthalmopathy.* Victoria, BC: SaraHealth Press.

Moore, E., and Wilkinson, S. 2009. *The Promise of Low Dose Naltrexone Therapy.* Jefferson, NC: McFarland.

Moses, Scott. 2012, May 31. "Antithyroid Drug." Family Practice Notebook, www.fpnotebook. com/endo/AnthyrdDrg.htm. Accessed July 10, 2012.

Mouritis, Maarten. 2000, April 29. "Radiotherapy for Graves' Orbitopathy: Randomised Placebo-Conrolled Study." *The Lancet* 355: 2505–09.

Nagata, K., Fukata, S., Kanai, K., Satoh, Y., Segawa, T., Kuwamoto, S., Sugihara, H., Kato, M., Murakami, I., Hayashi, K., and Sairenji, T. 2011, April. "The Influence of Epstein-Barr Virus Reactivation in Patients with Graves' Disease," *Viral Immunology* 24 (2): 143–49.

National Academy of Clinical Biochemistry (NACB). 2002. "Laboratory Support for the Diagnosis and Monitoring of Thyroid Disease. Washington, DC: NACB.

Neumann, S., Eliseeva, E., and McCoy, J. 2011. "A New Small-Molecule Antagonist Inhibits Graves' Disease Antibody Activation of the TSH Receptor." *The Journal of Clinical Endocrinology and Metabolism* 96 (2): 548–54.

Norman, James. 2012, July 30. "Thyroiditis," Endocrine Web, http://www.endocrineweb. com/conditions/thyroid/thyroiditis. Accessed August 30, 2012.

Nussey, Stephen, and Whitehead, Saffron. 2001. *Endocrinology: An Integrated Approach.* London: NCBI Bookshelf. Oxford: BIOS Scientific Publishers. http://www.ncbi.nlm.nih. gov/books/NBK22. Accessed July 5, 2012.

Ogedegbe, Henry. 2001, November. "Autoimmune Diseases: A Spectrum of Disease Processes," *Laboratory Medicine* 11 (32): 70–79.

Ontell, F., Moore, E., Shepard, J., and Shelton, D. 1997, May. "The Costal Cartilages in Health and Disease." *Radiographics* 17: 571–77.

O'Reilly, Kevin. 2011, December. "Proposal on Access to Labs Should Be Revised, Doctors Say," *Amednews,* http://www.ama-assn.org/ amednews/2011/12/12/prsb1212.htm. Accessed September 1, 2012.

Osborne, Sally. 1999. "Does Soy Have a Dark Side?" *Natural Health* 29 (2): 110–13.

Osda, E., Hiroi, N., Sue, M., Masai, N., Iga, R., Shigemitsu, R., Oka, R., Miyagi, M., Iso, K., Kuboki, K., and Yoshino, Gen. 2011. "Thyroid Storm Associated with Graves' Disease Covered by Diabetic Ketoacidosis: A Case Report." *Thyroid Research* 4:8 doi:10. 1186/1756–6614–4–8, http://www.thyroidre searchjournal.com/content/4/1/8. Accessed February 28, 2012.

Park, J., Kim, C., Nam, J., Kim, D., Yoon, S., Ahn, C., Cha, B., Lim, S., Kim, K., Lee, H., and Huh, K. 2004. "Graves' Disease Associated with Klinefelter's Syndrome." *Yonsei Medical Journal* 45 (2): 341–44.

Park, J., Kim, I., Lee, M., Seo, J., Suh, P., Cho, B., Ryu, S., and Chae, C. 1999. "Identification of the Peptides That Inhibit the Stimulation of Thyrotropin Receptor by Graves' IgG from Peptide Libraries." *Endocrinology* 138: 617–26.

Paunkovic, J., and Paunkovic, N. 2006, January. "Does Autoantibody-Negative Graves' Disease Exist? A Second Evaluation of the Clinical Diagnosis." *Hormone Metabolism Research* 38 (1): 53–56.

Pearce, E., Farwell, A., and Braverman, L. 2003, June 26. "Thyroiditis," *The New England Journal of Medicine* 348 (26): 2646–55.

Pineda, G., Arancibia, P., and Mejia, G. 1998, August. "Treatment of Basedow-Graves' Hyperthyroidism: Retrospective Analysis After 30 years." *Revista Medica de Chile* 126 (8): 953–62.

Porter, Lisa, and Mandel, Susan J. 2000. "The Blood in Thyrotoxicosis," in *Werner & Ingbar's The Thyroid: A Fundamental and Clinical Text,* 8th edition, edited by Lewis E. Braverman and Robert D. Utiger. Philadelphia: Lippincott Williams & Wilkins, 627–30.

Potenza, Matthew, Via, Michael, and Yanagisawa, Robert. 2009, April. "Excess Thyroid Hormone and Carbohydrate Metabolism," *Endocrine Practice* 15 (3): 254–262.

Prummel, M.F., Strieder, T., and Wiersinga, W. M. 2004, May. "The Environment and Autoimmune Thyroid Diseases," *European Journal of Endocrinology* 150 (5): 605–18.

Purtell, Kerry, Roepke, Thorsten, and Abbott, Geoffrey. 2010, November. "Cardiac Arrhythmia and Thyroid Dysfunction: A Novel Genetic Link," *The International Journal of Biochemistry and Cell Biology* 42 (11): 1776–70.

Pyne, D., and Isenberg, D. 2002. "Autoimmune Thyroid Disease in Systemic Lupus Erythematosus." *Annals of the Rhematic Diseases* 61 (1): 70–72.

Roberts, H.J. 2004. "Aspartame Disease," *Texas Heart Institute Journal* 31 (1): 105.

Rocchi, R. 2005, April. "Clinical Utility of Autoantibodies Directed against TSH-R," *Medical Laboratory Observer* 37 (4): 10–16.

Ron, E., Doody, M., Becker, D., Brill, B., Curtis, R., Goldman, M., Harris, B., Hoffman, D., McConahey, W., Maxon, H., Preston-Martin, S., Earshauer, E., Wong, L., and Boice, J., Jr. 1998. "Cancer Mortality Following Treatment for Adult Hyperthyroidism for the Cooperative Thyrotoxicosis Therapy Follow-up Study Group," *Journal of the American Medical Association* 280 (4): 347–55.

Rose, Noel, Bonita, Raphael, and Burek, Lynne. 2002, February. "Iodine, an Environmental Trigger of Thyroiditis," *Autoimmunity Reviews* 1 (1–2): 97–103.

Rose, Noel, Rasooly, Linda, Sabori, Ali, and Burek, C. Lynne. 1999, October. "Linking Iodine with Autoimmune Thyroiditis," *Environmental Health Perspectives* 107, Suppl 5: 749–52.

Rugger, R., Galetti, M., and Aragona, P. 2002. "Thyroid Hormone Autoantibodies in Primary Sjögren's Syndrome and Rheumatoid

Arthritis Are More Prevalent than in Autoimmune Thyroid Disease, Becoming Progressively More Frequent in These Diseases," *Journal of Endocrinological Investigation* 0391–4097 (7): 447–54.

Sabatini, L., Torricelli, M., and Scaccia, V. 2007, February. "Increased Plasma Concentrations of Antiprothrombin Antibodies in Women with Recurrent Spontaneous Abortions," *Clinical Chemistry* 53 (2): 228–32.

Sadigh, Micah, 2012. *Autogenic Training: A Mind-Body Approach to Treatment of Chronic Pain Syndrome and Stress-Related Disorders.* 2nd edition. Jefferson, NC: McFarland.

Sato, H., Harada, S., Yokoya, S., Tanaka, T., Asayama, K., Mori, M., and Sasaki, N. 2007, January. "Treatment for Childhood-Onset Graves' Disease in Japan: Results of a Nationwide Questionnaire Survey of Pediatric Endocrinologists and Thyroidologists." *Thyroid* 17 (1): 67–72.

Sato, A., Takemura, Y., Yamada, T., Ohtsuka, H., Sakai, H., Miyahra, Y., Aizawa, T., Teroa, A., Onuma, S., Junen, K., Kanamori, A., Nakamura, Y., Tejima, E., Ito, Y., and Kamijo, K. 1999, October. "A Possible Role of Immunoglobulin E in Patients with Hyperthyroid Graves' Disease." *Journal of Clinical Endocrinology and Metabolism* 84 (10): 3602–05.

Scheinman, Steven J., and Moses, Arnold M. 2000. "The Kidneys and Electrolyte Metabolism in Thyrotoxicosis," in *Werner & Ingbar's The Thyroid: A Fundamental and Clinical Text,* 8th edition, edited by Lewis E. Braverman and Robert D. Utiger. Philadelphia: Lippincott Williams & Wilkins, 617–21.

Schraga, Erik. 2012. "Hyperthyroidism, Thyroid Storm, and Graves' Disease," Medscape, http://emedicine.medscape.com/article/767130-overview. Accessed July 1, 2012.

Schwartz, Seymour. 1999. *Principles of Surgery.* Vol. 2. 7th edition. New York: McGraw-Hill.

Segni, M., Leonardi, E., Mazzoncini, B., Pucarelli, I., and Pasquino, A.M. 1999, September. "Special Features of Graves' Disease in Early Childhood." *Thyroid* 9 (9): 871–77.

Sellin, Joseph, and Vassilopoulou-Sellin, Rena. 2000. "The Gastrointestinal Tract and Liver in Thyrotoxicosis," in *Werner & Ingbar's The Thyroid: A Fundamental and Clinical Text,* 8th edition, edited by Lewis E. Braverman and Robert D. Utiger. Philadelphia: Lippincott Williams & Wilkins, 622–26.

Seo, S., Lee, B., Park, S., Kim, K., Kim, S., and Yun, M. 2003, April. "Thyrotoxic Autoimmune Encephalopathy: A Repeat Positron Emission Tomography Study." *Journal of Neurology and Neurosurgery and Psychiatry* 74 (4): 504–06.

Shimon, I., Pariente, C., Shomo-David, J., Grossman, Z., and Sack, J. 2003. "Transient Elevation of Triiodothyronine Caused by Triiodothyronine Autoantibody Associated with Acute Epstein-Barr-Virus Infection," *Thyroid* 13 (2): 211–24.

Shu, X., Ji, J., Li, X., Sundquist, J., Sundquist, K., and Hemminki, K. 2010. "Cancer Risk in Patients Hospitalised for Graves' Disease: A Population-Based Cohort Study in Sweden." *British Journal of Cancer* 102 (9): 1397–99.

Silva, J. Enrique. 2000. "Catecholamines and the Sympathoadrenal System in Thyrotoxicosis," in *Werner & Ingbar's The Thyroid: A Fundamental and Clinical Text*, 8th edition, edited by Lewis E. Braverman and Robert D. Utiger. Philadelphia: Lippincott Williams & Wilkins, 642–51.

Singer, Peter. 1991. "Thyroiditis, Acute, Subacute, and Chronic," in *The Thyroid, Medical Clinics of North America* 75 (1): 61–75.

Singh, Reetu. 2011, February 29. "Euthyroid Hyperthyroxinemia," Medscape, http://emedicine.medscape.com/article/118562-overview. Accessed June 6, 2012.

Snyder, Peter J. 2000. "The Pituitary in Thyrotoxicosis," in *Werner & Ingbar's The Thyroid: A Fundamental and Clinical Text*, 8th edition, edited by Lewis E. Braverman and Robert D. Utiger. Philadelphia: Lippincott Williams & Wilkins, 634–36.

Soparkar, C. 1999, October-November-December. "Thyroid Eye Disease — Surgical Options." *Thyroid USA*, 1.

Spiezia, S., Vitale, G., Di Somma, C., Assanti, A., Ciccarelli, A., Lombardi, G., and Colao, A. 2007. "Ultrasound-Guided Laser Thermal Ablation in the Treatment of Autonomous Hyperfunctioning Thyroid Nodules and Compressive Nontoxic Nodular Goiter." *Thyroid* 13 (10): 941–47.

Starr, Mark. 2011. *Hypothyroidism Type 2*. Columbia, MO: Mark Starr Trust.

Stevens, Alun. 2003. "Guidelines for Thyroid Function Tests." Thyroid Australia Ltd., http://www.thyroid.org.au/Information/NACBExtract.html. Accessed November 10, 2012.

Stocker, D., and Burch, H. 2003, September. "Thyroid Cancer Yield in Patients with Graves' Disease," Minerva Endocrinology 28 (3): 205–12.

Takeoka, K., Hidaka, Y., Hanada, H., Nomura, T., Tanaka, S., Takano, T., Amino, N. 2003, November. "Increase in Serum Levels of Autoantibodies After Attack of Seasonal Allergic Rhinitis in Patients with Graves' Disease," *International Archives of Allergy and Immunology* 132 (3): 268–76.

Tesavibul, N. 2007. "Multiple Autoimmune Diseases," The Ocular Immunology and Uveitis Foundation, http://www.uveitis.org/docs/dm/multiple_autoimmune_disease.pdf. Accessed March 20, 2012.

Teufel, A., Weinmann, A., Kahaly, G.J., Centner, C., Piendl, A., Wörns, M., Lohse, A.W., Galle, P.R., Kanzler, S. 2010, March. "Concurrent Autoimmune Diseases in Patients with Autoimmune Hepatitis." *Journal of Clinical Gastroenterology* 44 (3): 208–13.

Unsal, E., Oren, O., Salar, K., Makay, B., Abaci, A., Ozhan, B., and Bober, E. 2008, September-October. "The Frequency of Autoimmune Thyroid Disorders in Juvenile Idiopathic Arthritis." *Turkish Journal of Pediatrics* 50 (5): 462–65.

Upton, Arthur. 1998. "Ionizing Radiation," in *Environmental and Occupational Medicine*, 3rd edition, edited by W. Rom. Philadelphia: Lippincott-Raven.

Utiger, Robert. 2002, May. "Thyrotropin-Receptor Antibodies in Patients with Hyperthyroidism Inhibit Thyrotropin Secretion." *AllThyroid Newsletter*, The Thyroid Foundation of America.

Vadiveloo, T., Donnan, P., Cochrane, L., and Leese, G. 2011, May. "The Thyroid Epidemiology, Audit, and Research Study (TEARS): Morbidity in Patients with Endogenous Subclinical Hyperthyroidism," *Journal of Clinical Endocrinology and Metabolism* 96 (5): 1344–51.

Varanasi, Ajay, and Shakir, K.M. Mohamed. "Agent Orange," American Association of Clinical Endocrinologists 19th Annual Meeting. Abstract 1046. April 23, 2010.

Villanueva, R., Greenberg, D., Davies, T., and Tomer, Y. 2003. "Sibling Recurrence Risk in Autoimmune Thyroid Disease," *Thyroid* 13 (3): 761–64.

Vliet, Elizabeth. 1995. *Screaming to Be Heard: Hormonal Connections Women Suspect ... and Doctors Ignore*, New York: M. Evans and Company.

Vogel, H.C.A. 1991. *The Nature Doctor: A Manual of Traditional Complementary Medicine*. New York: Instant Improvement.

Wartofsky, Leonard. 2000. "Thyrotoxic Storm," in *Werner & Ingbar's The Thyroid: A Fundamental and Clinical Text*, 8th edition, edited by Lewis E. Braverman and Robert D. Utiger. Philadelphia: Lippincott Williams & Wilkins: 679–84.

Warwar, R. 1999, October. "New Insights into Pathogenesis and Potential Therapeutic Options for Graves' Orbitopathy." *Current Opinions in Ophthalmology* 10 (5): 358–61.

Weetman, Anthony. 2000, October 26. "Graves' Disease," *The New England Journal of Medicine* 343: 1236–48.

Weiss, R., and Retetoff, S. 1999. "Treatment of

Resistance to Thyroid Hormone — *Primum Non Nocere.*" *Journal of Clinical Endocrinology & Metabolism* 84 (2): 401–04.

Whybrow, Peter, and Bauer, Michael. 2000. "Behavioral and Psychiatric Aspects of Thyrotoxicosis," in *Werner & Ingbar's The Thyroid: A Fundamental and Clinical Text*, 8th edition, edited by Lewis E. Braverman and Robert D. Utiger. Philadelphia: Lippincott Williams & Wilkins, 673–78.

Woeber, K.A. 2005. "Observations Concerning the Natural History of Subclinical Hyperthyroidism," *Thyroid* 15: 687–91.

Xiao, H., Zhuang, W., Wang, S., Yu, B., Chen, G., Zhou, M., and Wong, Norman C. W. 2002. "Arterial Embolization: A Novel Approach to Thyroid Ablative Therapy for Graves' Disease." *The Journal of Clinical Endocrinology & Metabolism* 87 (8): 3583–89. http://jcem.endojournals.org/content/87/8/3583.full. Accessed March 1, 2012.

Yamada, T., Sato, A., Komiya, I., Nishimori, T., Ito, Y., Terso, A., Eto, S., and Tanaka, Yshiya. 2000, August. "An Elevation of Serum Immunoglobulin E Provides a New Aspect of Hyperthyroid Graves' Disease," *Journal of Clinical Endocrinology & Metabolism* 85 (8): 2775–78.

Yamamoto, M., Tatsuko, Y., Kojima, I., Yamashita, N., Togawa, K., Sawaki, N., and Ogata, E. 1983. "Outcome of Patients with Graves' Disease After Long-Term Medical Treatment Guided by Triiodothyronine (T3) Suppression Test." *Clinical Endocrinology* 19: 467–76.

Yeung, Sai-Ching Jim. 2011, September 30. "Graves' Disease," *Medscape Reference* http://emedicine.medscape.com/article/120619-overview. Accessed March 1, 2012.

Zha, LL. 1997, June. "Therapeutic effect and Its Mechanism Exploration on Mainly Using Traditional Chinese Medicine of Replenishing Qi and Nourishing Yin in Treating Graves' Disease," *Chung Juo Chung His I Chieh Ho Tsa Chih* 17 (6): 328–30.

Zimmermann-Belsing, T., Christensen, L., Hansen, H., Kirkegaard, J., Blichert-Toft, M., Feldt-Rasmussen, F., and U. 2000, March. "A case of Sarcoidosis and Sarcoid Granuloma, Papillary Carcinoma, and Graves' Disease in the Thyroid Gland," *Thyroid* 10 (3): 275–78.

Zuraw, Bruce. 1997. "Urticaria, Angioedema, and Autoimmunity," in *Progress and Controversies in Autoimmune Disease Testing, Clinics in Laboratory Medicine,* Philadelphia: W.B. Saunders, 559–70.

Resources

Recommended Books

Arem, Ridha. 1999. *The Thyroid Solution: A Mind-Body Program for Beating Depression and Regaining Your Emotional and Physical Health.* New York: Ballantine. Written by an endocrinologist, this book focuses on the emotional aspects of thyroid disease.

Barnes, Broda, and Galton, Lawrence. 1976. *Hypothyroidism: The Unsuspected Illness.* New York: Harper & Row. This book explains how thyroid disorders often escape diagnosis when laboratory tests are used as the sole diagnostic criteria and describes the Barnes basal temperature test as a diagnostic tool.

Baskin, H. Jack. 1991. *How Your Thyroid Works*, 3rd edition. Chicago: Adams Press. This book provides a good introduction to basic thyroid function.

Christenson, Alan, and Bender, Hy. 2011. *The Complete Idiot's Guide to Thyroid Disease.* New York: Penguin. Provides basic information on hypothyroidism and hyperthyroidism, goiter, Graves' disease, Hashimoto's disease, thyroid cancer, and adrenal gland diseases. The official website for the book is www.CIGThyroid.com.

Colborn, Theo, Dumanoski, Diane, and Myers, John Peterson. 1997. *Our Stolen Future: Are We Threatening Our Fertility, Intelligence, and Survival? A Scientific Detective Story.* New York: Penguin. Discusses the environmental influences, particularly industrial chemicals, that contribute to autoimmune disease.

Fagin, Dan, Lavelle, Marianne, and the Center for Public Integrity. 1997. *Toxic Deception: How the Chemical Industry Manipulates Science, Bends the Law, and Endangers Your Health*, 2nd edition. Monroe, ME: Common Courage Press. Discusses the environmental influences, particularly industrial chemicals, that contribute to autoimmune disease.

Krimsky, Sheldon. 2000. *Hormonal Chaos: The Scientific and Social Origins of the Environmental Endocrine Hypothesis.* Baltimore, MD: Johns Hopkins University Press. Discusses the hormonal disturbances caused by environmental agents.

Langer, Stephen. 1984. *Solved: The Riddle of Illness.* New Canaan, CT: Keats Publishing. This book provides excellent information on nutrient deficiencies that may induce or exacerbate symptoms of both hypothyroidism and hyperthyroidism.

Rom, William, editor. 1998. *Environmental & Occupational Medicine*, 3rd edition, Philadelphia, Lippincott-Raven. Discusses the health consequences of radiation.

Shames, Richard, and Shames, Karilee. 2002. *Thyroid Power: Ten Steps to Total Health.* New York: HarperCollins. This book describes the treatment of thyroid disorders.

Shames, Richard, and Shames, Karilee. 2005. *Feeling Fat, Fuzzy, or Frazzled?: A 3-Step Program to: Restore Thyroid, Adrenal, and Reproductive Balance, Beat Hormone Havoc, and Feel Better Fast!.* New York: Penguin. This book describes the treatment of thyroid disorders.

Shomon, Mary. 2000. *Living Well with Hypothyroidism: What Your Doctor Doesn't Tell You That You Need to Know.* New York: Avon Books. This book, written by a Hashimoto's thyroiditis patient who is a journalist and thyroid educator, is a must for Graves' patients who have become hypothyroid.

Shomon, Mary. 2007. *Living Well with Graves' Disease and Hyperthyroidism: What Your Doctor Doesn't Tell You ... That You Need to Know.* New York: HarperCollins. Describes the symptoms and complications of hyperthyroidism.

Teitlebaum, Jacob. 2007. *From Fatigued to Fantastic.* New York: Penguin. This book describes the immune system disturbances that contribute to chronic fatigue syndrome and hypothyroidism.

Recommended Journals

Advance for Medical Laboratory Professionals. Bimonthly journal dealing with advances in laboratory testing. http://laboratorian.advanceweb.com/

British Medical Journal. Prestigious United Kingdom medical journal; website offers some full-text articles. http://www.bmj.com/

Journal of Clinical Endocrinology and Metabolism. Monthly medical journal focused on current endocrinology issues. http://jcem.endojournals.org/

Journal of the American Medical Association (JAMA), http://jama.jamanetwork.com/journal.aspx

The Lancet, http://www.thelancet.com/.

New England Journal of Medicine. The NEJM is a medical journal intended for physicians and other health professionals that presents full-text articles based on peer-reviewed clinical studies. http://www.nejm.org/

Thyroid. Medical journal affiliated with the Thyroid Foundation of America (TFA); contains conventional thyroid-related articles contributed from worldwide sources. Sample issues and subscription information can be found at TFA website, http://www.tsh.org/

Websites and Additional Resources

About.com thyroid disease page. This site provides a wealth of thyroid-related information and has numerous links to articles and forums. http://thyroid.about.com/

About.com thyroid forum. A forum focused on the exchange of thyroid-related information. http://forums.about.com/ab-thyroid

Columbia University Medical Center; New York Thyroid Center. This site provides information on disorders of the thyroid gland. Referrals available. http://columbiathyroidcenter.org/

Dear Thyroid. This site provides a forum for thyroid patients and their families to write love and hate letters to their thyroids. This site also includes links to columns and podcasts. http://dearthyroid.org/

Elaine Moore's Graves' Disease and Autoimmune Education. My personal Graves' disease site has pages dedicated to environmental concerns, pregnancy, childhood Graves' disease, and many other points of interest. http://www.elaine-moore.com/

Endocrineweb. http://www.endocrineweb.com/

Graves' Disease and Thyroid Foundation forum. http://www.gdatf.org/forum/

Graves' Disease and Thyroid Foundation News. Offers tips on dealing with eye and hair changes, news about the foundation's educational conventions, and basic information geared toward the newly diagnosed Graves' patient. The foundation also provides a number of excellent informational bulletins on topics related to Graves' hyperthyroidism and Graves' ophthalmology. http://www.gdatf.org/news/

Graves' Disease Yahoo support group. This list is for people with Graves' disease and family and friends who are interesting in supporting them. http://health.groups.yahoo.com/group/graves_support/

InFocus Newsletter. The newsletter of the American Autoimmune Related Diseases Association, Inc. (AARDA) provides a wealth of information on autoimmune diseases. http://www.aarda.org/infocus_newsletter.php.

iThyroid. Founded by John Johnson, a Graves' patient who treated his symptoms of hyperthyroidism using a natural approach, this group focuses on correcting the nutritional imbalances that contribute to the development of thyroid disorders. http://www.ithyroid.com/

Mary Shoman's Thyroid Info website. Includes a directory of doctors. http://www.thyroid-info.com/

The Mayo Clinic. The Mayo Clinic is a nonprofit worldwide leader in medical care, research and education. Through the clinic, doctors from various medical specialties work together to care for patients and share information. Mayo Clinic is governed by a 33-member board of trustees. The site includes thyroid-related articles. http://www.mayoclinic.com/

Paula Free Heart. Paula Ehler's blog about her personal experiences with Graves' disease and her subsequent development of fibromyalgia. http://paulaspaininthepancreas.blogspot.com/2012/02/here-it-is.html

Sticking Out Our Necks. Mary Shomon's e-mail newsletter for thyroid patients. This newsletter contains current information regarding medication interferences, dieting tips, environmental concerns and treatment issues. http://www.thyroid-info.com/

Thyroid boards. Links to message boards related to Graves' disease, radioiodine ablation, thyroid cancer, Hashitoxicosis, and Hashimoto's disease. http://www.thyroidboards.com/

Thyroid Coaching. Thyroid coaching site run by Mary Shoman, a thyroid patient, advocate, and author. http://www.thyroidcoaching.com/

Thyroid Disease Manager. This site comprises a complete thyroid textbook that is frequently updated by its authors, all internationally acclaimed thyroid experts. Although this site is primarily intended for physicians, the chapters relating to Graves' disease contain valuable information relating to both the autoimmune nature of Graves' disease and treatment concerns. http://www.thyroidmanager.org/

Thyroid Friends and Family on Facebook. http://www.facebook.com/thyroidfamily

Thyroid Research. This site posts extracts from thyroid-related medical research. http://thyroidresearch.com/

Thyroid Sexy. This is the Facebook page of celebrity Gena Lee Nolin. It is designed to create thyroid awareness. http://www.facebook.com/thyroidsexy

Thyroid Support on Facebook. http://www.facebook.com/thyroidsupport

UpToDate. This site provides a collection of medical articles written and peer reviewed by doctors. http://www.uptodate.com/home

National and International Organizations

AllThyroid.org. This site includes information on thyroid research, patient groups, thyroid disorders and treatments. http://www.allthyroid.org/

The American Academy of Medical Acupuncture. This site has a searchable database of acupuncture physicians. http://medicalacupuncture.org/

The American Association of Acupuncture and Oriental Medicine. Provides a search tool to find acupuncture practitioners. http://www.aaaomonline.org/

American Association of Clinical Endocrinologists. This professional organization for endocrinologists allows for searches of U.S. and international members based on location and specialty (choose thyroid dysfunction). https://www.aace.com/

The American Association of Naturopathic Physicians. Provides information on natural health, natural medicine, and a search engine for finding a physician. http://www.naturopathic.org/

American Autoimmune Related Diseases Association. This site provides information on autoimmune disorders. http://www.arda.org/arda/home.aspx

American Board of Medical Specialties. This site can be used to research the certification of doctors. http://www.abms.org/

American Holistic Health Association. This site provides resources for wellness and healing.

The organization's purpose is to offer impartial holistic health resources — both alternative and traditional. http://ahha.org/

American Medical Association. This site has a database of more than 814,000 physicians, which can be searched by location, name, and/or specialty. http://www.ama-assn.org/

American Thyroid Association. This organization promotes thyroid health and the understanding of thyroid biology. http://www.thyroid.org/

Australian Thyroid Foundation, https://www.thyroidfoundation.com.au/

British Thyroid Foundation, http://www.btf-thyroid.org/

Broda O. Barnes Research Foundation. This is a nonprofit organization dedicated to education, research and training in the field of thyroid and metabolic balance. http://brodabarnes.org/

Coalition for Better Thyroid Care. This is a U.S.–based, patient-oriented organization dedicated to promoting improvements in thyroid care. http://betterthyroidcare.org/

The Endocrine Society. This group works to foster better understanding of endocrinology among the public and practitioners of complementary medical disciplines and to promote endocrinologists' interests at the national scientific research and health policy levels of government. http://www.endo-society.org/

European Thyroid Association. The association's purpose is to promote knowledge in the thyroid field (fundamental and clinical) and improve knowledge of the thyroid gland and its diseases. http://www.eurothyroid.com/

Herb Research Foundation. The mission of this foundation is to foster improved world health and well-being through the informed use of herbs. http://www.herbs.org/herbnews/

Hormone Foundation. This site provides information on hormones and health as well as information on various thyroid disorders. http://www.hormone.org/Thyroid/index.cfm

Hypoparathyroidism Association, Inc. This association was founded in 2004 to share information about hypoparathyroidism. The associated is directed by a volunteer board of directors and is overseen by a medical advisory board. https://www.hypopara.org/

International Thyroid Eye Disease Society. This is a nonprofit society dedicated to educating the public and physicians about thyroid eye disease as well as conducting research to understand the disease that may lead to prevention and cures. http://thyroideyedisease.org/

Maharishi Ayurveda. This organization serves as an educational resource for the Ayurvedic products it manufactures. It offers a newsletter, *Total Health News,* and answers questions regarding therapies. http://mapi.com/

Major Aspects of Growth in Children (The MAGIC Foundation). This is a national non-profit organization created to provide support services for the families of children afflicted with a wide variety of chronic and/or critical disorders, syndromes and diseases that affect a child's growth. http://www.magicfounda tion.org/www

Medicine in Germany. Provides information on thyroid doctors in Germany. http://www.med knowledge.de/germany/hospitals/surgery/thy rodi-gland-surgery.htm

National Organization for Rare Disorders (NORD). NORD is committed to the identification, treatment, and cure of rare disorders through programs of education, advocacy, research, and service. http://www.rarediseases. org/

Society of Nuclear Medicine. This site may be useful for researching radioiodine ablation. http://www.snm.org. See also http://interac tive.snm.org/index.cfm?PageID=11031.

Thyroid Change. A web-based initiative to share information among the international thyroid community. http://www.thyroidchange.org/

Thyroid Eye Disease (TED). Informational site affiliated with the University of Dundee. http://www.dundee.ac.uk/medther/tayendoweb/ thyroid_eye_disease.htm

Thyroid Federation International. Established in Toronto and now registered in Sweden, this organization is a network of patient support organizations from many countries. http:// thyroid-fed.org/

Thyroid Foundation. Provides a wide variety of information about thyroid disorders. http://www.thyroidfoundation.org/

Thyroid Foundation International. This is an umbrella organization for thyroid patient organizations worldwide. http://www.thyroid-fed.org/tfi-wp/about/

Thyroid Foundation of Canada, http://www.thyroid.ca/

Thyroid Info.com. Directory of international and U.S. thyroid doctors. http://www.thy roid-info.com/topdrs/index.htm

Government Funded Medical Resources

Medline Plus. The U.S. government's National Institutes of Health run this site, which is designed to be patient friendly. It provides information about major illnesses, including thyroid disease. www.medlineplus.gov

National Institutes of Health; Office of Dietary

Supplements. This site contains fact sheets on vitamins and minerals. http://ods.od.nih.gov/

PubMed.gov. The U.S. National Library of Medicine, National Institutes of Health search service that provides access to over 22 million biomedical literature from Medline, life science journals, and online books. Citations may include links to full-text content from PubMed Central and publisher websites. http://www.ncbi.nlm.nih.gov/pubmed.

Womenshealth.gov. This is a basic women's health information site provided by the Office of Women's Health, U.S. Department of Health and Human Services. This site has basic thyroid information. http://womens health.gov/

Laboratory Resources

The Afirma Thyroid FNA Biopsy Evaluation. Afirma is developing molecular tests designed to improve the diagnostic accuracy of cytology samples, thereby helping to increase the utility of these minimally invasive procedures as an alternative to surgical biopsy. http://www.veracyte.com/afirma

American Society for Clinical Pathology, http://www.ascp.org/

The Canary Club. This organization conducts saliva-based testing. http://www.canaryclub. org/

Diagnos-Techs, Inc. Clinical and Research Laboratory. This organization conducts saliva-based testing. http://diagnostechs.com/

Lab Test Online. http://labtestsonline.org/

MyMedLab. Through this site, various thyroid, hormonal, and other blood tests can be ordered. https://thyroid-info.mymedlab.com/ mary-shomon-profiles/shomon-thyroid-basic

National Institutes of Health. "How Medications Affect Thyroid Function." http://www.ncbi.nlm.nih.gov/pmc/articles/PMC1070767/

ZRT Laboratory. ZRT tests for a number of hormones and values. http://www.zrtlab.com/

Alternative Medicine Resources

Acupuncture.com. This site provides a list of licensed acupuncturists by state. http://www.acupuncture.com/

Alternative Medicine at About.com. This site provides general information about alternative medicine. Within this site, you can search under "thyroid disease" and find links to information on alternative therapy for thyroid disease. http://altmedicine.about.com/

American Botanical Council Online. This site provides information about the safe and effective use of herbs. http://abc.herbalgram.org/site/PageServer

Ballentine, Rudolph. 1999. *Radical Healing*, New York, Harmony Books. The author, an integrative physician, has a background in psychiatry, herbalism, homeopathy and Ayurveda.

Blumentahl, Mark, editor. 1998. *The Complete German Commission E Monographs Therapeutic Guides to Herbal Medicine*, Boston: The American Botanical Council in cooperation with Integrative Medicine Communications. Center for Mind-Body Healing. The center teaches mind-body medicine techniques that enhance each person's capacity for self-awareness and self-care to health professionals around the world, including those in traumatized communities in the greatest need. http://www.cmbm.org/

The Chopra Center for Wellbeing. Deepak Chopra, M.D., and David Simon, M.D., opened the Chopra Center for Wellbeing in 1996 to help people experience physical healing, emotional freedom, and higher states of consciousness. http://www.chopra.com/

The Continuum Center for Health and Healing. Provides information on health conditions and integrative health care. This site is associated with the Department of Integrative Medicine at Beth Israel Hospital in New York City. http://healthandhealingny.org/

Eleven Eleven Wellness Center. The center offers patient-centered care to help people become and stay healthy. Its treatment strategies take an integrative approach, combining Western medicine with alternative therapies. http://www.drfranklipman.com/eleven-eleven-wellness-center/

Environmental Working Group. This is a non-profit organization devoted to protecting consumers from environmental toxins, the cause of most thyroid disease. http://ewg.org/

Gao, Duo. 1997. *Chinese Medicine*, New York, Thunder Mouth's PressGreen Guide for Everyday Living. This site from the National Geographic Society is filled with simple tips for going green. thegreenguide.com

Health Central. This site contains articles, questions and answers, information on the 50 most common herbs, and an archive of newspaper columns. http://www.healthcentral.com/

HerbMed. This site contains an interactive database that provides information on herbs. http://herbmed.org/

Institute for Health and Healing. The Institute for Health and Healing is an integrative medicine center. It was created to support healing and healthier ways of living, for both individuals and communities. The institute was founded in 1994 by joining three long-standing programs at California Pacific Medical Center in San Francisco. California Pacific Medical Center is the largest private, not-for-profit medical center in California and is a Sutter Health affiliate. http://www.cpmc.org/services/ihh/

Let's Live. An online wellness community; includes a health library, recipes, and health products. http://www.letslive.co.nz/

Life Extension. An online source of natural health products. http://www.lef.org/index.htm

Local Harvest. Provides information on local family farms and farmers' markets. http://www.localharvest.org/

Lockie, Andrew, and Geddes, Nicola. 1995. *The Complete Guide to Homeopathy*, New York, DK Publishing.

Patients Medical Center. Patients Medical is a holistic wellness center dedicated to health and vitality. The center focuses on the root causes of secondary medical conditions, integrating modern medicine, holistic practices, and natural supplements to spark healing and prevent disease. http://www.patientsmedical.com/center/default.aspx

USDA Agricultural Marketing Service. Provides information on U.S. farmers market locations, directions, operating times, product offerings, and accepted forms of payment. http://search.ams.usda.gov/farmersmarkets/

A Woman's Time. Provides options in the management of menopause issues, women's health, and the prevention and treatment of chronic diseases. http://www.awomanstime.com/

Thyroid Drugs and Their Manufacturers

Armour Thyroid, Thyrolar, Levothroid
Forest Pharmaceuticals, http://forestpharm.com/; http://www.armourthyroid.com/; http://www.thyrolar.com/; http://w.levothyroid.com/

Synthroid
Abbott Laboratories, http://abbott.com/index.htm; http://www.synthroid.com/default.aspx

Tapazole, Levoxyl, and Cytomel
Pfizer/King Pharmaceuticals Division, http://www.pfizer.com/kingpharmaceuticals/. See http://www.pfizer.com/products/#A

Thyrogen
Genzime Therapeutics, http://www.genzyme.com/; http://www.thyrogen.com/home/thy_home.asp

Thyroid®
Erfa, http://erfa-sa.erfa.net/english_fr.htm

Tirosint
Akrimax, http://akrimax.com/; http://www.tirosint.com/index.php?page=gelcaps

Unithroid
Lannett Pharmaceuticals, http://lannett.com/; http://www.unithroid.com/

Westhroid/Nature-Throid
RLC Laboratories, http://rlclabs.com/; http://nature-throid.com/; http://www.westhroid.com/

Index

Numbers in **_bold italics_** indicate pages with illustrations.

acetyl-l-carnitine 184–5
acne 97, 146, 162, 167, 179, 228
acropachy 15, 230–2, **_231_**
acupressure 182
acupuncture 182
Adams and Purves 48
Adderall *see* amphetamines
Addison's disease 57, 61, 88, 90, 92, 93–4
adenoma, thyroid 31–3, **_32_**
adenovirus 81
adipocytes 232
adrenal failure 91
adrenal glands 6, 18
adrenal insufficiency 93–4
age-related symptoms 12–3, 14–5
Agent Orange 82–3
agitation 20, 21, 25, 172
agranulocytosis 137, 138, 154
AITD *see* autoimmune thyroid disease
alanine transaminase 15, 97
alcohol 16, 21
alkaline phosphatase 15, 97, 106, 144
allergies 50, 77, 78–80, 85, 86, 176, 186
alopecia areata 17, 57, 89, 90, 92, 93, 179, 226, 229
amenorrhea 6, 188
American Association of Clinical Endocrinologists 131
American Thyroid Association 1, 131
Americans with Disabilities Act 52
amiodarone 23, 41, 77, 85, 122, 162
amnesia 67
amphetamines 77, 122, 219
ANA *see* antinuclear antibodies
ANCA *see* antineutropilic cytoplasmic antibodies
angioedema 57, 60
anorexia 13, 85, 113

antibodies *see* autoantibodies
anticardiolipin antibodies 100, 102
antigens 60, 75
antineutropilic cytoplasmic antibodies (ANCA) 68, 137, 138
antioxidants 77, 227
antiparietal cell antibodies 68, 96
antiphospholipid antibodies 100, 102
antiphospholipid syndrome 65, 92, 99–103
antithyroid drugs 21, 86, 123, 136–42, 191–2
anxiety 15, 17, 22, 55, 66
apathetic hyperthyroidism 13, 51, 66–7
apathy 20, 66
APECED 91
aplastic anemia 104
apoptosis 70, 71, 81
appetite 17, 56
Arnica montana 178
arrhythmia 14, 15
arterial embolization 157–8
Askanazy cells 10
aspartame 77, 85, 161
aspartate transaminase 15, 97
aspirin *see* salicylates
ATD's *see* antithyroid drugs
atrial fibrillation 14, 19–20, 25, 57
atrophic autoimmune thyroiditis 52, 87
atrophic gastritis 57, 92, 96
attention deficit hyperactivity disorder (ADHD) 13, 23, 203
autoantibodies 177, 179, 182, 189
autogenic training 183–4
autoimmune disease 60, 87, 89
autoimmune endocrine disorders 6, 57, 59, 91, 92, 93
autoimmune polyglandular syndromes 91–3
autoimmune thyroid disease (AITD) 12–3, 55–6, 57, 59, 69–70, 85, 93

autoimmunity 70, 74
autonomously functioning nodules 32, 105, 120, 194, 203, 210
autoreactive cells 71, 74, 82, 177, 182, 213, 221
autoregulation 155
axial proptosis 217
Ayurveda 168, 180–1

B lymphocyte cells 73, 74, 80
bacterial antigens 41, 44, 73, 77, 79, 82, 84
basal metabolism rate 97
Basedow's disease 48
bee pollen 227–8
behavior 20, 21
beta adrenergic blocking agents 21, 51, 122, 123, 153–4, 192, 208–9
beta blockers see beta adrenergic blocking agents
beta–HCG see beta human chorionic gonadotropin
beta human chorionic gonadotropin (beta–HCG) 29, 37–8, 187, 189, 193, 194
Bihari, Bernard 167, 227–8
bilateral proptosis 38, 217
biopsy, thyroid 123–4
bipolar disorder 21, 66
blisters 62, 63
block and replace therapy 140–1
blocking TSH receptor antibodies 54
blood clots 65, 99, 100, 101
blood urea nitrogen (BUN) 101
BMR see basal metabolism rate
bone changes 70, 166
Borrelia burgdoferi 77
bowel movements 17, 64
breast cancer 105, 151
breast enlargement see gynecomastia
bruit 8, 15
bugleweed see Lycopus virginicus
BUN see blood urea nitrogen
Burch, Henry 131
Burman, Kenneth 131

C cells see parafollicular cells
C1 inhibitor deficiency 60
C-reactive protein (CRP) 64
Calcitonin 8, 10
Calcium 10, 34, 70, 106, 122, 144, 162, 165
cAMP see cyclic adenosine monophosphate
CAMPATH 84
Candida 91
Carbamazepine 121
Carbimazole 132, 136, 139, 140, 201, 202
cardiovascular symptoms 19, 20, 70, 95
catecholamines 20, 23, 28
cedar pollen 80
celiac disease see gluten sensitivity
chi 161
childbirth 25
children 13, 203–10

cholesterol 16, 106
choriogonadotropin-mediated thyrotoxicosis 37–8
chromosomes 147–8
chronic active hepatitis 76, 84, 90, 97
cigarettes 76, 84, 220–1
coenzyme Q10 (CoQ10) 16, 164, 186
co-existing conditions 87–9
cognitive function 20, 66, 67
collagen 90, 124
colloid 8, 124, 135, 136, 198
coma 21
computed tomography (CT) 129, 219
congestive heart failure 20, 25, 51, 52, 154, 164
congestive ophthalmopathy 212–27, 213
Cooper, David 131
Cooperative Thyrotoxicosis Follow-up Study 151
Cooperative Thyrotoxicosis Therapy Study 146
copper 166
CoQ10 see coenzyme Q10
corneal ulcer 214
corticosteroids 68, 202, 222–3
cortisol 22–3, 79
craniosynostosis 205
CT see computed tomography
Cushing's disease 217, 219
cyclic adenosine monophosphate 35
cyclosporine A 223
cyclothymia 21
cytokines 50, 53, 55, 79, 81, 213
cytomegalovirus (CMV) 89, 93, 102
cytotoxic lymphocyte antigen 50, 71, 76

DeGroot, Leslie 13, 69, 84
deiodinase enzymes 166
deiodination 193
deoxyribonucleic acid (DNA) 11, 20, 95, 119, 145, 181
depression 15, 17, 20, 21, 51, 55, 56
De Quervain's thyroiditis see subacute thyroiditis
dermatitis herpetiformis 61–2, 76, 90
dermopathy 58; see also hyperpigmentation; skin changes in hyperthyroidism
DES see diethylstilbesterol
Dexamethasone 152–3
diabetes 18; see also insulin dependent diabetes mellitus
dietary influences 161–2, 163
diethylstilbesterol (DES) 77
diets 85
digestive problems 64, 181
diiodotyrosine (DIT) 9
dioxin 77, 82; see also Agent Orange
diplopia 214
disorders associated with Graves' disease 57, 88

DNA *see* deoxyribonucleic acid
DNA antibodies 62, 123
dopamine 55, 114, 121, 186
double vision *see* diplopia
Down's syndrome 45
DRL *see* drug related lupus
drug interferences 10, 121–2
drug metabolism 16, 140
drug related lupus 123

ectopic thyroid tissue 197–8
edema 17, 18, 25
elderly patients 12–3, 14–5, 20, 51, 66
emotions 17, 21; *see also* mood changes; psychiatric symptoms
encephalopathy 67–8
endocrine changes 6; *see also* autoimmune polyglandular syndromes
endocrine disruptors 77, 82
endocrine glands 6, 55
Endocrine Society 1, 131
energy healing 181–2
enlarged thyroid gland *see* goiter
environmental influences 11
eosinophil derived neurotoxin (EDN) 80
epiphora 221
Epstein-Barr virus (EBV) 77, 102
erectile dysfunction 22
erythema annulare centrifugum 62
erythrocyte sedimentation rate 44, 64
essential fatty acids *see* free fatty acids
estrogens 23, 46, 76, 77, 78, 188
ethanol injection 77, 155
European Thyroid Association 131
euthyroid Graves' disease 212
euthyroid hyperthyroxinemia 23–4
euthyroid thyrotoxicosis 5, 24
euthyroidism 21, 51, 111, 113, 141, 152, 153, 154, 155, 157
exercise intolerance 19
exogenous thyroid hormone 14, 203
exophthalmic ophthalmoplegia 221, 222, 223
exophthalmos 34, 117, 217, 219, 224, 226, 229, 232; causes 219
extraocular muscle 16, 214, 215, 216, 217, 218, 210, 220, 221
eye disorder *see* Graves' ophthalmopathy
eye muscle surgeries 225
eyelid retraction 205, 214, 216, 225
eyelid surgery 225–6

Factor VIII 65
familial autoimmune hyperthyroidism 35
familial dysalbuminemic hyperthyroxinemia 123
familial hypersensitivity to beta HCG 35–6
familial non-autoimmune hyperthyroidisim 35
fas ligand 81
fatigue 17, 21, 51, 97

females 15, 48, 76; *see also* gender
fertility 22, 188–9
fetal cell microchimerism 81–2
fetal hyperthyroidisim 191, 196, 199–200
fetal pituitary-thyroid axis 199
fever 24, 44, 97
fibrocytes 71
fibrosis 34
Flajani, Giuseppe 47
fluoride 82, 153
follicle sacs 8, 198
follicular adenoma 32–3
follicular cells 9
formaldehyde 85
free (essential) fatty acids 6, 10, 167
free T3 (FT3) 16, 28
free T4 (FT4) 18, 28, 110–11
FT3 *see* free T3
FT4 *see* free T4
GAG *see* glycosaminoclycan
gender 15, 48, 76
gene mutations 27, 28, 33, 34, 35, 46, 93, 156, 200–3
genes in Graves' disease 70–3, 76, 123
genetic susceptibility 71
German Commission E 169, 171
Gershengorn, Arvin 158
gestational thyrotoxicosis 189, 190
gliadin antibodies 123
glomerular filtration rate 18
glucocorticoids *see* corticosteroids
glucose 18, 63
gluten sensitivity enteropathy 62, 64, 76, 80, 85, 98, 161, 163, 164
glycosaminoglycan (GAG) 213, *213*, 221, 223, 230, 231, 232

GO *see* Graves' ophthalmopathy
Gofman, John 128
goiter 7, 14, 16, 17, 46
goitrogens 135, 162–3, 202
Gong, Joseph 147
Graves, Robert 48
Graves' disease 16–7, 47–54, 56–9, 91, 175–6
Graves' ophthalmopathy 15, 66, 71, 150, 185, 211–227, *213*, *220*; alternative medicine in 227–8; classification by Werner 218
Graves' rage 21–2
GSE *see* gluten sensitivity enteropathy
gynecomastia 6, 17, 22, 188

hair changes 17, 89, 228–9
hallucinations 66, 67
haplotypes 72–3, 76, 92
Hashimoto's encephalopathy 56, 67–8
Hashimoto's thyroiditis 10, 44–5, 56, 57, 88, 91, 212; hyperthyroid phase 5, 45
hashitoxicosis 10, 45, 56–7, 212
hCG *see* beta human chorionic gonadotropin

headache 15, 17, 67
Health Insurance Portability & Accountability Act (HIPAA) 133
heart attack *see* cardiovascular symptoms
heart rate 15, 20, 26, 57, 191, 192, 208
heat intolerance 17
heat shock proteins 81, 84
Helicobacter pylori 77, 79, 96
Heparin 23
herbal medicine 168, 169–75
hereditary hyperthyroidism *see* familial autoimmune hyperthyroidism
heroin 23, 122
herpes gestationis 62, 90
Hertel exophathalmometry 217
Hirata's disease 18
Hispanics 69–70
histamine 59
hives 57, 58, 59, 61
HLA genes *see* human leukocyte antigens
homeopathy 177–9
hormonal disruptors *see* endocrine disruptors
hormones 6, 58
HT *see* Hashimoto's thyroiditis
human chorionic gonadotropin *see* beta human chorionic gonadotropin
human leukocyte antigens (HLA) 54, 72–4, 75–6, 92
human parvovirus B19 77, 102
Hürthle cells 10
hygiene hypothesis 50, 81
hypercalcemia 165, 167
hyperemesis gravidarum 29, 35, 36, 42
hypereosinophilic syndrome 62
hyperglycemia 25, 63
hyperkinesis 16
hyperparathyroidism 142
hyperpigmentation 17, 228
hyperplasia 16, 49
hypersensitivity reactions 59–60, 62
hypertension 16, 20, 37
hyperthyroidism: causes 27–8, 30–41; definition 5, 12, 14; diagnosis 51, 108–12, 113–30; disease course 12–3, 31, 51, 52; phases 12; in teenagers 13, 203–10
hypertrophy 9, 49
hypoglycemia 18, 63
hypogonadism 92
hypokalemic periodic paralysis *see* thyrotoxic periodic paralysis
hypomania 21, 66
hypoparathyroidism 91
hypophysis *see* pituitary gland
hypophysitis 90
hypothalamus 28, *30*, 106, *107*
hypothyroidism 41, 51

I-123 128
I-131 128, 147, 151
iatrogenic causes 85

ICAM-1 52
IDDM *see* insulin dependent diabetes mellitus
idiopathic thrombocytopenic purpura (ITP) 57, 65, 90, 102–3
IFN *see* interferon
IFN-alpha 84, 85
IFN-gamma 50, 213
Ig *see* immunoglobulins
IL *see* interleukins
IL-1 54, 74
IL-2 74
IL-6 17, 52, 71
IL-8 17, 52
IL-13 80
IL-17 84
IL-22 84
IL-23 84
imaging studies 143, 219, 221, 231
immune complexes 17, 59, 65
immune response 71, 74
immune system 54–5
immunoglobulin E 59, 60, 79–80, 86
immunoglobulins 60, 201, 223
immunomodulators 175–6
inattention 17, 21
infection 76–7, 85, 93
infectious thyroiditis *see* suppurative thyroiditis
inflammation 64, 81, 214
injury 77, 79
insomnia 20, 172, 173, 175, 179, 185, 223
insulin dependent diabetes mellitus 58, 76, 84, 91–3
insulin growth factor 232
insulin resistance 18, 63
integrative medicine 174
interferon (IFN) 50, 77, 84, 85
interleukins (IL) 50, 52, 77, 84, 85
intrinsic factor antibodies 96
iodine 9, 62, 78, *146*; deficiency 78, 162; excess 25, 40–1, 78, 127, 162; imaging contrast media *see* Ipodate; uptake 17
ionic transport inhibitors 152–3
ionizing radiation 81, 128, 145, 147, 148
Ipodate 153, 201
irradiated thyroid tissue 10
irritability 17, 20, 67
isthmus 8
ITP *see* idiopathic thrombocytopenia purpura
IVIG *see* intravenous immunoglobulins

Japan Thyroid Association 131

KCNQ1 14
KDNE2 14
kelp 170
keratitis 216–7
kidney function 18–9, 101

Klinefelter syndrome 103
Koop, Peter 14

laboratory test interferences 121–2
laboratory tests 13, 121, 125, 141, 202
Lacri-Lube 221
lactation 193
Lactuca virosa 170
lemon balm *see Melissa officinalis*
Leonurus cardiac 170–1
leucopenia (leukopenia) 95, 102
levothyroxine 156
libido 22, 188
lichen planus 89
lid lag 16, 38, 211, 216, 217, 218, 221
light sensitivity *see* photophobia
linkage disequilibrium 72–3
lipids 165
lithium 85, 122, 126, 136, 153, 217
Lithospermum ruderale 171
liver enzymes 15, 64, 97, 185
liver function 19, 97
liver membrane antibodies 123
long acting thyrid stimulator (LATS) 48
long QT syndrome 14
low dose naltrexone (LDN) 3, 167–8, 227, 229
Lugol's solution 26, 143, 154–5
Lupus anticoagulant 100
Lycopus virginicus 170, 171
lymph nodes 16, 64, 208, 209
lymphatic system, thyroid 8–9
lymphocytes 53, 74, 75, 77, 95, 136, 213, 224
lymphocytic infiltration 95
lymphoma, thyroid 39, 105

magnetic resonance imaging (MRI) 129–30, 219
major histocompatibility complex (MHC) 72, 79
malabsorption 16, 64, 87, 95
males with Graves' disease 62, 64, 76, 77, 103, 188, 204, 229, 231
mania 20, 21, 66
Marine-Lenhart syndrome 31
McCune-Albright syndrome 201
meditation 183, 221
megalin antibodies 16, 119
Melissa officianalis 170, 171–2
menstrual problems 17, 22
mental problems 17, 20–1, 66; *see also* psychiatric symptoms
metabolism 18, 122, 139, 140, 163, 164, 165, 166
methadone 23
methimazole 3, 136–8, 139–40, 190–1
methylation defects 186–7
methylcellulose 221
MHC *see* major histocompatibility complex

microcephaly 201
microsomal antibodies *see* thyroid peroxidase antibodies
milk thistle *see Silybum marianum*
minerals 166
miscarriages 65, 100
mitral valve prolapse 17, 65
molecular mimicry 81, 82
monoiodtyrosine (MIT) 9
mood disturbances 17, 21, 55, 66
Mourits, criteria 218
MRI *see* magnetic resonance imaging
MS *see* multiple sclerosis
multiple autoimmune disorders 57–8, 88–90
multiple sclerosis (MS) 84, 90
muscle wasting 18, 70
muscle weakness *see* myopathy
myasthenia gravis 57, 92
myoclonus 67
myopathy 16, 17, 25, 55, 63–4, 67, 164
myxedema 52, 93; *see also* pretibial myxedema

nail changes 17, 57, 229
Natrum muriaticum 179
natural killer cells 189
nausea 18, 25, 36, 57
neonatal Graves' disease 200–2
neonatal hyperthyroidism 36–7, 200–2
nephropathy 101
nervous system 55, 70
nervousness 15, 57
Neumann, Susanne 158
neural therapy 184
neurotransmitters 55
NK cells *see* natural killer cells
nodules, thyroid 31–2, 123, 208–11
non-steroidal anti-inflammatory drugs (NSAIDs) 10, 122, 186–7
nonthyroidal illness 110, 111, 112
NOSPECS 217
novel molecule 158
NSAIDs *see* non-steroidal anti-inflammatory drugs
nursing mothers *see* lactation
nutrient deficiencies 16, 64, 87, 164, 203
nystagmus 67

obsessive compulsive disorder 20–1, 66
ocreotide 222
onchylosis 17
optic neuropathy 218, 220, 222, 223, 224
oral contraceptives 23, 67
oral tolerance 176–7
orbital decompression 214–5, 226
orbital fibroblasts 232
organification 9
organotherapy 179–80
osteoarthropathy 232
osteoporosis 165, 166
oxyphil cells 10

PA *see* pernicious anemia
painless sporadic thyroiditis 42
palpitations 19, 57
panic disorder 20, 22
pancreas 6, 58, 150, 197
parafollicular cells 9, 10
paranoia 21, 66
parathyroid glands 143, 150
parathyroid hormone 165, 167
Parry, Caleb 47, 79
Passiflora incarnate 172
pemphigus 90, 91
pentoxyphylline 223
peptides 159
perchlorate 82, 152
periorbital edema 216, 217, 225
peripheral neuropathy 55, 95
pernicious anemia (PA) 57, 61, 88, 92, 95–6
    128
pertechnetate 128
phagocytes (monocytes) 73, 104, 213
phenobarbital 121
phenytoin (Dilantin) 10, 121
phobia 20
photophobia 214, 216, 221
pituitary hormones 12
pituitary tumors 39–40, 134
placenta 199
plasmapheresis 26, 223
platelet antibodies 65–6, 102–3
Plummer's nails 17
PNI *see* psychoneuroimmunology
polychlorinated biphenyl (PCB) 77, 82
postpartum depression 192
postpartum Graves' disease 78, 79
postpartum thyroiditis 41, 42, 195
potassium 14, 19, 64–5
prednisone *see* corticosteroids
pregnancy 22, 187, 195; lab tests in 187–8
premature ejaculation 22
pretibial myxedema 15, 150, 190, 212, 228,
    229–30
primary biliary cirrhosis 90, 92, 97
primary sclerosing cholangitis 97
prisms 221, 222
propranolol 51, 111, 122, 123, 143, 154, 192,
    202
proptosis *see* exophthalmos
propylthiouracil (PTU) 3, 136–8, 139, 190,
    202
protein C 100, 102
protein S 102
pseudoadenoma, thyroid 8
psychiatric symptoms 20–1, 22, 66–7, 95
psychoneuroimmunology 55
psychosis 21, 25, 152
PTM *see* pretibial myxedema
PTU *see* propylthiouracil
pulse pressure 19
pyramidal lobe 8

radiation thyroiditis 151
radiotherapy *see* orbital supervoltage radio-
    therapy
RAI *see* radioiodine ablation
RAI-U *see* radioiodine uptake test
rapid consciousness distrurbance 66
rashes 58
Raynaud's phenomena 102
red blood cell volume 20
redness, skin 17, 44
reflexes 16, 64
relapse 52, 77, 80, 112, 134, 140, 152
remission 52
reproductive system in hyperthyroidism 22,
    188–9
resistance to thyroid hormone (RTH) 14, 45–
    6, 156–7
resorcinol 127, 136
respiratory symptoms 20
reverse T3
RF *see* rheumatoid factor
rhabdomyoysis 16, 25, 64
rheumatoid arthritis 57, 87, 88, 90, 94, 98
rheumatoid factor 121
Rhodiola rosea 186
Riedel's thyroiditis 42–3

salicylates 115, 122, 127
salivary glands 150, 196
sarcoidosis, thyroid 34, 93, 105
saturated solution potassium iodide (SSKI)
    26, 143, 154–5, 192; *see also* Lugol's solution
schizophrenia 66
scleroderma 90
seizures 16, 21
selenium 76, 86, 122, 166–7
self-reactivity 76
self-tolerance 74–5
sensory therapies 186–7
Silybum marianum 172–3
Sjögren's syndrome 60, 62, 92
SLE *see* systemic lupus erythematosus
sleep disturbances 18, 20
somatostatin 222
soy 127, 163, 202
speech 17, 21
spleen 64, 97, 201
SSKI *see* saturated solution potassium iodide
staring 205, 213, 218
steatorrhea 16, 64
steroid responsive encephalopathy (SREAT)
    67–8
stimulants 21
stress 6, 21–2, 51, 55, 62, 66, 76, 79, 86,
    182–3, 221
stroke 67
struma ovarii 38–9, 105
subacute thyroiditis 42–3
subclinical Graves' disease 48–9
subclinical hyperthyroidism 22, 23, 39

superantigens 79
superfamily of receptors 11–12
surgery *see* thyroidectomy
sweating 17, 25
systemic lupus erythematosus (SLE) 57, 60, 62, 88

T helper cells (CD8) 50, 74
T lymphocytes 71, 74–5, 177
T suppressor cells (CD4) 50, 74
T3 *see* triiodothyronine
T3 antibodies 99
T3 response events (TREs) 11
T3 suppression test 140
T3 thyrotoxicosis 39, 112
T3 uptake test 110, 115
T4 *see* thyroxine
T4 antibodies 99
tachycardia 19, 20, 24, 46
tai chi 221
Tapazole *see* methimazole
TBG *see* thyroxine binding globulin
TBII *see* thyrotropin binding inhibiting immunoglobulins
TCM *see* traditional Chinese medicine
Technetium 128
Testa, Antonio 47
testosterone 22
tetraiodothyronine *see* thyroxine
Th cells 50
Th1 cells 50, 53, 84, 167
Th2 cells 50, 53, 80, 84, 167
Th17 cells 83–4
thiocyanate 127, 152
thrill 8, 16
thymoma 89
thymus gland 16
thyroglobulin 9; antibodies 16, 68, 120
thyroglossal duct 197, 198, 208
thyroid antibodies 49–50, 54–5, 61, 116, 120; in pregnancy 191–2
thyroid cancer 39, 105, 123, 151
thyroid cells **8**, 9–10
thyroid eye disease (TED) *see* Graves' ophthalmopathy
thyroid failure 52, 87, 151, 152
thyroid gland 7, **32**, *107*, 196–7
thyroid growth stimulating immunoglobulins 119
thyroid hormone production 9, 12, 53, 58, 70
thyroid hormone receptors 11–2
thyroid hormone resistance *see* resistance to thyroid hormone
thyroid lobes 7–8
thyroid lobules 8
Thyroid Manager 13, 84
thyroid nodules in Graves' disease 8; *see also* Marine-Lenhart syndrome
thyroid peroxidase (TPO) 9; antibodies 16, 42, 67, 80, 120

thyroid-pituitary-hypothalamic axis 28, 31, 39, 106, *107*, 108, 117, 166, 202
thyroid stimulating hormone (TSH)
thyroid stimulating immunoglobulins (TSI); *see also* TSH receptor antibodies, stimulating
thyroid storm 5, 16, 21, 24–6, 132, 137, 145, 151, 153, 154, 155, 185
thyroidal sodium/iodide symporter antibodies 16, 119
thyroidectomy 25, 142–4, 207
thyroidinium 179–80
thyroiditis 12–3, 15–6
Thyrosoothe 170
thyrotoxic autoimmune encephalopathy 104
thyrotoxic myopathy 16, 38, 63, 93, 226
thyrotoxic periodic paralysis 19, 65, 219
thyrotoxicosis: causes 41–6; definition 5, 13
thyrotoxicosis factitia 41, 45
thyrotropin *see* thyroid stimulating hormone (TSH)
thyrotropin binding inhibiting immunoglobulins 118–9
thyrotropin releasing hormone (TRH) 28–9, 40
thyroxine 20, 24, 28, 83, 92, 97, 110
thyroxine binding globulin (TBG) 46
TNF *see* tumor necrosis factor
toxic diffuse goiter 47, 49
toxic multinodular goiter 27, 33
TPO *see* thyroid peroxidase
traditional Chinese medicine 168, 173–5
transport proteins 6, 23, 70
trauma 25, 77, 79
treatment: alternative 160–186; conventional 132–159; in pregnancy 190–3
tremor 16, 18, 55, 67
TRH *see* thyrotropin releasing hormone
Triiodothyronine 28, 111–2
TSH *see* thyroid stimulating hormone
TSH antibodies 99
TSH receptor 52–3, 80–1; antibodies 16, 79, 80, 105, 108, 116–7; receptor mutations 34–5
TSI *see* thyroid stimulating immunoglobulins
tumor necrosis factor alpha (TFN-alpha) 71
tumors 38
Turner's syndrome 102–3
tyrosine 9, 28

ultrasonography 128–9, 155–6
unilateral proptosis 217, 219
uric acid 18
urination 17, 18
urticaria 59, 60–1

vaccines 50, 55
Valeriana officinalis 173
Varanasi, Ajay 83
vasculitis 60, 68

viruses *see* infection
vitamin A derivatives 11–12, 61, 86, 165
vitamin B12 deficiency 87, 94–5
vitamin C 86, 165, 181
vitamin D 11, 34, 70, 165, 186
vitamins 164–5, 186
vitiligo 57, 61, 88, 89, 92
Vogel, H.C.A. 78, 169
von Basedow, Carol Adolph 48

Waheed, Shamal 70
wasting *see* muscle wasting

Weetman, Anthony 51
weight gain 14, 18, 19, 58, 63
weight loss 18, 19, 25, 79
Wolff-Chaikoff effect 155

Yamamoto, M. 140, 157
Yersinia enterocolitica 77, 79
yin and yang 168
yoga 184, 221

zinc 166